# Orofacial Pain:

*Guidelines for Assessment, Diagnosis, and Management,* Fourth Edition

# American Academy of Orofacial Pain
# Guidelines for Assessment, Diagnosis, and Management

*Contributors*

### Reny de Leeuw, DDS, PhD
### Editor

Peter M. Baragona, DMD

Peter M. Bertrand, DMD, MS

David F. Black, MD

Charles R. Carlson, PhD

J. Richard Cohen, DDS

Dorothy C. Dury, DDS, PhD

Donald A. Falace, DMD

Steven B. Graf Radford, DDS

Gary M. Heir, DMD

Jules R. Hesse, PT, PhD

Andrew S. Kaplan, DMD

Steven L. Kraus, PT, OCS

Jeffrey Mannheimer, PT, PhD

Richard Ohrbach, DDS, PhD

Jeffrey P. Okeson, DMD

Richard A. Pertes, DDS

Jerry W. Swanson, MD

Alan Stiles, DMD

Mark V. Thomas, DMD

Corine Visscher, PT, PhD

Edward F. Wright, DDS, MS

# Orofacial Pain

*Guidelines for Assessment,
Diagnosis, and Management*

## Fourth Edition

American Academy of Orofacial Pain

**Reny de Leeuw,** DDS, PhD
Editor

Quintessence Publishing Co, Inc
Chicago, Berlin, Tokyo, London, Paris, Milan, Barcelona,
Istanbul, São Paulo, Mumbai, Moscow, Prague, and Warsaw

**Library of Congress Cataloging-in-Publication Data**

Orofacial pain : guidelines for assessment, diagnosis, and management. --
4th ed. / Reny de Leeuw, editor.
     p. ; cm.
  Rev. ed. of: Orofacial pain : guidelines for assessment, diagnosis, and
management / the American Academy of Orofacial Pain ; edited by Jeffrey P.
Okeson. c1996.
  "Three publications have preceded this current edition of what commonly is
referred to as the *AAOP Guidelines*"--Pref.
  Includes bibliographical references and index.
  ISBN 978-0-86715-413-9 (softcover)
  1. Orofacial pain. 2. Temporomandibular joint--Diseases. I. De Leeuw,
Reny. II. American Academy of Orofacial Pain. III. American Academy of
Orofacial Pain. Orofacial pain.
  [DNLM: 1. Facial Pain--Practice Guideline. 2. Headache--Practice
Guideline. 3. Temporomandibular Joint Disorders--Practice Guideline. WE
705 O74 2008]
  RC815.A67 2008
  617.5'2--dc22
                        2007049961

quinte//ence
book/

© 2008 Quintessence Publishing Co, Inc

Quintessence Publishing Co, Inc
4350 Chandler Drive
Hanover Park, IL 60133
www.quintpub.com

Editor: Bryn Goates
Design: Dawn Hartman
Production: Sue Robinson


Printed in China

# Table of Contents

# Preface

The American Academy of Orofacial Pain (AAOP) was founded in 1975 with the goal to improve the understanding and quality of education in temporomandibular disorders (TMDs) and orofacial pain. The AAOP remains an organization of dedicated health care professionals with a mission of alleviating pain and suffering through the promotion of excellence in education, research, and patient care within the field of orofacial pain and associated disorders. Three publications have preceded this current edition of what commonly is referred to as the *AAOP Guidelines*. Dr Charles McNeill spearheaded the first two editions: *Craniomandibular Disorders: Guidelines for Evaluation, Diagnosis, and Management* (published in 1990) and *Temporomandibular Disorders: Guidelines for Classification, Assessment, and Management* (published in 1993). These publications focused predominantly on TMDs. As health care professionals and researchers became more conscious of the relationship between TMDs and other disorders of the head and neck, there was a need to expand the *Guidelines* to include disorders presenting as or related to TMDs. These disorders comprised not only headaches and neck disorders but several neuropathic pain conditions as well. Hence, a committee was appointed to develop a document to broaden the scope of orofacial pain conditions and related disorders. In 1996, under the editorship of Dr

Jeffrey Okeson, the third version of the *AAOP Guidelines* was published: *Orofacial Pain: Guidelines for Assessment, Diagnosis, and Management*. The third edition used the term *orofacial pain* to echo the changes within the field of orofacial pain as well as to underscore the idea that TMDs and orofacial pain should not be regarded as separate conditions; rather, TMDs should be considered a substantial part of the disorders that fall under the umbrella of orofacial pain.

In this fourth edition of the *AAOP Guidelines*, again entitled *Orofacial Pain: Guidelines for Assessment, Diagnosis, and Management*, the field of orofacial pain has expanded to more completely express the current evidence-based concepts. Though the structure of the current *Guidelines* resembles that of the third edition, every chapter contains important updates, and some chapters have undergone drastic revision. When available, evidence-based literature has been presented to provide the reader with scientifically sound and effective diagnostic procedures and treatment options. Whereas in the previous edition information on cervical disorders was dispersed among several chapters, in this edition an entire chapter has been dedicated to cervical disorders to emphasize the close relationships between some orofacial pain disorders and cervical pain disorders, while calling attention to the differences and similarities associated with these disorders.

It is important for the reader to understand that this work is not intended to be an all-encompassing textbook comprehensively detailing all aspects of orofacial pain. Instead, it is meant to provide insight into and assist the reader with the procedures of evidence-based assessment, diagnosis, and management of orofacial pain conditions, based on the latest scientific knowledge. Because TMDs are considered the major part of orofacial pain and the majority of practitioners will, in all likelihood, focus on its assessment, diagnosis, and treatment, this area is described in the greatest detail. In addition, TMDs are also the major focus of the chapter on classification. Other chapters, such as the ones on neuropathic pain conditions and on odontogenic pain and mucogingival disorders, also contain more detailed information. The chapter on head-aches describes the primary headaches and will help seasoned as well as less-experienced professionals recognize and distinguish headaches that may or may not be related to TMDs. The chapter on cervical spine disorders predominantly describes the neuro-anatomic connection between the cervical spine and the trigeminal system and highlights some of the more common cervico-genic disorders that can cause or present as orofacial pain. Other related conditions such as intracranial and mental disorders are described with adequate detail to provide insight into such disorders and their relationship with and potential impact on other orofacial pain conditions.

*Reny de Leeuw, DDS, PhD*
*Chair, Guidelines Committee*

# Acknowledgments

More than 10 years have passed since the previous edition of the *AAOP Guidelines* was published. It is hard to describe the many hours that AAOP members have dedicated to producing this fourth edition. Numerous members have served on the Guidelines Committee over the years, and I wholeheartedly thank them for their valuable opinions and insights.

The main contributors to this edition of the *AAOP Guidelines* are listed across from the title page; however, they are not the only people who have put in significant efforts over the course of the past 10 years. Many individuals worked on an earlier version of what ultimately has become this edition of the *AAOP Guidelines*. Unfortunately, because of a subsequent significant reorganization, the work of several authors could not be included in this version. Nevertheless, these people put in considerable effort and time and therefore deserve credit. Robert Rosenbaum deserves special recognition in this regard. Prior to the reorganization, he spearheaded a much broader version of this edition. Sincere thanks are extended to him for all of his dedication, diligence, and hard work. Other people who were involved in the making of the earlier draft are Romulo Albuquerque, Francisco Alençar, Ronald Attanasio, Dennis Bailey, Elizangela Bertoli, Hong Chen, Glenn Clark, Harold Cohen, Jeffrey Crandall, Karen Decker, Jim Fricton, Henry Gremillion, Sheldon Gross, Steve Harkins, Lisa Heaton, Maureen Lang, Matthew Lark, Pei Feng Lim, John Look, James Luderitz, Bruce Lundgren, Jeannette McNeill, Robert Merrill, Somsak Mitrirattanakul, Mariona Mulet, Cibele Nasri, Hieu Nguyen, Elaine Nicholson, Richard Niedermann, Donald Nixdorf, Diane Novy, John O'Brien, Kathy Robbins, Mariano Rocabado, Eric Schiffman, Anthony Schwartz, Donald Tanenbaum, Ed Truelove, and Eduardo Vazquez Delgado.

Finally, I would like to express my appreciation to several individuals who worked hard behind the scenes: Jenna Klingenberg, Dewayne Martin, Lisa McCoy, and Tipton Moody. I thank them for their administrative support.

# Introduction to Orofacial Pain

*Orofacial pain* refers to pain associated with the hard and soft tissues of the head, face, and neck. These tissues, whether skin, blood vessels, teeth, glands, or muscles, send impulses through the trigeminal nerve to be interpreted as pain by brain circuits that are primarily responsible for processing complex behavior.[1] Headaches, neurogenic, musculoskeletal, and psychophysiologic pathology, as well as cancer, infection, autoimmune phenomena, and tissue trauma represent the diagnostic range for the complaint of orofacial pain. The diverse potential for pain arising from trigeminal receptive fields is why evaluation and management of orofacial pain require collaboration among all fields of medicine.

The quest to better manage pain involving the trigeminal nerve, such as temporomandibular disorders (TMDs) and headaches, has led to the establishment of orofacial pain as a discipline in the field of dentistry. There are residency training programs in orofacial pain, board certification processes, and increasing cooperation among advocacy groups, universities, professional organizations, and federal agencies.

This revised edition is a collaborative effort derived from reviews of refereed literature spanning the spectrum of conditions at the root of orofacial pain. It is intended for health care professionals who evaluate and treat patients with orofacial pain and face the daunting task of "keeping up with the literature" in the rapidly emerging arena of pain management in clinical practice.

## The Health Care Professional's Responsibility in Orofacial Pain

The capacity to remain unbiased during evaluation and differential diagnosis is every clinician's responsibility. Due to the diverse, complex physiologic interrelationships involved in orofacial pain complaints, all clinicians must be able to judge when their diagnostic acumen requires consultation;

otherwise, treatment may not target the appropriate source.

The clinician's responsibility is threefold. First, the clinician must combine a current working knowledge of the basic and clinical science of orofacial pain with an ability to elaborate a relevant history. Appropriate questions must be asked, answers must be analyzed, and findings must be synthesized into an initial differential diagnosis.

Second, the clinician must perform a thorough clinical assessment, including a physical examination and indicated laboratory testing, imaging studies, neurologic testing, and consultations. Accurate diagnosis may require insight from other health care professionals.

Third, the clinician must be able to explain all findings to the patient as well as the details of the treatment plan, which must be consistent with standards of care based on scientific literature. When the scope of care falls beyond individual expertise, a team approach may be developed. The clinician should discuss appropriate referral options with the patient.

# Epidemiology of Orofacial Pain

The 1986 Nuprin Pain Report[2] reported that most Americans experience an average of three or four different kinds of pain every year. Crook et al[3] reported that 16% of a general population had experienced pain within the past 2 weeks. More than 81% of the general population report at least one significant pain experience in their lifetime.[4] Brattberg et al[5] reported that 66% of 827 randomly selected individuals from a general population reported pain or discomfort in different parts of their bodies, with approximately 10% describing pain in the head, face, or neck. Von Korff et al[6] surveyed 1,016 members of a large health maintenance organization (HMO) and found that, while 12% reported facial pain in the previous 6 months, rates for other types of pain were 41% for back pain, 26% for headaches, 17% for abdominal pain, and 12% for chest pain. In addition, 40% of individuals reported missing one or more workdays because of pain.

Lipton et al[7] surveyed 45,711 American households and reported that nearly 22% of the general population experienced at least one of five types of orofacial pain in the past 6 months. The most common type of orofacial pain was toothache, reported by 12.2% of the population. Temporomandibular joint (TMJ) pain was reported by 5.3%, with face or cheek pain being reported by 1.4%.

However, orofacial pain seldom appears to be an isolated complaint. More than 81% of patients reporting to an orofacial pain center had pain sources beyond the trigeminal system,[8] but few patients mentioned these other pain sources.[9] Conditions such as fibromyalgia, chronic fatigue syndrome, headache, panic disorder, gastroesophageal reflux disorder, irritable bowel syndrome, multiple chemical sensitivity, and posttraumatic stress disorder seem to coexist with TMDs.[10] Symptoms for such comorbid conditions differentiate orofacial pain patients from patients seeking routine dental care.[11,12] If all pain sources are not revealed during the evaluation, prognosis for an orofacial pain problem may be due to the barrage of brain circuits from unaddressed sources of chronic nociception.

Pain is a common experience that has profound societal effects. Bonica estimated that nearly a third of the population of industrialized nations suffers to some extent from chronic pain.[13] Chronic pain costs billions of dollars annually for health care services, loss of work, decreased productivity, and disability compensation.

## Pain Constructs

Pain is defined as "an unpleasant sensory and emotional experience associated with actual or potential tissue damage, or described in terms of such damage."[14] Nociceptors are polymodal, high-threshold nerve endings that send tissue damage impulses on slow Aδ fibers and even slower C-fibers to the central nervous system (CNS). Although pain is an interpretation of nociception, many orofacial pain patients lack apparent tissue damage, and anatomic changes such as TMJ disc displacement without reduction do not predict continuing pain.[15,16]

About 25% of the free nerve endings in skeletal muscle that transmit impulses to the CNS on Aδ and C-fibers are chemo- and mechanoreceptive but not nociceptive.[17] Some of these low-threshold receptors, called metaboreceptors, appear to be uniquely stimulated by metabolic products generated during muscle activity,[18,19] while others sense the relative distension of postcapillary bed venules.[20] These receptors display background activity at rest, accelerate impulse transmission as behavior intensity increases,[20–22] and may affect the same central modulatory systems affected by nociception.[23] The CNS uses such input to sequence respiratory and cardiac changes during dynamic muscle behavior.[18,20–22] Future consideration of the role of these receptors in pain etiology may help us better understand pain conditions in which there is no apparent visible tissue damage.

## Anatomic and Physiologic Considerations in Orofacial Pain

Orofacial pain may be defined as pain and dysfunction affecting motor and sensory transmission in the trigeminal nerve system.[24] From a sensory perspective, the trigeminal system oversees the efficacy and tissue integrity of highly integrative orofacial behaviors that are controlled by the cranial nerves and modulated by the autonomic nervous system (ANS) and the greater limbic system.[25] Orofacial tissues transmit impulses about touch, position, temperature, and pain to the trigeminal nuclei, which have extensive bidirectional connections throughout the brain.[26–28] These trigeminal connections affect the sensory, motor, and autonomic-endocrine changes that occur during orofacial behaviors, and, when these behaviors are impaired, orofacial pain may result. The next sections briefly discuss peripheral and central trigeminal neuroanatomy to elucidate how the trigeminal system affects physiology and pain.

### Neuroanatomy of the orofacial structures

Cranial nerves are extensions of the brain that innervate tissues involved with the trigeminal system directly or indirectly.[13] The specialized neurons of the olfactory, optic, and vestibulocochlear nerves that send smell, sight, sound, and balance impulses to the CNS do not travel through the trigeminal nuclei. However, nose, eye, and ear tissues do transmit proprioceptive, pressure, and potential pain impulses into the trigeminal nuclei. These cranial nerves, along with the occulomotor, trochlear, abducens, and the hypoglossal nerves, will not be reviewed here. The remaining five cranial nerves and upper cervical nerves will be briefly discussed. However, a comprehensive orofacial pain evaluation should include a basic assessment of the function of all cranial nerves (see chapter 2).

## The trigeminal nerve

The *trigeminal nerve* is the largest cranial nerve, consisting of three peripheral branches: the ophthalmic, the maxillary, and the mandibular. Figure 1-1a shows the regions where these branches collect the sensory input that is conveyed by first-order neurons through the trigeminal ganglion, where most neuron cell bodies are located, to the brainstem. Although these neurons enter the ganglion on three branches, they exit in one large sensory root that enters the brainstem at the level of the pons before reaching the trigeminal nuclei.[29]

### The ophthalmic branch ($V_1$)

This branch of the trigeminal nerve leaves the skull through the superior orbital fissure and transmits sensory information from the scalp and forehead, upper eyelid, conjunctiva and cornea of the eye, nose (including the tip of the nose), nasal mucosa, frontal sinuses and parts of the meninges (the dura and blood vessels), and deep structures in these regions. It also carries postganglionic parasympathetic motor fibers to the glands and sympathetic fibers to the pupillary dilator muscles.[29]

### The maxillary branch ($V_2$)

This branch exits the skull at the foramen rotundum. It has a sensory function for the lower eyelid and cheek, the nares and upper lip, the maxillary teeth and gingiva, the nasal mucosa, the palate and roof of the pharynx, the maxillary and ethmoid and sphenoid sinuses, and parts of the meninges. Near its origin, it divides to form the middle meningeal nerve, which supplies the middle meningeal artery and part of dura mater. The terminal $V_2$ branches—the anterior and greater palatine nerves and the superior, middle, and anterior alveolar nerves—innervate the soft palate, uvula, hard palate, maxillary gingiva and teeth, and mucous membranes of the cheek.[29]

### The mandibular branch ($V_3$)

This branch leaves the skull through the foramen ovale and functions in sensory and motor transmission. $V_3$ carries sensory information from the lower lip, mandibular teeth and gingiva, floor of the mouth, anterior two-thirds of the tongue, chin and jaw (except the angle of the jaw, which is supplied by C2 and C3), parts of the external ear, parts of the meninges, and deep structures. A branch of $V_3$, the auriculotemporal nerve, innervates most of the TMJ.

The motor nuclei use $V_3$ to provide motor fibers to the muscles of mastication (ie, masseter, temporalis, medial pterygoid, lateral pterygoid, anterior digastric, and mylohyoid), the tensor veli palatini involved with eustachian tube function, and the tensor tympani, which attaches to the malleus bone in the eardrum.[29]

### The trigeminal nuclei

The trigeminal sensory nuclei lay in bilateral columns on either side of the brainstem that originate in the midbrain and terminate in the dorsal horn of the cervical spinal cord (Fig 1-1c). They are, in a rostrocaudal orientation, the mesencephalic nucleus, the main sensory nucleus, and the spinal trigeminal nucleus. All touch, position, and tempera-

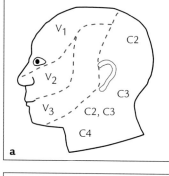

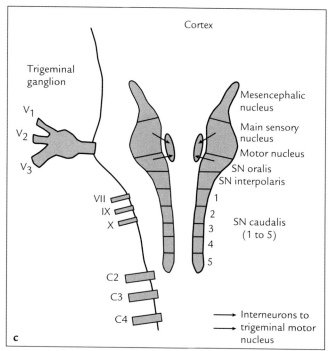

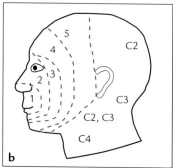

**Fig 1-1** Basic neuroanatomy. *(a)* Receptive fields for the ophthalmic ($V_1$), maxillary ($V_2$), and mandibular ($V_3$) branches of the trigeminal nerve and the upper cervical nerves. *(b)* The "onion skin" facial dermatomes. Impulses are carried on $V_1$, $V_2$, and $V_3$ through the trigeminal ganglion to the bilateral trigeminal nuclear columns in the pons. *(c)* The trigeminal nuclear columns and converging nerves. Note the subnucleus caudalis and the rostral caudal arrangement of its laminae (1 to 5), which receive nociceptive impulses from the respectively numbered facial dermatomes whether they originate on $V_1$, $V_2$, or $V_3$. Also note where cranial nerves VII, IX, X, and C2, C3, and C4 can provide pathways for convergence onto trigeminal nuclei. SN = subnucleus.

ture sensory input from the face plus potential pain input from the face, head, and neck is sent to the trigeminal nuclei.[13]

The mesencephalic nucleus, which is more a ganglion than a nucleus, houses the cell bodies of the proprioceptive neurons that convey input from the apical periodontal ligament and the muscle fibers that contract during the jaw-closing reflex. These proprioceptive neurons, and possibly the blink reflex nerves, represent the only peripheral nerves with cell bodies located within the CNS.[13,30] The neurons are monosynaptic and pass through the mesenceph-

alic nucleus to synapse in the trigeminal motor nuclei located medially to the much larger main sensory nucleus. The main sensory nucleus receives the facial proprioceptive and pressure input for orofacial behaviors (eg, chewing, kissing, smiling, and light touch) other than the jaw-closing reflex. These neurons have their cell bodies in the trigeminal ganglion and synapse in the main sensory nucleus where input is conveyed to the motor nuclei by arrays of small interneurons.[13]

The spinal trigeminal nucleus, sometimes referred to as the *medullary dorsal horn* because it extends into the spinal cord, consists of three subnuclei: subnucleus oralis, subnucleus interpolaris, and subnucleus caudalis. The subnucleus oralis and subnucleus interpolaris receive some peripheral nociceptive fibers, but mostly they receive temperature on Aδ fibers and touch impulses on Aβ fibers from the periphery and convey this input via interneurons to the motor nuclei.[13] Partly because of their temperature and tactile reception, the subnucleus oralis and subnucleus interpolaris play a significant role in the symptoms indicating central sensitization.[31,32]

The subnucleus caudalis is the main terminus for most slow first-order neurons that convey potential pain from trigeminal receptive fields. Figures 1-1b and 1-1c illustrate the "onion peel" somatotopic organization of the face (areas 1 to 5) and the corresponding laminae (1 to 5) in the subnucleus caudalis, where first-order nociceptive neurons terminate regardless of their division of origin.[13] For instance, Aδ and C-fiber neurons from area 5 in the face, whether they start in $V_1$, $V_2$, or $V_3$, all synapse with second-order nociceptive neurons in the most caudal aspect of the subnucleus caudalis, lamina 5. Such convergence means that a dural blood vessel, masseter muscle, or a tooth or tongue nociceptive afferent could excite the same second-order neurons. This convergence, the anatomic basis for referred pain, is not just a facial phenomenon. Cervical spine nociceptive afferents also synapse in the subnucleus caudalis, meaning that trapezius or sternocleidomastoid nociceptive afferents can excite second-order neurons that also receive input from facial tissues (Fig 1-2).[27,28,33]

Besides the convergence of the peripheral input, the trigeminal nuclei also receive extensive neuronal and interneuronal connections from sites throughout the CNS, including the motor cortex, which also sends afferents to the other cranial nerve motor nuclei,[13] and structures of the reticular formation, the limbic system, and the hypothalamus.[26,32,34-36] The nuclei are also rich in receptors for the spectrum of neurotransmitters through which sensory input and motor behaviors are modulated.[37]

In addition, second-order nociceptive neurons from the subnucleus caudalis arborize throughout the reticular formation and limbic structures and connect with the subnucleus interpolaris, subnucleus oralis, and main sensory nucleus (see Fig 1-2). These nuclei also receive descending motor input from the cortex and circuits involved with pain interpretation.[38-40] These ascending second-order neuronal and descending corticospinal connections show that nociception, before *and* after it is interpreted as pain, affects ongoing behavior.

Another construct to consider is that all of the CNS structures affected by trigeminal nociceptive input are also contacted by second-order neurons from the dorsal horn of the spinal cord.[13] Therefore, potential pain input from regions outside trigeminal receptive fields may excite CNS structures that heavily communicate with trigeminal nuclei and modulate their functions.

## The facial nerve

The seventh cranial nerve is a mixed nerve that has five branches (temporal, zygomatic, buccal, mandibular, and cervical) that course through the parotid gland but do not innervate the gland. Its main function is motor control of most of the muscles of facial expression and the stapedius muscle of the middle ear. The facial nerve supplies parasympathetic fibers to the sublin-

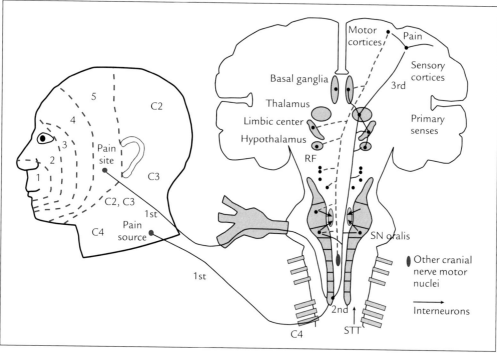

**Fig 1-2** Sensory pathways and motor response to referred pain. The first-order neurons from a pain site in facial lamina 5 and from the pain source in the C4 receptive field each converge on lamina 5 of the subnucleus caudalis and excite the same second-order neurons. As these second-order neurons ascend, they arborize with the subnucleus oralis and subnucleus interpolaris (not shown) and many reticular formation structures before synapsing with third-order neurons in the thalamus. The third-order neurons are thalamo-cortico-basal ganglia-limbic circuits that interpret pain and generate the descending motor and pain modulatory reactions to pain interpretation. The descending motor neurons also arborize with reticular formation locations and connect, via interneurons, to the trigeminal motor nucleus and to all cranial nerve motor nuclei. Note that trigeminal input is never analyzed in isolation as primary sensory; spinal thalamic tract input is also always being presented to the brain for analysis. RF = reticular formation structure, SN = subnucleus, STT = spinal thalamic tract.

gual and submandibular glands via the chorda tympani and to the lacrimal gland via the pterygopalatine ganglion. It also sends taste sensations from the anterior two-thirds of the tongue to the solitary tract nucleus and carries some cutaneous sensation from the skin in and around the ear lobe via the nervus intermedius.[29]

### The glossopharyngeal nerve

The ninth cranial nerve is composed of somatic, visceral, and motor fibers. Sensory fibers transmit from the posterior third of the tongue, the tonsils, the pharynx, the middle ear, and the carotid body. Taste sensation from the posterior third of the tongue and carotid body baroreceptor and chemoreceptor input is transmitted to the solitary tract nucleus. Nociceptive input from the ear is sent to the trigeminal spinal nucleus. From the inferior salivatory nucleus, the glossopharyngeal nerve delivers parasympathetic control to the parotid and mucous glands throughout the oral cavity. From the nucleus ambiguus, it sends motor fibers to the stylopharyngeus muscle and upper pharyngeal muscles. An altered gag reflex indicates glossopharyngeal nerve damage.[29]

## The vagus nerve

The tenth cranial nerve originates in the brainstem and extends to the abdomen, innervating virtually all organs from the neck to the transverse colon except the adrenal glands. It supplies visceral afferent fibers to the mucous membranes of the pharynx, larynx, bronchi, lungs, heart, esophagus, stomach, intestines, and kidneys, and distributes efferent or parasympathetic fibers to the heart, esophagus, stomach, trachea, bronchi, biliary tract, and most of the intestines. Also, the vagus nerve affects motor control of the voluntary muscles of the larynx, pharynx, and palate and carries somatic sensory fibers that supply the skin of the posterior surface of the external ear and the external acoustic meatus.[29] Through these connections, the vagus affects activities as varied as respiration, cardiac function, sweating, digestion, peristalsis, hearing, and speech.

## The spinal accessory nerve

The eleventh cranial nerve innervates the cervical muscles, the sternocleidomastoid and trapezius, which are coactivated during masticatory behaviors. Like the trigeminal motor nucleus, the accessory motor nuclei are rich in norepinephrine receptors, which can facilitate vigilant behaviors.[37] Nociceptive afferents from the cervical muscles converge onto the spinal trigeminal nucleus. It is notable that cervical myofascial pain seems to be prominent in patients with orofacial pain.

## The upper cervical nerves

Spinal nerves C1 to C4 and possibly C5 are important considerations in orofacial pain because their sensory fibers converge onto the trigeminal subnucleus caudalis.[27,28,33] As C1 to C4 leave the spine, they combine to form the cervical plexus, which yields cutaneous, muscular, and mixed branches. C1 forms the suboccipital nerve that supplies motor control to the muscles of the suboccipital triangle. The cutaneous branches are the lesser occipital (C2, C3), the greater auricular (C2, C3), the transverse cervical (C2, C3), and the supraclavicular (C3, C4). These nerves innervate the back of the head and neck, the auricle and external auditory meatus, the anterior neck and angle of the mandible and the shoulders, and the upper thoracic region. The muscular branch, the ansa cervicalis, innervates the sternohyoid, the sternothyroid, and the omohyoid muscles and is composed of a superior root (C1, C2) and an inferior root (C2, C3). The mixed branch is the phrenic nerve (C3, C4, and C5), which innervates the diaphragm.[29]

## The autonomic nervous system

The ANS comprises three divisions: the sympathetic, parasympathetic, and enteric nervous systems, which work to maintain homeostasis.[29] The peripheral ANS is controlled by the central ANS, composed of cortical, limbic, and reticular formation structures and nuclei.[41] Stimuli that activate the central ANS induce increased sympathetic activity initially in the brainstem and then in the periphery.[41,42] The sympathetic system is involved in vigilance, energy expenditure, and the "flight or fight" response, and the parasympathetic system counterbalances sympathetic arousal with "rest and digest" actions.[43]

The sympathetic and parasympathetic systems have preganglionic neurons that originate in different parts of the CNS and postganglionic neurons that deliver impulses to target tissues. Preganglionic neurons release acetylcholine at the autonomic ganglia, and postganglionic sympathetic and parasympathetic neurons release norepinephrine and acetylcholine, respectively, at the target sites.

The enteric system provides local sensory and motor fibers to the gastrointestinal tract, the pancreas, and the gallbladder. This system can function autonomously but is regulated by CNS reflexes. Its control of gastrointestinal vascular tone, motility, secretions, and fluid transport plays a vital role in homeostasis. Persistent sympathetic arousal that impairs parasympathetic function and leads to disturbances of the enteric system may be relevant to orofacial pain, since functional disorders of visceral organs controlled by the ANS seem to be common comorbid conditions.[10–12,43]

### Sympathetic input to the orofacial region

Sympathetic preganglionic neurons originate in the spinal cord. Their cell bodies are found in the intermediolateral gray matter at the level of all 12 thoracic and the upper 3 lumbar vertebrae. They exit the spinal cord via the ventral horn at the segmental level, where their cell bodies are located, but can synapse with any of the sympathetic ganglia

in the bilateral paravertebral chains. The superior portion of the sympathetic chain contains four cervical ganglia. In a rostrocaudal orientation, they are the superior cervical, middle cervical, intermediate cervical, and stellate ganglia. Postganglionic fibers leaving these sympathetic ganglia transmit motor input to the blood vessels in the head and neck, various glands, and the eyes. The skin of the face and scalp receive sympathetic innervation from the superior cervical ganglia via plexuses extending along the branches of the external carotid artery.[29,43]

### Parasympathetic input to the orofacial region

Parasympathetic preganglionic neurons originate in the brainstem nuclei where their cell bodies are located or in the lateral gray columns of the sacral spinal cord (S2-S4). Cranial nerves III, VII, IX, X, and the splanchnic nerve in the pelvic region carry parasympathetic preganglionic neurons, which are considerably longer than the postganglionic fibers because ganglia are generally located close to or embedded in the target organ. This close proximity to target sites and the parasympathetic preganglionic to postganglionic neuron ratio of 1:3 compared with a 1:10 ratio for the sympathetic system reflect the more specific cholinergic actions of parasympathetic postganglionic neurons and the more diffuse sympathetic noradrenergic effect on physiology.[43] Parasympathetic activity is purely neural, rapid, and short in duration, while sympathetic activity has a longer duration because of an additional humoral component. The secretion of catecholamines into the blood by the adrenal medulla is also a significant factor that explains why persistent sympathetic activity can override parasympathetic activity.

# Neurophysiology of Orofacial Pain

## Orofacial pain pathways

Nociceptive impulses generated by potential or actual tissue damage are just one type of input that different levels of the CNS continuously assess. The senses (smell, sight, hearing, touch, and taste) alert the brain to stimuli through thalamic-amygdala and thalamic-cortical-amygdala circuits, and those data streams are analyzed and compared with what the brain already knows in order to sequence efficient behavior.[44,45] Ongoing proprioceptive, nociceptive, thermoreceptive, baroreceptive, chemoreceptive, and vestibular input tells the brain how effectively its tissues are conducting responses and enables the brain to make ongoing behavioral adjustments aimed at maintaining efficiency. Nociception provides the brain an opportunity to interpret pain and make behavioral adjustments to avoid further, potentially damaging stimuli.

First-order nociceptive neurons, whether they synapse in the trigeminal subnucleus caudalis or in the dorsal horn, excite both nociceptive-specific and wide-dynamic range neurons. These neurons conduct nociception and/or other sensations through the brainstem and display varying degrees of arborization with structures throughout the reticular formation, where baseline physiologic processes are controlled before reaching the third-order neurons in the thalamus (see Fig 1-2).[13,38–40] Second-order neurons, stimulated by the faster-conducting Aδ fibers that release glutamate, arborize less than those receiving impulses from the slower-conducting C-fibers that release a wide variety of neurotransmitters.[13,46,47] Aδ input informs the brain about the onset of potential pain, while C-fiber input is used to coordinate the reparative and behavioral responses.

With sufficient temporal and/or spatial summation, third-order circuits, which start in the thalamus and connect the sensory cortex with the basal ganglia and the limbic system, interpret nociceptive input and pain is perceived.[1,13] While pain can often be felt, it is sometimes difficult to locate the actual source. Cutaneous stimuli are easier to recognize than stimuli from the muscles and visceral organs because the dermis has more nociceptive free nerve endings than are found in the deep tissues in order to assess integument integrity.[13]

In response to pain interpretation, multilevel behavioral responses are coordinated, and descending motor commands are created. Whether nociception is delivered to the CNS through the spinothalamic tract or the trigeminal thalamic tract, pain perception evokes ANS-modulated cranial nerve responses.[13,48,49] Since tissues under cranial nerve control will continue to excite trigeminal nociceptive pathways, an orofacial pain prognosis may be poor if ongoing pain sources beyond trigeminal receptive fields cannot be controlled.

## Nociception and pain modulation

The thinking brain needs to be able to recognize and avoid pain, but it does not want to be bothered by minor volleys of potential tissue damage. Therefore, nociception has a biphasic effect in the CNS. Initial low-intensity nociceptive impulses are facilitated through the CNS by serotonin. Only once stimulation of cortical circuits occurs, and pain is actually interpreted, does serotonin released from brainstem regions induce inhibition.[50,51] This action in combination with norepinephrine, which is the primary mediator of antinoception, cause a net inhibitory effect on transmission.[50,52,53] If nociception is relatively minor, inhibition minimizes the impact that transient nociceptive barrages have on thinking and task performance. Simultaneously, low-intensity nociception via second-order neuron arborization stimulates reticular formation structures to coordinate adjustments in motor and vascular behavior.[49] Such adjustments, because of net inhibition, can occur almost below the level of consciousness, and we continue to behave efficiently.

When nociception persists to excite third-order neurons and pain is realized, the brain's inhibitory capacity, called *stimulation-produced analgesia* (SPA), must work harder to counteract facilitation. SPA, by both noradrenergic and serotonergic pathways, inhibits nociceptive transmission first where the first-order and second-order neurons synapse in the subnucleus caudalis or in the dorsal horn and then at many other sites.[13] This descending inhibition is mediated by endogenous opioids, gamma-aminobutyric acid (GABA), and various inhibitory amino acids. Regions such as the periaqueductal gray serve as reservoirs for such compounds. These same inhibitory compounds are activated when stressors induce anxiety, fear, or depression.[54]

Brain circuits that interpret pain and direct descending inhibition also send commands to alter motor behavior and ANS functions. These descending commands reach structures throughout the reticular formation and, by vast pools of interneurons, stimulate all cranial nerve motor nuclei to alter behavior in response to pain (see Fig 1-2).[34-36] Alternative motor pathways are recruited, and protective changes

in respiration and cardiovascular mechanisms are engaged.[55] In the case of trigeminal motor activity, premotor interneurons deliver messages to the main sensory nucleus, the subnucleus oralis, and the subnucleus interpolaris, which, through interneurons, alter $\alpha$ motor neuron sequencing in the motor nuclei. These same nuclei mediate the minor motor adjustments[38-40] when net inhibition minimizes minor nociceptive volleys from intruding on circuits where pain is perceived.

## Sensitization

When persistent nociceptive facilitation exceeds inhibitory capacity, a spectrum of neuroplastic changes occur, first peripherally and then centrally. These changes are known as *sensitization*. Nerve thresholds are lowered, receptive fields are enlarged, gene expression is changed, and pain is persistent, evoked even by nonpainful stimuli.[46-48]

High-threshold peripheral nociceptors do not fire unless exposed to noxious stimuli. However, repeated stimulation can rapidly reduce firing thresholds through a variety of inflammatory molecules acting on various receptors. The antidromic release of neurogenic inflammatory compounds by perivascular afferents at the location of the pain also enhances peripheral nociceptive sensitization. This increase in the transmission frequency of noxious action potentials to second-order neurons is called *wind-up* and, if persistent, leads to central sensitization.[46,47]

Sensitization is a time- and intensity-dependent progression. Initially, low-intensity nociceptive volleys carried on A$\delta$ neurons release glutamate and activate postsynaptic $\alpha$-amino-3-hydroxy-5-methyl-4-isoxazole-propionic acid (AMPA) receptors in the subnucleus caudalis or dorsal horn. Higher-intensity stimuli induce C-fibers to fire, and a variety of neurotransmitters are released. At this point, in addition to the AMPA receptor activation, magnesium blocks to N-methyl-D-aspartic acid (NMDA) receptors are removed, and calcium channels are opened, producing central sensitization. Besides lowering thresholds for second-order neurons, NMDA receptor activation governs sensitization in areas such as the insular and anterior cingulate cortices, resulting in significant alterations in the interpretation of visceral sensation.[56,57]

In nonpainful states, Aβ fibers release only glutamate and deliver tactile sensations, which are important for the coordination of motor behaviors, to the subnucleus oralis and subnucleus interpolaris or dorsal horn lamina III and IV. But as central sensitization develops, thresholds are lowered where second-order neurons arborize to the subnucleus oralis and subnucleus interpolaris,[31,32] and Aβ fibers can begin to sprout axons into the adjacent nociceptive lamina.[58,59] Thus, nonpainful stimuli that converge onto a sensitized CNS will be interpreted as painful (Fig 1-3).[60] This mechanism is vital in acute pain states, such as posttraumatic wounds, to help avoid contact that would slow wound healing.

However, in chronic pain states, with glial cell activation augmenting CNS cytokine release, maintenance of central sensitization requires minimal nociceptive input.[13,61] Patients may have *allodynia*, pain exacerbations induced by stimuli that normally would not be perceived as painful, and *hyperalgesia*, exaggerated pain responses to mildly painful stimuli.[13] Understanding central sensitization is elemental to pain practice, as it explains light-touch pain symptoms that once were considered psychosomatic. Increasingly, sensitization is viewed as affecting symptoms associated with a variety of diagnoses, such as migraine, gastroesophageal reflux disease, irritable bowl syndrome, and fibromyalgia, which are often comorbid with facial pain.[48,62,63] It is vital to abort acute pain and eliminate pain sources as quickly as possible because once central sensitization is firmly established, it becomes exceedingly difficult to diminish.

**Heterotopic pain**

A common phenomenon associated with orofacial pain that may confuse both patient and clinician is heterotopic pain. When reporting chief complaints, patients often describe the site where they feel the pain rather than the actual pain source.[64] Clinicians must determine the sources of pain for treatment to be effective. *Primary pain* is that which occurs at the source, as is often the case in acute injury or infection.[64] It is not a difficult problem to diagnose and treat when other pain sources are absent.

Diagnostic difficulties may be encountered when the source of pain is not located in the region of pain perception. Such pain is said to be *heterotopic*. In the spinal system, heterotopic pain commonly involves impulses projected along the same nerve distribution.[64] For instance, in the L4 distribution, a patient may feel big toe pain when the source is a hip muscle impingement or foraminal stenosis. Projected nerve pain also occurs in the trigeminal system. A good example is the pain related to trigeminal neuralgia, which is felt throughout the peripheral distribution of the affected nerve. Another diagnostic challenge is *referred pain*, in which the pain is felt at a location served by one nerve but the source of nociception arrives at the subnucleus caudalis on a different nerve (see Fig 1-2). A common example is temple pain in the $V_1$ distribution

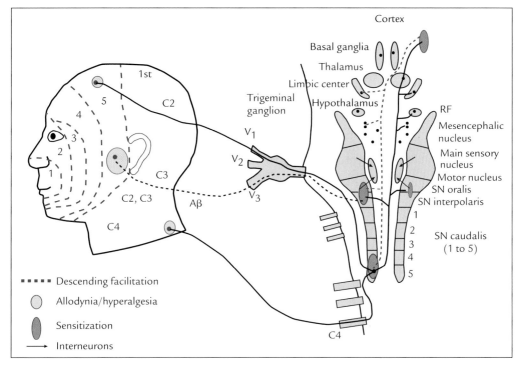

**Fig 1-3** Sensitization. First-order nociceptive neurons from facial lamina 5 transmitted via $V_1$ and C4 converge onto lamina 5 of the subnucleus caudalis. The pain sources are not controlled, summation exceeds descending inhibition, and progressive levels of central sensitization occur, first at the subnucleus caudalis, then at the ipsilateral subnucleus oralis/interpolaris, where A$\beta$ fibers carried on $V_3$ synapse. With continued summation, sensitization occurs at higher brain sites and at the contralateral subnucleus oralis/interpolaris. Nonpainful thermal and tactile inputs are experienced as painful (allodynia) or a more intense pain is felt (hyperalgesia) because of the effects of central sensitization. RF = reticular formation structure, SN = subnucleus.

caused by trapezius input delivered to the subnucleus caudalis on C4.[65]

Convergence by multiple sensory nerves carrying input to the trigeminal spinal nuclei from cutaneous and deep tissues located throughout the head and neck is the neuroanatomic basis for referred pain. As opposed to dermatomal-projected pain in the spinal system, primary nociceptive afferents from tissues served by $V_1$, $V_2$, $V_3$, C2, C3, and C4 can excite some of the same second-order neurons in the trigeminal sub-nucleus caudalis. In addition, first-order nociceptive neurons carried by C5, C6, and C7 and cranial nerves VII, IX, and X can synapse in trigeminal spinal nuclei as well as para-trigeminal nuclei.[13,27,28] Further, data clearly show that trigeminal second-order neurons converge on multiple brainstem locations involved in motor, ANS, and hypothalamic-pituitary-adrenal (HPA) axis activity.[26,27] Convergence explains how intracranial, neck, shoulder, or throat nociception may excite second-order neurons receiving input from facial structures. This convergence of input from tissues controlled by multiple motor nerves and delivered by multiple different sensory nerves to trigeminal nuclei also illustrates that the trigeminal system plays an integrative role in the behaviors of head, neck, and shoulder tissues.

As important as convergence of peripheral afferents is to understanding orofacial behaviors and referred pain, it is perhaps even more significant to appreciate descending convergence from cortical, limbic, hypothalamic, and ANS regions into the vast interneuronal pools of the brainstem. These interneurons reach the trigeminal motor nuclei through the subnucleus oralis, subnucleus interpolaris, and main sensory nucleus, and simultaneously convey directives to the other cranial nerve motor nuclei.[34–36] When pain is felt, the brain adapts, trying to minimize continued nociceptive barrages by altering patterns of movement[55] involving the highly integrative behaviors controlled by the cranial nerve. Reduced jaw range of motion or cocontraction as the brain restricts jaw movement in response to a trigger point in the sternocleidomastoid is an example of such adaptive behavior that is familiar to orofacial pain practitioners.

The muscles of the jaw, tongue, face, throat, and neck work synergistically to execute multiple orofacial functions, but pain in these areas alters the movements.[25] Neck or shoulder pain may result in impaired jaw or neck movement just as a sore tooth alters chewing and swallowing or a severe headache compels retreat from light and sound. But these sources will also contribute to central sensitization. While convergence is the anatomic construct for referred pain, sensitization with its allodynic and hyperalgesic responses underlies the neurophysiologic changes that make diagnosis and treatment of persistent pain involving the trigeminal system challenging.

## The Biopsychosocial Model: Allostasis and the Emotional Motor System

*Mind/body dualism* is a concept that views the mind and mental phenomena as being nonphysical, something apart from the body. Descartes' views on dualism, presented in 1641, still pervade today as many physicians and patients believe that disease and pain must be the result of a detectable physical malady or injury.[13] This mechanistic or biomedical model of medicine discounts the effects of the mind and society on disease processes. It views pain as the result of tissue damage, and if such organic disease or injury cannot be detected, then pain is explained as psychosomatic.

Engel[66] challenged the traditional biomedical model of disease as shortsighted in its assumptions that correcting the somatic parameters of disease defined the scope of physicians' responsibilities and that the psychosocial elements of human malfunction lay outside the domain of medicine's responsibility and authority. He rejected the biomedical approach, which asserted that all clinicians need to do to resolve pain is to find and repair the offending tissues, and developed the *biopsychosocial model*. This model views biologic, psychologic, and sociologic issues as body systems, just like the musculoskeletal or cardiovascular systems, with no separation of mind and body. Pain arises as a symptom that results from the combination of biologic, psychologic, and sociologic factors that continuously affect all individuals, and no two people experience the same spectrum of factors. Psychologic and sociologic differences are why equal degrees of nociception, a measurable biologic parameter, can produce vastly different pain and behavioral responses.

The biopsychosocial model also makes a distinction between disease associated with demonstrable pathology and illness in which poor health is perceived but biologic parameters do not show disease pathology. As science evolves, imaging techniques[67] and biologic markers continue to be discovered that show the adverse effects of psychologic and sociologic issues on physiology, thus redefining disease.[68,69] The mechanisms for central sensitization or the modification of neuroendocrine parameters that have been found to characterize abuse victims, who often suffer from many comorbid illnesses, are examples of science revealing markers for conditions previously considered to lack biologic basis.[70,71]

*Allostasis* is the adaptation of neural, neuroendocrine, and immune mechanisms in the face of stressors. *Allostatic load* refers to the physiologic changes that continued stressors produce as organisms attempt to maintain homeostasis. The changes in HPA axis function and brain cytokine activity that underlie cardiac disease and diabetes are examples of allostatic load.[72,73] Allostasis intersects with the controversial concept known as the *emotional motor system*. Proponents of the emotional motor system maintain that thoughts and emotions create neuroendocrine-mediated motor responses.[74,75] When an organism hears, sees, or smells, its limbic system (amygdala and hippocampus) acquires primary sensory stimuli and compares their relevance with prior knowledge in a matter of 15 to 30 milliseconds to help sequence dynamic behavior.[44] Input analysis and the emotional motor system facilitation

of autonomic and cranial nerve motor behavior involve the full spectrum of brain neurochemistry and endocrine function.[45,76]

Two scenarios not uncommon in orofacial pain practice illustrate how sociologic experiences may alter supraspinal physiology and pain experience. Consider an excessively worried patient who awakes with neck pain, the same initial complaint reported by his uncle who died from cancer, or a headache patient experiencing a panic attack when a smell rekindled the fear physiology associated with an assault 7 years earlier. For these patients, investigating only acute biomedical parameters may not help and may contribute to a deepening state of illness as the pathologic processes continue without recognition and treatment. These are patients for whom the biopsychosocial approach may prevent increased allostatic load. Taking sufficient time to obtain a thorough history and explain the physiologic effects related to psychosocial problems can help patients control factors that affect illness symptoms.

Although there is an increasing awareness of the need to assess all three systems outlined by Engel,[66] many barriers described in a 2005 study prevent its widespread utilization.[77] The study found that physicians and residents avoided approaching psychosocial issues because of inadequate training, lack of time, insufficient monetary incentive, and a large cultural ethos that favors "quick fixes."[77] The Research Diagnostic Criteria (RDC) for TMDs represent an attempt to apply both biologic (Axis I) and psychosocial (Axis II) factors to better understand a patient's condition.[78] However, the RDC have met resistance, because Axis I fails to account for how referred pain and central sensitization affect physical findings and Axis II is perceived by many as indicating that TMDs are psychosomatic despite evidence of disease. Yet, a 5-year follow-up study showed that in the 49% of TMD patients whose pain remitted, baseline psychologic measures were the same as those found in the general population.[79] Of the remaining 51%, the 14% who experienced high levels of pain improvement had improved psychologic parameters but minimal change in physical findings. In the 37% who did not get better, neither psychologic nor physical findings improved. Such data, which suggest that psychologic issues affect prognosis, demand that the physiology of psychosocial parameters be better addressed. Otherwise, advances in managing chronic orofacial pain and the possible comorbid conditions may not be achieved.

Although a great deal of effort is dedicated toward understanding genetic predisposition for disease, it is equally if not more important to realize that environmental stressors alter the expression of genetic codes and behavior. An animal model has shown that placing an identical twin in a harsher environment causes downregulation of GABA receptors and increases locus coeruleus (noradrenergic)-modulated stress behaviors.[80] It is important to understand that each brain, dependent on what that brain has previously experienced and what type of allostatic adaptations have been forced, will interpret nociception differently.

## Suffering and Pain: Comorbid Conditions

*Suffering*, a term notably absent in most medical dictionaries, and *pain* are different. Fordyce[81] defined *suffering* as the negative emotional/psychologic state that occurs in response to or in anticipation of nociception, while *pain* was defined as perceived nociception. But suffering is not exclusive to pain, as it is a state characterized by sadness, sorrow, and/or grief. The anticipation of intense and protracted pain or sadness or grief does affect the intensity of suffering. Moral and societal premises such as secondary gain also influence how much suffering an individual may demonstrate. In the realm of sadness, time may improve some wounds. But in the case of pain from uncontrolled sources, sensitization of the anterior cingulate cortex with limbic system and endocrine modulation[82] may make suffering a progressive experience to the individual and those who are touched by that person's struggle.

*Acute pain* is associated with a quick onset and short duration. It may be very intense, as in postsurgical pain, but usually the cause and effect relationship is apparent and the stimuli are not repeated. Central sensitization is induced but as a protective element to protect wound sites. As tissues heal, pain improves, sensitization resolves, and suffering is of short duration.

Periods of pain lasting 3 to 6 months, or the time it would take connective tissue to heal, have been presented as factors that distinguish *acute* from *chronic* pain. *Chronic pain* is persistent pain that becomes part of the patient's daily routine and is resistant to medical treatment because of neuroplastic changes throughout the CNS.[83] Although chronic pain may present with psychopathologic symptoms, such as depression, it is not always the case.[13] What seems to be true in patients with chronic pain is persistent central sensitization and an increased possibility of comorbid conditions. Although conditions like conversion disorders may exist, new evidence showing the links between stressor effects on the CNS and the digestive, respiratory, musculoskeletal, cardiovascular, endocrine, and immune systems are redefining what used to be called *somatoform disorders*.[68,84–87] As does chronic nociception, unrelenting stressors or horrific experiences can induce central sensitization, sympathetic upregulation, and endocrine abnormalities. These factors help explain why comorbid conditions such as posttraumatic stress disorder, headaches, TMDs, irritable bowel syndrome, gastroesophageal reflux disease, and fibromyalgia may evolve in patients afflicted by chronic pain.[88–90]

The role of the clinician is changing as science clarifies how CNS processes evolve when patients are exposed to chronic stressors. It is incumbent on practitioners to get a glimpse of the whole story, not just the portion seen through the biomedical model. The reality is that exposure to violence in our society is a common experience. In patients with chronic pain, exposure to abuse may be threefold greater than that experienced in the general population.[91] The taboos associated with being a victim of abuse or the repression induced by the sheer horror of abuse or some other catastrophic event can prevent patients from revealing these experiences. Clinicians must realize that severe pain and comorbid conditions due to disturbed CNS function may be the only indications of psychosocial distress. It is often a delicate subject to approach, but clinicians must be able to open the door to extremely skilled therapists for patients with problematic psychosocial histories if pain improvement is to be achieved.

# Chronic Orofacial Pain Disorders: TMDs and Comorbid Conditions

The 1996 National Institutes of Health (NIH) Technology Assessment Conference defined *TMDs* as "a collection of medical and dental conditions affecting the [TMJ] and/or the muscles of mastication, as well as contiguous tissue components."[92] This definition was similar to that published in the 1996 guidelines of the American Academy of Orofacial Pain,[93] which referred to "contiguous tissue components" as "associated structures." What constitutes "contiguous tissue components" for TMDs, a question as yet not answered, strongly influenced the NIH Conference's major conclusions, summarized as: "diagnostic classifications for TMDs are flawed as they were based on signs and symptoms and not etiology, etiology was not known, no consensus on what or when to treat existed, and no therapies had proven efficacy although behavioral approaches offered the best outcomes with the least risks." Since then, consensus on TMD etiology and the scope of signs and symptoms has not been achieved, but more is understood.

Many if not most patients with TMDs will recover with no or minimal care.[15,16] A minority of TMD cases become chronic,[94] and of those that do, one-third seemed to resolve over an 8- to 10-year period.[95] TMD patients who significantly improve may have minimal psychologic issues,[79] while patients with chronic TMDs,[96,97] like those with chronic musculoskeletal pain,[98] have psychologic comorbidity similar to other chronic pain patients.[99] Chronic TMD pain, like headache and most other chronic pains, seems more prevalent among women,[100–102] especially when multiple symptoms are present.[103] Recently, it was shown that female patients with orofacial pain displayed more medical problems than female controls.[11]

Over a 12-month period, 73% of adults experienced headaches, 56% had back pain, 46% had stomach pain, and 27% had dental pain.[104] These findings are in concert with data suggesting that preexisting headache or back, abdominal, or chest pain were better predictors than depression for the onset of facial pain experienced by 12% of the population.[6] Patients with facial pain rarely mention other conditions and yet, more than 81% of such patients have pain in regions below the head.[8,9] TMD patients frequently have symptoms of fibromyalgia, chronic fatigue syndrome, headaches, panic disorder, gastroesophageal reflux disease, irritable bowel syndrome, multiple chemical sensitivity, posttraumatic stress disorder, and interstitial cystitis.[10] Mazzeo and co-workers[12] found that self-report of symptoms of such conditions, in addition to greater measures of anxiety, depression, and sleep disturbance, differentiate those with orofacial pain from controls. They also found that 88% of study subjects reported a TMD plus at least one additional set of symptoms, and 31% reported six or more conditions. Among controls, 34% were symptom free, and none reported more than five conditions. Interestingly, symptoms of irritable bowel syndrome, panic disorder, and posttraumatic stress disorder did not differentiate study subjects from controls because of the high occurrence of these symptoms reported by controls. These findings support data showing that people may avoid care when symptoms carry psychosomatic stigma.[105]

Heart rate variability is a measure of the beat-to-beat time interval that reflects CNS control of ANS tone.[41] Low heart rate variability, when the beat-to-beat time interval becomes inflexible, occurs when high sympathetic tone impedes parasympathetic (vagal) dampening of cardiac activity. Low heart rate variability is a common finding for conditions seemingly as diverse as cardiovascular disease, diabetes, depression, anxiety, cognitive problems, irritable bowel syndrome, gastroesophageal reflux disease, posttraumatic stress disorder, migraine, fibromyalgia, and sleep apnea.[41,106–116] High heart rate variability, when parasympathetic control modulates a variable beat-to-beat time interval, is associated with good health and improved cognitive capacity.[41,106]

TMD patients have been differentiated from controls by pain, anxiety, depression, sleep disturbance, and measures of ANS reactivity,[117] and behavioral therapies have been shown to treat these conditions more successfully than traditional dental therapies.[118,119] Recently, orofacial pain patients with TMDs and other comorbid conditions, such as headaches, gastroesophageal reflux disease, and fibromyalgia, demonstrated low heart rate variability compared with controls when subjected to stressors[120] (also M Welder et al, unpublished data, 2007). Three months after patients were exposed to self-regulation skills aimed at controlling stress, associated jaw, neck, and breathing behaviors by pain scores improved, and measures of heart rate variability no longer differentiated patients from pain-free controls. The improved heart rate variability scores correlated with decreased pain interference scores, suggesting enhanced self-efficacy in the face of stressors.

Patients with orofacial pain report a high degree of exposure to traumatic events and significant disability.[89,90] In the past, disabling chronic pain was attributed to the failure of coping skills[121] related to personality type.[122] The heart rate variability study data suggest that, for some orofacial pain patients with multiple comorbid conditions, specific self-regulation skills may enable patients to cope with previously unrecognized and therefore uncontrolled physiologic disturbances associated with the pain (M Welder et al, unpublished data, 2007). Patient acceptance of the biopsychosocial approach may largely be dependent on previous psychosocial experience.[123]

Persistent elevation of sympathetic tone and impaired parasympathetic tone may be responsible for many of the comorbid conditions that affect patients with orofacial pain. Heart rate variability may be a noninvasive measurable parameter that could track the physiology of ANS problems in patients with trigeminal pain and shed light on its cause.[124] Reducing upregulated sympathetic activation, which may drive an out-of-control emotional motor system, may reduce the central sensitization that underlies the refractory nature of the spectrum of conditions seen in orofacial pain practice.

## Headache and Orofacial Pain Disorders

Recurrent headaches may occur in as many as 80% of TMD patients[125-129] compared with a 20% to 23% occurrence rate in a general population.[130,131] One in three persons has been estimated to suffer from a severe headache at some point in his or her life,[132]

a lifetime incidence similar to the 34% rate estimated for TMDs.[6] Yet, only 5% to 10% of the North American population has sought medical advice for severe headache.[133] Although earlier studies have shown associations between TMDs and headaches, causal interrelationships between the two conditions have not been demonstrated.[101,134-136] However, in a recent study in which 61% of orofacial pain patients had headache complaints and 38% fulfilled the criteria for migraine, higher migraine disability assessment (MIDAS) scores correlated with masticatory and cervical myalgia but did not correlate with the presence or absence of intracapsular TMJ problems.[129]

Headaches and TMDs are major trigeminal pain complaints that lead to significant suffering and absenteeism from work or school[2,104] and for which traumatic stressors may play a significant etiologic role.[89,90] The myalgia correlation[129] suggests that head and neck muscles, which orient organisms to collect primary sensory input and execute orofacial behaviors, may affect barrages of input that might contribute to states of ANS dysfunction and central sensitization that characterize headaches[48,115,137-139] as well as the host of other problems that afflict patients with orofacial pain.

## References

1. Groenewegen HJ, Uylings HBM. The prefrontal cortex and the integration of sensory, limbic and autonomic information. Prog Brain Res 2000;126:3–28.
2. Sternbach RA. Pain and "hassles" in the United States: Findings of the Nuprin Pain Report. Pain 1986;27:69–80.
3. Crook J, Rideout E, Browne G. The prevalence of pain complaints in a general population. Pain 1984;18:299–314.
4. James FR, Large RG, Bushnell JA, Wells J. Epidemiology of pain in New Zealand. Pain 1991;44:279–283.

5. Brattberg G, Thorslund M, Wikman A. The prevalence of pain in a general population. Pain 1989; 37:215–222.

6. Von Korff M, Dworkin SF, Le Resche L, Kruger A. An epidemiologic comparison of pain complaints. Pain 1988;32:173–183.

7. Lipton JA, Ship JA, Larach-Robinson D. Estimated prevalence and distribution of reported orofacial pain in the United States. J Am Dent Assoc 1993;124:115–121.

8. Türp JC, Kowalski, O'Leary NO, Stohler CS. Pain maps from facial pain patients indicate a broad pain geography. J Dent Res 1998;77:1465–1472.

9. Türp JC, Kowalski CJ, Stohler CS. Temporomandibular disorders—Pain outside the head and face is rarely acknowledged in the chief complaint. J Prosthet Dent 1997;78:592–595.

10. Aaron LA, Burke MM, Buchwald D. Overlapping conditions among patients with chronic fatigue syndrome, fibromyalgia, and temporomandibular disorder. Arch Intern Med 2000;160:221–227.

11. de Leeuw R, Klasser GD, Albuquerque RJ. Are female patients with orofacial pain medically compromised? J Am Dent Assoc 2005;136:459–468.

12. Mazzeo N, Colburn SW, Ehrlich AD, et al. Co-morbid conditions, sleep quality, pain measures, and psychometric parameters differentiate orofacial pain and general dentistry patient populations. Submitted to J Orofac Pain (in press).

13. Loeser JD, Butler SH, Chapman R, Turk DC (eds). Bonica's Management of Pain, ed 3. Philadelphia: Lippincott Williams & Wilkins, 2001.

14. Merskey H, Bogduk N (eds). Classification of Chronic Pain, ed 2. Seattle: IASP Press, 1994:209–214.

15. Kurita K, Westesson PL, Yuasa H, Toyama M, Machida J, Ogi N. Natural course of untreated symptomatic temporomandibular joint disc displacement without reduction. J Dent Res 1998;77:361–365.

16. Sato S, Kawamura H, Nagasaka H, Motegi K. The natural course of anterior disc displacement without reduction in the temporomandibular joint: Follow-up at 6, 12, and 18 months. J Oral Maxillofac Surg 1997;55:234–238.

17. Mense S. Group III and IV receptors in skeletal muscle: Are they specific or polymodal? Prog Brain Res 1996;113:83–100.

18. Houssiere A, Najem B, Ciarka A, Velex-Roa S, Naeije R, van de Borne P. Chemoreflex and metaboreflex control during static hypoxic exercise. Am J Physiol Heart Circ Physiol 2005;288:H1724–H1729.

19. Sinoway LI, Li J. A perspective on the muscle reflex: Implications for congestive heart failure. J Appl Physiol 2005;99:5–22.

20. Haouzi P, Chenuel B, Huszczuk A. Sensing vascular distension in skeletal muscle by slow conducting afferent fibers: Neurophysiologic basis and implication for respiratory control. J Appl Physiol 2004;96:407–418.

21. Adreani CM, Hill JA, Kaufman MP. Responses of group III and IV muscle afferents to dynamic exercise. J Appl Physiol 1997;82:1811–1817.

22. Adreani CM, Kaufman MP. Effect of arterial occlusion on responses of group III and IV afferents to dynamic exercise. J Appl Physiol 1998;84:1827–1833.

23. Adreani CM, Hill JA, Kaufman MP. Intrathecal blockade of both NMDA and non-NMDA receptors attenuates the exercise pressor reflex in cats. J Appl Physiol 1996;80:315–322.

24. Bertrand PM. Management of facial pain. In: Piecuch JF (ed). OMS Knowledge Update. Rosemont, IL: AAOMS, 2001:ANS77–107.

25. Ter Horst GJ, Copray J, Leim R, Van Willigen J. Projections from the rostral parvocellular reticular formation to pontine and medullary nuclei in the rat: Involvement in autonomic regulation and orofacial motor control. Neuroscience 1991;40:735–758.

26. Malick A, Strassman A, Burstein R. Trigeminohypothalamic and reticulohypothalamic tract neurons in the upper spinal cord and caudal medulla of the rat. J Neurophysiol 2000;84:2078–2112.

27. Marfurt CF, Rajchert DM. Trigeminal primary afferent projections to "non-trigeminal" areas of the rat central nervous system. J Comp Neurol 1991;303:489–511.

28. Saxon DW, Hopkins DA. Efferent and collateral organization of paratrigeminal nucleus projections: An anterograde and retrograde fluorescent tracer study in the rat. J Comp Neurol 1998;402:93–110.

29. Gray H. Developmental and gross anatomy of the central nervous system. In: Clemente C (ed). Anatomy of the Human Body, American ed 13. Philadelphia: Lea and Febiger, 1985.

30. Byers MR, Dong WK. Comparison of trigeminal receptor location and structure in the periodontal ligament of different types of teeth from the rat, cat, and monkey. J Comp Neurol 1989;279:117–127.

31. Wang H, Wei F, Dubner R, Ren K. Selective distribution and function of primary afferent nociceptive inputs from deep muscle tissue to the brainstem trigeminal transition zone. J Comp Neurol 2006;498:390–402.

32. Ikeda T, Terayama R, Jue SS, Sugiyo S, Dubner R, Ren K. Differential rostral projections of caudal brainstem neurons receiving trigeminal input after masseter inflammation. J Comp Neurol 2003;465:220–233.

33. Sessle BJ, Hu JW. Mechanisms of pain arising from articular tissues. Can J Physiol Pharmacol 1991;69:617–626.

34. Fay RA, Norgren R. Identification of rat brainstem multisynaptic connections to the oral motor nuclei using pseudorabies virus. I. Masticatory muscle motor systems. Brain Res Rev 1997;25:255–275.

35. Fay RA, Norgren R. Identification of rat brainstem multisynaptic connections to the oral motor nuclei in the rat using pseudorabies virus. II. Facial muscle motor systems. Brain Res Rev 1997;25:276–290.

36. Fay RA, Norgren R. Identification of rat brainstem multisynaptic connections to the oral motor nuclei using pseudorabies virus. III. Lingual muscle motor systems. Brain Res Rev 1997;25:291–311.

37. Paxinos G. Human Nervous System. San Diego: Academic Press, 1990.

38. Westberg KG, Olsson KA. Integration in trigeminal premotor interneurones in the cat. 1. Functional characteristics of neurones in the subnucleus-γ of the oral nucleus of the spinal trigeminal tract. Exp Brain Res 1991;84:102–114.

39. Olsson KA, Westberg KG. Integration in trigeminal premotor interneurones in the cat. 2. Functional characteristics of neurones in the subnucleus-γ of the oral nucleus of the spinal trigeminal tract with a projection to the digastric motoneurone subnucleus. Exp Brain Res 1991;84:115–124.

40. Westberg KG, Sandström G, Olsson KA. Integration in trigeminal premotor interneurones in the cat. 3. Input characteristics and synaptic actions of neurones in the subnucleus-γ of the oral nucleus of the spinal trigeminal tract with a projection to the masseteric motoneurone subnucleus. Exp Brain Res 1995;104: 449–461.

41. Thayer JF, Siegel GJ. Neurovisceral integration of cardiac and emotional regulation. IEEE Eng Med Biol Mag 2002;21(4):24–29.

42. Lachuer J, Gaillet S, Barbagli B, Buda M, Tappaz M. Differential early time course activation of the brainstem catecholaminergic groups in response to various stresses. Neuroendocrinology 1991;53:589–596.

43. Kandel ER, Schwartz JH, Jessell TM (eds). Principles of Neural Science, ed 3. New York: Elsevier Science, 1991.

44. Li XF, Stutzmann GE, LeDoux JE. Convergent but temporally separated inputs to lateral amygdala neurons from auditory thalamus and auditory cortex use different postsynaptic receptors: In vivo intracellular and extracellular recordings in fear conditioning pathways. Learn Mem 1996;3:229–242.

45. Stutzmann GE, McEwen BS, LeDoux JE. Serotonin modulation of sensory inputs to the lateral amygdala: Dependency on corticosterone. J Neurosci 1998;18: 9529–9538.

46. Mannion RJ, Woolf CJ. Pain mechanisms and management: A central perspective. Clin J Pain 2000;16: S144–S156.

47. Bolay H, Moskowitz MA. Mechanisms of pain modulation in chronic syndromes. Neurology 2002;59(5 suppl 2):S2–S7.

48. Yamamura H, Malick A, Chamberlin NL, Burstein R. Cardiovascular and neuronal responses to head stimulation reflect central sensitization and cutaneous allodynia in a rat model of migraine. J Neurophysiol 1999;81:479–493.

49. Benarroch EE. Pain-autonomic interactions. Neurol Sci 2006;27(suppl 2):S130–S133.

50. Zhuo M, Gebhart GF. Biphasic modulation of spinal nociceptive transmission form the medullary raphe nuclei. J Neurophysiol 1997;78:746–758.

51. Terayama R, Dubner R, Ren K. The roles of NMDA receptor activation and nucleus reticularis gigantocellularis in the time-dependent changes in descending inhibition after inflammation. Pain 2002;97:171–181.

52. Wei F, Ren K, Dubner R. Inflammation-induced fos protein expression in the rat spinal cord is enhanced following dorsolateral or ventrolateral funiculus lesions. Brain Res 1998;782:136–141.

53. Cahusac PMB, Morris R, Hil RG. A pharmacological study of the modulation of neuronal and behavioral nociceptive responses in the rat trigeminal region. Brain Res 1995;700:70–82.

54. Graeff F, Guimarães FS, De Andrade TG, Deakin JF. Role of 5-HT in stress, anxiety and depression. Pharmacol Biochem Behav 1996;54:129–141.

55. Lund JP, Donga R, Widmer CG, Stohler CS. The pain-adaptation model: A discussion of the relationship between chronic musculoskeletal pain and motor activity. Can J Physiol Pharmacol 1991;69:683–694.

56. Wu LJ, Toyoda H, Zhao MG, et al. Upregulation of forebrain NMDA NR2B receptors contributes to behavioral sensitization after inflammation. J Neurosci 2005;25:11107–11116.

57. Sami SA, Rossel P, Dimcevski G, et al. Cortical changes to experimental sensitization of the human esophagus. Neuroscience 2006;140:269–279.

58. Woolf CJ, Shortland P, Coggeshall RE. Peripheral nerve injury triggers central sprouting of myelinated afferents. Nature 1992;355:75–78.

59. Coggeshall RE, Leakan HA, Doubell TP, Allchorne A, Woolf CJ. Central changes in primary afferent fibers following peripheral nerve lesions. Neuroscience 1997;77:1115–1122.

60. Baron R, Baron Y, Disbrow E, Roberts TP. Activation of the somatosensory cortex during A beta-fiber mediated hyperalgesia. A MSI study. Brain Res 2000; 871:75–82.

61. Watkins LR, Milligan ED, Maier SF. Glial cell activation: A driving force behind pathologic pain. Trends Neurosci 2001;24:450–455.

62. Price DD, Zhou Q, Moshiree B, Robinson ME, Verne G. Peripheral and central contributions to hyperalgesia in irritable bowel syndrome. J Pain 2006;7:529–535.

63. Van Handel D, Fass R. The pathophysiology of non-cardiac chest pain. J Gastroenterol Hepatol 2005; 20(suppl):S6–S13.

64. Okeson JP. Bell's Orofacial Pains, ed 6. Chicago: Quintessence, 2005.

65. Simons DG, Travell JG, Simons LS. Myofascial Pain and Dysfunction: The Trigger Point Manual, vol 1: Upper Half of Body, ed 2. Baltimore: Williams & Wilkins, 1999.

66. Engel GL. The need for a new medical model: A challenge for biomedicine. Science 1977;196:129–136.

67. Chugani H, Behen M, Muzik O, Juhasz C, Nagy F, Chugani D. Local brain functional activity following deprivation: A study of postinstitutionalized Romanian orphans. Neuroimage 2001;14:1290–1301.

68. Monnikes H, Tebbe JJ, Hildebrandt M, et al. Role of stress in functional gastrointestinal disorders. Evidence for stress-induced alterations in gastrointestinal motility and sensitivity. Dig Dis 2001;19:201–211.

69. Mayer EA, Naliboff BD, Chang L. Basic pathophysiologic mechanisms in irritable bowel syndrome. Dig Dis 2001;19:212–218.

70. Heim C, Newport DJ, Bonsall R, Miller AH, Nemeroff CB. Altered pituitary-adrenal axis responses to provocative challenge tests in adult survivors of childhood abuse. Am J Psychiatry 2001;158:575–581.

71. Kaufman J, Plotsky P, Nemeroff C, Charney D. Effect of early adverse experiences on brain structure and function: Clinical implications. Biol Psychiatry 2000; 48:778–790.

72. McEwen BS. Stress, adaptation, and disease. Allostasis and allostatic load. Ann N Y Acad Sci 1998;840: 33–44.

73. Schulkin J, McEwen B, Gold P. Allostasis, amygdala, and anticipatory angst. Neurosci Behav Rev 1994; 18:385–396.

74. Holstege G, Bandler R, Saper CB. The emotional motor system. Prog Brain Res 1996;107:3–6.

75. Nieuwenhuys R. The greater limbic system, the emotional motor system and the brain. Prog Brain Res 1996;107:551–580.

76. de Kloet E, Oitzl M, Joels M. Stress and cognition: Are corticosteroids good or bad guys? Trends Neurosci 1999;22:422–426.

77. Astin JA, Goddard TG, Forys K. Barriers to the integration of mind-body medicine: Perceptions of physicians, residents, and medical students. Explore (NY) 2005;1:278–283.

78. LeResche L, Dworkin SF, Sommers E, Truelove EL. An epidemiologic evaluation of two diagnostic classification schemes for temporomandibular disorders. J Prosthet Dent 1991;65:131–137.

79. Ohrbach R, Dworkin SF. Five-year outcomes in TMD: Relationship of changes in pain to changes in physical and psychological variables. Pain 1998;74:315–326.

80. Fish EW, Shahrokh D, Bugot R, et al. Epigenetic programming of stress responses through variations in maternal care. Ann N Y Acad Sci 2004;1036:167–180.

81. Fordyce WE. Pain and suffering. A reappraisal. Am Psychol 1988;43:276–283

82. Price DD. Psychological and neural mechanisms of the affective dimension of pain. Science 2000;288: 1769–1772.

83. Flor H. Cortical reorganisation and chronic pain: Implications for rehabilitation. J Rehabil Med 2003;(41 suppl):66–72.

84. Esler M, Alvarenga M, Pier C, et al. The neuronal noradrenaline transporter, anxiety and cardiovascular disease. J Psychopharmacol 2006;20(4 suppl):60–66.

85. Bennett R. Fibromyalgia: Present to future. Curr Rheumatol Rep 2005;7:371–376

86. Wilhelmsen I. Somatization, sensitization, and functional dyspepsia. Scand J Psychol 2002;43:177–180.

87. Herman JP, Ostrander MM, Mueller NK, Figueiredo H. Limbic system mechanisms of stress regulation: Hypothalamo-pituitary-adrenocortical axis. Prog Neuropsychopharmacol Biol Psychiatry 2005;29:1201–1213.

88. Heim C, Newport DJ, Heit S, et al. Pituitary-adrenal and autonomic responses to stress in women after sexual and physical abuse in childhood. JAMA 2000;284:592–597.

89. De Leeuw R, Schmidt JE, Carlson CR. Traumatic stressors and post-traumatic stress disorder symptoms in headache patients. Headache 2005;45:1365–1374.

90. De Leeuw R, Bertoli E, Schmidt JE, Carlson CR. Prevalence of post-traumatic stress disorder symptoms in orofacial pain patients. Oral Surg Oral Med Oral Pathol Oral Radiol Endod 2005;99:558–568.

91. Curran SL, Sherman JJ, Cunningham LL, Okeson JP, Reid KI, Carlson CR. Physical and sexual abuse among orofacial pain patients: Linkages with pain and psychologic distress. J Orofac Pain 1995;9:340–346.

92. The Integrated Approach to the Management of Pain. NIH Consensus Statement 1986 May 19-21;6(3):1–8.

93. Okeson JP. Orofacial Pain: Guidelines for Assessment, Diagnosis, and Management. Chicago: Quintessence, 1996.

94. Von Korff M, LeResche L, Dworkin SF. First onset of common pain symptoms: A prospective study of depression as a risk factor. Pain 1993;55:251–258.

95. Magni G, Marchetti M, Moreschi C, Merskey H, Luchini SR. Chronic musculoskeletal pain and depressive symptoms in the National Health and Nutrition examination. I. Epidemiologic follow-up study. Pain 1993;53:163–168.

96. Sanders SH. Chronic pain: Conceptualization and epidemiology. Ann Behav Med 1985;7:3–5.

97. Kinny RK, Gatchel RJ, Ellis E, Holt C. Major psychological disorders in chronic TMD patients: Implications for successful management. J Am Dent Assoc 1992;123:49–54.

98. Merskey H. Classification of chronic pain: Descriptions of chronic pain syndromes and definitions of pain terms. Pain 1986;(suppl 3):1–225.

99. Bush FM, Harkins SW. Pain-related limitations in activities of daily living in patients with chronic orofacial pain: Psychometric properties of a disability index. J Orofac Pain 1995;9:57–63.

100. Agerberg G, Bergenholz A. Craniomandibular disorders in adult populations of West Bothnia, Sweden. Acta Odontol Scand 1989;47:241–250.

101. Schokker RP, Hansson TL, Ansink BJJ. The result of treatment of the masticatory system of chronic headache patients. J Craniomandib Disord Facial Oral Pain 1990;4:126–130.

102. Agerberg G, Inkapööl I. Craniomandibular disorders in an urban Swedish population. J Craniomandib Disord Facial Oral Pain 1990;4:154–164.

103. Glass EG, McGlynn FD, Glaros AG, Melton K, Romans K. Prevalence of temporomandibular disorder symptoms in a major metropolitan area. J Craniomandib Pract 1993;11:217–220.

104. Sternbach RA. Survey of pain in the United States: The Nuprin Pain Report. Clin J Pain 1986;2:49–53.

105. Hoge CW, Lesikar SE, Guevara R, et al. Mental disorders among US military personnel in the 1990's: Association with high levels of health care utilization and early military attrition. Am J Psychiatry 2002;159:1576–1583.

106. Thayer JF, Friedman BH. Stop that! Inhibition, sensitization, and their neurovisceral concomitants. Scand J Psychol 2002;43:123–130.

107. Dobrek L, Nowakowski M, Mazur M, Herman RM, Thor PJ. Disturbances of the parasympathetic branch of the autonomic nervous system in patients with gastroesophageal reflux disease (GERD) estimated by short-term heart rate variability recordings. J Physiol Pharmacol 2004;55(suppl 2):77–90.

108. Chen CL, Orr WC, Yang CC, Kuo TB. Cardiac autonomic regulation differentiates reflux disease with and without erosive esophagitis. Scand J Gastroenterol 2006;41:1001–1006.

109. van Orshoven NP, Andriesse GI, Smout AJ, Akkermans LM, Oey PL. Subtle involvement of the parasympathetic nervous system in patients with irritable bowel syndrome. Clin Auton Res 2006;16:33–39.

110. Tillisch K, Mayer EA, Labus JS, Stains J, Chang L, Naliboff BD. Sex specific alterations in autonomic function among patients with irritable bowel syndrome. Gut 2005;54:1396–1401.

111. Schroeder ED, Chambles LE, Liao D, et al. Atherosclerosis Risk in Communities (ARIC) study. Diabetes, glucose, insulin, and heart rate variability: The Atherosclerosis Risk in Communities (ARIC) study. Diabetes Care 2005;28:668–674.

112. Furlan R, Colombo S, Perego F, et al. Abnormalities of cardiovascular neural control and reduced orthostatic tolerance in patients with primary fibromyalgia. J Rheumatol 2005;32:1787–1793.

113. Stein PK, Domitrovich PP, Ambrose K, et al. Sex effects on heart rate variability in fibromyalgia and Gulf War illness. Arthritis Rheum 2004;51:700–708.

114. Thompson JJ, Elsenbruch S, Harnish MJ, Orr WC. Autonomic functioning during REM sleep differentiates IBS symptom subgroups. Am J Gastroenterol 2002;97:3147–3153.

115. Shechter A, Stewart WF, Silberstein SD, Lipton RB. Migraine and autonomic nervous system function: A population-based, case-control study. Neurology 2002;58:422–427.

116. Guilleminault C, Poyares D, Rosa A, Huang YS. Heart rate variability, sympathetic and vagal balance and EEG arousals in upper airway resistance and mild obstructive sleep apnea syndromes. Sleep Med 2005;6:451–457.

117. Carlson CR, Reid KI, Curran SL, et al. Psychological and physiological parameters of masticatory muscle pain. Pain 1998;76:297–307.

118. Carlson CR, Bertrand PM, Ehrlich AD, Maxwell AW, Burton RG. Physical self-regulation training for the management of temporomandibular disorders. J Orofac Pain 2001;15:47–55.

119. Dworkin SF, Turner JA, Mancl L, et al. A randomized clinical trial of a tailored comprehensive care treatment program for temporomandibular disorders. J Orofac Pain 2002;16:259–276.

120. Schmidt JE. A controlled comparison of emotional reactivity and physiological response in chronic orofacial pain patients [thesis]. Lexington, KY: Univ of Kentucky, 2006.

121. Turk DC, Rudy TE. Towards a comprehensive assessment of chronic pain patients. Behav Res Ther 1987;25:237–249.

122. Swimmer GI, Robinson ME, Geisser ME. Relationship of MMPI cluster type, pain coping strategy, and treatment outcome. Clin J Pain 1992;8:131–137.

123. Browne AL, Schug SA, Ray P, French D. A biopsychosocial approach to pretreatment assessment of patients with persistent pain: Identifying factors associated with pain-related disability. Pain Med 2006;7:466–467.

124. Lewis MJ. Heart rate variability analysis: A tool to assess cardiac autonomic function. Comput Inform Nurs 2005;23:335–341.

125. Yap AU, Chua EK, Dworkin SF, Tan HH, Tan KB. Multiple pains and psychosocial functioning/psychologic distress in TMD patients. Int J Prosthodont 2002;15:461–466.

126. Liljeström MR, Le Bell Y, Anttila P, et al. Headache children with temporomandibular disorders have several types of pain and other symptoms. Cephalalgia 2005;25:1054–1060.

127. Jokstad A, Mo A, Krogstad BS. Clinical comparison between two different splint designs for temporomandibular disorder therapy. Acta Odontol Scand 2005;63:218–226.

128. Nilsson IM, List T, Drangsholt M. The reliability and validity of self-reported temporomandibular disorder pain in adolescents. J Orofac Pain 2006; 20:138–144.

129. Dando WE, Branch MA, Maye JP. Headache disability in orofacial pain patients. Headache 2006;46: 322–326.

130. Lyngberg AC, Rasmussen BK, Jorgensen T, Jensen R. Has the prevalence of migraine and tension-type headache changed over a 12-year period? A Danish population survey. Eur J Epidemiol 2005;20:243–249.

131. Wiendels NJ, Neven AK, Rosendaal F, et al. Chronic frequent headache in the general population: Prevalence and associated factors. Cephalalgia 2006;26: 1434–1442.

132. Göbel H, Petersen-Braun M, Soyka D. The epidemiology of headache in Germany: A nationwide survey of a representative sample on the basis of the headache classification of the International Headache Society. Cephalalgia 1994;14:97–106.

133. Campbell JK. Headache in adults: An overview. J Craniomandib Disord 1987;1:11–15.

134. Wänman A, Agerberg G. Headache and dysfunction of the masticatory system in adolescents. Cephalalgia 1986;6:247–255.

135. Forssell H. Mandibular dysfunction and headache. Proc Finn Dent Soc 1985;81(suppl 1–2):1–91.

136. Schokker RP, Hansson TL, Ansink BJ. Craniomandibular disorders in patients with different types of headache. J Craniomandib Disord Facial Oral Pain 1990;4:47–51.

137. Jensen R. Mechanisms of tension-type headache. Cephalalgia 2001;21:786–789.

138. Bartsch T, Goadsby PJ. The trigeminocervical complex and migraine: Current concepts and synthesis. Curr Pain Headache Rep 2003;7:371–376.

139. Goadsby P. Migraine pathophysiology. Headache 2005;45(suppl 1):S14–S24.

# General Assessment of the Orofacial Pain Patient

In his course lectures, Weldon Bell would state that when examining and managing orofacial pain patients, it was important to set goals to achieve an acceptable degree of success. Bell maintained that the first goal was to establish a specific diagnosis. This statement, made more than 20 years ago, remains true. Diagnosis cannot be based solely on the patient's description of pain; it depends on an accurate assessment of the the history combined with appropriate clinical examination, radiographic, and laboratory findings. Even when information from the history is pathognomonic for a disorder, it is necessary to rule out comorbid disorders with a physical examination and further evaluations if indicated. Bell continued that having missed the first goal—diagnosis—the treating doctor cannot logically establish the second, third or fourth goals. The result is that all patients are treated the same and we are merely technicians or methodologists. When an accurate diagnosis is made, the correct treatment often becomes apparent.

The expanding field of orofacial pain has increased the scope of practice for dental practitioners. Evaluation of orofacial pain must go beyond the oral cavity, teeth, temporomandibular joints (TMJs), and the muscles of mastication. Knowledge of orofacial pain disorders allows clinicians to obtain a complete history with targeted questions and thorough documentation, to perform indicated examinations, and to obtain consultations and referrals when necessary. This chapter will guide the informed clinician in history gathering, physical examination, and testing, using techniques that have achieved scientific validity.

## Screening Evaluation

It has become integral to current dental practice to screen all patients for temporomandibular disorders (TMDs) and other orofacial pain disorders. The results of the screening should help the clinician determine whether a more comprehensive evaluation is necessary.[1] The screening may consist of a short questionnaire (Box 2-1), a brief history, and a limited examination. Although the value of questionnaires may be

**Box 2-1**  Example of screening questions for TMDs*

1   Do you have difficulty, pain, or both when opening your mouth, for instance, when yawning?
2   Does your jaw "get stuck," "locked," or "go out"?
3   Do you have difficulty, pain, or both when chewing, talking, or using your jaws?
4   Are you aware of noises in the jaw joints?
5   Do your jaws regularly feel stiff, tight, or tired?
6   Do you have pain in or near the ears, temples, or cheeks?
7   Do you have frequent headaches, neck aches, or toothaches?
8   Have you had a recent injury to your head, neck, or jaw?
9   Have you been aware of any recent changes in your bite?
10  Have you been previously treated for unexplained facial pain or a jaw joint problem?

*All patients should be screened for TMDs and other orofacial pain disorders. The decision to perform a comprehensive history and clinical examination will depend on the number of positive responses and the apparent severity of the problem. A positive response to any question may be sufficient to warrant a comprehensive examination if it is of concern to the patient or viewed as clinically significant.

**Box 2-2**  Example of screening examination procedures for TMDs*

1   Measure range of motion of the mandible on opening and right and left lateral movement. (Note any incoordination in the movements.)
2   Palpate for preauricular or intrameatal TMJ tenderness.
3   Auscultate and/or palpate for TMJ sounds (ie, clicking or crepitation).
4   Palpate for tenderness in the masseter and temporalis muscles.
5   Note excessive occlusal wear, excessive tooth mobility, buccal mucosal ridging, or lateral tongue scalloping.
6   Inspect symmetry and alignment of the face, jaws, and dental arches.

*All patients should be screened for TMDs and other orofacial pains using this or a similar, cursory clinical examination. The need for a comprehensive history and clinical examination will depend on the number of positive findings and the clinical significance of each finding. Any one positive finding may be sufficient to warrant a comprehensive examination.

challenged, a questionnaire can facilitate the clinical examination by focusing on specific complaints.[2]

The TMD screening (Box 2-2) usually consists of observation of the mandibular range of motion, palpation of the TMJs, and palpation of the masseter and temporalis muscles for tenderness. Palpation and/or auscultation of the joints may reveal sounds, and observation of mandibular function may disclose uncoordinated movements that may indicate biomechanical problems.[3] Caution should be observed when evaluating the results of the screening process; however, the clinical findings and the patient's complaints may not be consistent. The results of the screening evaluation should not be the only rationale to pursue a more thorough evaluation. For example, a clicking TMJ may represent a stable, nonpainful condition that does not require treatment.

**Box 2-3** Comprehensive history format for orofacial pain patients*

| | |
|---|---|
| Chief complaint | Date and event of onset |
| | Location of signs and symptoms |
| | Frequency and duration, intensity, quality of signs and symptoms |
| | Remissions or change over time |
| | Modifying factors (alleviate, precipitate, or aggravate) |
| | Previous treatment results |
| Medical history | Current or preexisting relevant physical disorders or disease (specifically, systemic arthritides or other musculoskeletal/rheumatologic conditions) |
| | Previous treatments, surgeries, and/or hospitalizations |
| | Trauma to the head and face |
| | Medications (prescription and nonprescription) |
| | Allergies to medications |
| | Alcohol and other substances of abuse |
| Dental history | Current or preexisting relevant physical disorders or diseases |
| | Previous treatments and patient's attitude toward treatment |
| | History of trauma to the head and neck (include iatrogenic trauma) |
| | Parafunctional history, both diurnal and nocturnal |
| Psychosocial history | Social, behavioral, and psychologic |
| | Occupational, recreational, and family |
| | Litigation, disability, or secondary gain issues |

*The sequence of a comprehensive history should parallel the traditional medical history and review of systems format including the patient's chief complaint(s), the history of present illness, medical and dental histories, and a psychosocial history.

## Comprehensive Evaluation

A comprehensive evaluation should be performed when a patient's chief complaints of pain are not of dental origin or when a patient's screening evaluation results are positive for an orofacial pain disorder. A comprehensive evaluation starts with a detailed patient history (Box 2-3). The examination process that follows may include some or all of the components listed in Box 2-4. Many patients have a lengthy list of complaints that, when reviewed, can lead the astute clinician to a differential diagnosis. A meticulous history will often guide the clinician to the most likely diagnoses and which, if any, additional diagnostic procedures are appropriate.

### History taking

The interview, or history, is usually the first contact between clinician and patient and, as such, a sympathetic approach by the clinician can quickly create a bond critical to successful communication.

### Chief complaint(s)

The patient must be allowed to express the symptoms that prompted the consultation, although the clinician must take control of

---

**Box 2-4** Comprehensive orofacial pain physical examination procedures

| | |
|---|---|
| General inspection of the head and neck | Note unusual symmetry, size, shape, consistency, posture, and involuntary movement or tenderness. |
| Neurologic evaluation | Conduct cranial nerve screening, noting signs and symptoms. Conduct vascular compression of the temporal and carotid arteries. |
| Evaluation of the associated muscles, TMJs, and cervical spine | Palpate the muscles of mastication and cervical muscles. Palpate the TMJ intrameatally and/or preauricularly. Measure range of motion, quality of movement, and association with pain. Auscultate and palpate for joint noises in all movements. Guide mandible movement, noting pain, end feel, and joint noise. Note any tenderness, swelling, enlargement, or unusual texture. |
| Ear, nose, and throat evaluation | Inspect the ears and nose for pathology, discharge, swelling, and enlargement. Inspect the oropharynx for pathologic changes. |
| Intraoral evaluation | Note hard and soft tissue conditions or disease. Analyze occlusion, both static and dynamic. |

---

the interview to gather information in an organized manner. Adequate time is necessary to allow the patient to fully describe each of the complaints. The complaints are documented in the order of severity as indicated by the patient, and details of each complaint are elicited in a systematic manner.

### History of chief complaint(s)

A description of each chief complaint usually includes its location, onset, frequency and duration, intensity, quality and associated symptoms, as well as alleviating, triggering, and exacerbating factors. The combination of these features often reveals recognizable patterns that can help the clinician to categorize the complaint.

#### Location

Very often, the patient will complain of pain in a part of the face or head in terms consistent with how he or she may understand the anatomy. Therefore, it is helpful to have the patient identify the exact location of the pain using one finger to either point to or circumscribe the area of the pain. The location of the pain does not always correspond to the source of the pain; therefore, finding the source, if different from the location, becomes a process of further investigation.

#### Onset

It is important to understand the circumstances that precipitated the pain. Trauma is a frequent cause of pain and should be differentiated from pain secondary to systemic disease or psychologic stressors. It is also important to know how the pain begins at each episode, for instance, whether it arises gradually or suddenly. The time of day the pain occurs may render additional clues.

#### Frequency and duration

The frequency of painful episodes yields information such as whether the pain comes in clusters, has periods of remission, or is

**Table 2-1** Pain quality descriptors and secondary symptoms associated with different pain categories*

| Pain Category | Quality | Secondary Symptoms |
|---|---|---|
| Musculoskeletal | Dull<br>Aching<br>Pressure<br>Depressing<br>Occasionally sharp | Flushing<br>Hyperalgesia<br>Allodynia<br>Can be referred from distant sites<br>Worse with function |
| Neurovascular | Throbbing<br>Stabbing<br>Pounding<br>Rhythmic | Worsened by increasing intracranial pressure<br>(ie, Valsalva, bending over, physical activity)<br>Sensitivity to light and/or sound<br>Nausea, vomiting |
| Neuropathic | Bright<br>Stimulating<br>Burning<br>Itchy<br>Electric shock–like<br>Cutting | Numbness<br>Hyperalgesia<br>Paresthesia<br>Allodynia |
| Psychogenic | Descriptive | Complaint patterns often do<br>not match anatomic sensory supply |

*Although the descriptive qualities are different for each pain category, there is much overlap, and clear communication between the clinician and the patient is essential for an accurate history.

continuous. The duration of pain is often recorded in days, weeks, or months. The daily duration of pain is categorized as constant or intermittent. If intermittent, the pain can be rated as brief, momentary, persisting for minutes, or lasting for hours. The frequency and duration of periods of remission are also recorded.

### Intensity

The level of pain is subjective and very often is augmented by the emotional status of a patient. It is important for the clinician to understand the patient's interpretation of the level or intensity of his or her pain. The intensity of the pain can be measured by a verbal rating (ie, mild, moderate, or severe), numeric rating (ie, a number between 0 and 10, where 0 represents no pain and 10 represents the most extreme pain), or a visual

analog scale (ie, a 10-cm line labeled at one end with "no pain" and at the other end with "most extreme pain").

### Quality

Different diagnostic categories of pain may be distinguished based on the quality of pain (Table 2-1). However, the clinician must be cautious when categorizing pain quality, because pain related to certain musculoskeletal disorders can mimic neurovascular or neuropathic disorders, and the reverse may also be true.

### Associated symptoms

Very often, a symptom associated with the patient's chief pain complaint can help the clinician narrow his or her diagnostic focus. Sensory and motor changes, as well as autonomic features should be recorded. For example, the presence of neurosensory disturbances such as scintillating scotoma or hemianopsia may be indicative for migraine with aura.

*Aggravating and alleviating factors*

Sensory changes such as diminished or increased perception of touch or pain may relate to neuropathic disorders. Aggravating and alleviating factors yield important information as well. Seemingly minor details that may not impress the patient as important may have tremendous diagnostic value. Examples include precipitating factors such as light wind, touch, or shaving, and aggravating factors such as emotional stress. Similarly, discovering that mandibular movement does not precipitate or aggravate the pain is of equivalent diagnostic importance.

## Previous treatments

Prior medical and dental treatment interventions for each complaint should be listed, along with the patient's perception of the results. Results of previous treatment can offer insight into the nature of the complaint. For instance, if an anti-inflammatory drug alleviated the pain, it is not likely that the cause is neuropathic. The patient's recall of medications, dosages, and length of medication trials should also be recorded to avoid re-treatment with a failed therapy or to determine whether certain medications were tried at an appropriate dose and for an appropriate period of time. This part of the interview may also give insight into patient compliance with treatment.

## Medical and dental history

Past illnesses, surgeries, long- and short-term use of medications (including over-the-counter medications and herbal preparations), developmental or genetic abnormalities, and any sequelae should be documented. Use of tobacco and alcohol and caffeine consumption should be noted, as well as past or present substance abuse. In addition, the patient should be questioned about physical and/or emotional trauma.

A complete dental history should be obtained, particularly as it relates to the chief complaint. Complications of therapies are important to document as are any behaviors such as clenching, bruxism, or other parafunctional activities (eg, gum chewing, nail biting).

## Review of systems

Because the patient's complaints may be a manifestation of systemic disease, he or she should be questioned regarding any symptoms that might relate to systemic disorders, such as those affecting connective tissue as well as autoimmune disorders, fibromyalgia, diabetes, cardiovascular disorders, or Lyme disease. Poor sleep habits and sleep disorders are often present in the chronic pain population; therefore, a discussion of sleep quality, quantity, snoring, and sleep walking is also important.

## Psychosocial history

An evaluation for the presence of stressors and the patient's response to stress is extremely relevant to the diagnostic process. Whether the patient has depression and/or anxiety, which are often comorbid and complicating factors related to chronic pain, needs to be determined. Specific inquiries should be directed to disclose any sexual abuse or domestic violence.

Litigation, the expectation of monetary reward for disability, or secondary gain can also be complicating factors for the patient's prognosis.

The psychosocial history may provide insight regarding the patient's mental status and coping skills, interactions with others, and the presence of any psychologic overlay. In addition, an appreciation of how pain affects the patient's life can help direct treatment.

## Physical examination

### Vital signs

Baseline blood pressure, pulse rate, respiration rate, temperature, and weight are recorded. Evaluating vital signs is important for every patient but especially for those who are medically compromised or who are taking medications.

### Neurologic examination

Orofacial pain complaints may be the result of a neurologic problem. As part of the orofacial pain examination, an evaluation of cranial nerves is performed to assess the function (ie, strength, sensation) of the corresponding right and left nerves.

Cranial nerve dysfunction may manifest as changes in either motor or sensory function. Abnormal movement of muscles stimulated by one of the cranial nerves can indicate pathology along the motor pathways. A patient reporting sensory alterations should be tested for anesthesia, paresthesia, dysesthesia, allodynia, and hyperalgesia. Areas of altered sensation can be mapped to demonstrate pathology and may help to determine whether the patient's condition is progressive. Abnormal findings should prompt a more detailed neurologic evaluation, and, if indicated, the patient should be referred to an appropriate specialist. Table 2-2 lists the cranial nerves and

the most common methods of screening these nerves for dysfunction. Other tests are recommended for a complete neurologic and cranial nerve assessment.

### Palpatory examination

#### Muscular

The muscles of mastication are palpated bilaterally not only to determine equality of size and firmness, but, more importantly, to check for pain or tenderness to palpation, and pain referral. The clinician may also palpate for *myofascial trigger points*, which are hyperirritable sites in taut bands of muscle. Provocation of a myofascial trigger point will cause discomfort at the site and referred pain to a predictable zone of reference.[4,5] The temporalis, deep and superficial masseter, medial pterygoid, and suprahyoid muscles are also palpated. The lateral pterygoid is difficult to approach intraorally,[6,7] but the inferior lateral pterygoid may be accomplished with functional manipulation by challenging the muscle to contract against resistance or by observing for symptom changes with stretching.[8,9] Myalgia may be exacerbated during this maneuver. Similar procedures of functional manipulation may be used for the superior lateral pterygoid and medial pterygoid muscles.[8] Muscles that can be palpated intraorally include the medial pterygoid and the anterior digastric. The temporal tendon can be palpated intraorally as well.

#### Cervical

It is common for orofacial pain to be caused by, and referred from, primary pain sites in the cervical structures.[9] Therefore, examination of the cervical structures is included in the comprehensive evaluation (see chapter 9).

**Table 2-2** Overview of cranial nerves and tests to evaluate their functions

| No. | Cranial nerve | Test |
|-----|---------------|------|
| I | Olfactory | Sense of smell (use, for example, camphor, coffee, vanilla) |
| II | Optic | Visual acuity, visual fields (confrontation); ophthalmoscopy |
| III | Oculomotor | Pupillary symmetry |
| IV | Trochlear | Pupillary light reflexes |
| V | Trigeminal | Sensation of light touch to face in all three divisions; motor innervation of muscles of mastication (strength); corneal reflex |
| VI | Abducens | Observation of palpebral fissures; position and alignment of eyes on straight-ahead gaze; eye movement in six directions |
| VII | Facial | Observation of facial expressions during spontaneous activity; voluntary strength of facial muscle of expression; taste to the anterior two-thirds of the tongue |
| VIII | Acoustic vestibular | Hearing (eg, ability to hear a watch tick), Weber and Rinne tests; observation for nystagmus on extraocular muscle testing; caloric testing |
| IX | Glossopharyngeal | Listening to patient's voice; observing the palate rise when patient says "ah" |
| X | Vagus | Gag reflex |
| XI | Accessory | Examination of the sternocleidomastoid and trapezius muscles for bulk and strength (press against resistance) |
| XII | Hypoglossal | Tongue bulk, strength, and movement (protrude and wiggle, press against resistance) |

**Arterial**

The temporal arteries are palpated for tenderness, consistency, and provocation of pain in all patients who complain of headache. Pain to palpation of the temporal artery may be a sign of giant cell arteritis, particularly in the elderly patient (see chapter 4). If giant cell arteritis is suspected, additional diagnostic tests are indicated.

**Temporomandibular joints**

The TMJs are palpated bilaterally for tenderness, pain, swelling, and patterns of movement. Palpation during mandibular movements is a common and accurate method of detecting joint sounds. The presence and timing of early, middle or late opening and/or closing, clicking, crepitation, and other interferences with smooth mandibular movement should be noted.[10]

Joint sounds can be signs of an intracapsular abnormality such as internal derangement, degenerative processes, or architectural defects of articulating surfaces. They may correlate with pain or pathologic conditions or may be due to functional adaptations not associated with pain or dysfunction. Joint sounds are common in the general population and should be evaluated within the context of other signs and symptoms.[11] While the predictive value of joint palpation is low in nonpatient populations,[12,13] positive findings may have clinical significance in symptomatic patients.[14]

## Mandibular range of motion

Normal mandibular opening is estimated to range from 40 to 55 mm, and excursive movements of at least 7 mm are considered normal.[15] While these are generally accepted ranges, opening distance may vary depending on many factors, such as stature, craniofacial form, and other variables.[16,17] The normal opening range or active range of motion is less in women than in men, and decreases with increasing age.[18] Three vertical opening measurements are suggested: maximum comfortable opening; full, unassisted opening; and assisted opening.[19] Maximum comfortable opening is defined by the range of motion that can be attained without pain. Full, unassisted opening or active range of motion is defined by the maximal range of motion a patient can attain regardless of pain. Assisted opening, also called passive range of motion, is defined as the maximal opening that can be attained with gentle stretching after the patient has reached his or her active range of motion. Several techniques for assessing the mandibular range of motion are available, including the use of a millimeter ruler and elaborate electrodiagnostic measuring systems. The range of vertical and horizontal movements should be recorded, as should the location of pain provoked by these movements. The patient's perception of re-

duced movement or change in movement may be more useful than actual measurements.[18]

## Ear, nose, and throat

Patients who complain of TMJ pain, or pain in the teeth or face, may be suffering from diseases or infections of the ear, nose, or throat. It is common for patients to report ear pain when, in fact, that pain is related to the affected TMJ. A patient may complain of maxillary tooth pain when that pain is being caused by sinus disease. The reverse can also be the case.

Examination of the external ear, the external auditory canal, and the tympanic membrane is performed using an otoscope.[20] When the complaint of ear pain is in the outer ear, the area should be examined for redness or swelling, which could indicate an infection or inflammatory process. The external auditory canal may be examined by pulling the ear upwards and backwards to straighten the canal for inspection. The canal is then observed for signs of infection, inflammation, discharge, or blockage. The properly trained clinician can observe the eardrum for any gross pathology that could explain the complaint of ear pain.

When evaluating the nose and sinuses, the skin overlying the nose is first inspected for abnormalities, such as unexplained ulcers, dark moles, or tissue growths. The skin over the maxillary and frontal sinuses is palpated, and tenderness noted. The trained clinician may inspect the nostrils using adequate light and a nasal speculum.

Each major salivary gland, including the parotid, submandibular, and sublingual glands is be palpated. Salivary gland duct exits can be inspected intraorally to confirm normal function. Salivary flow from each major duct exit should be palpated. If no spontaneous flow is seen after drying the area of the exit, the gland can be massaged, noting color and consistency of the fluid, if any, and the size of the gland or duct. If indicated, the saliva should be cultured.

The oropharynx is readily visualized by retraction of the tongue with a tongue depressor or dental mirror; this area should not be overlooked. Neoplastic disease may present in any of these structures. The palatine tonsils and posterior pharyngeal walls should be inspected. No special instrumentation is required.

As part of the head and neck examination, the clinician should palpate lymph nodes, including the submental, submandibular, superficial, and deep cervical chains. The latter group may be examined with relative ease by palpating the relaxed sternocleidomastoid muscle. Disease states of the oral cavity are most often reflected in changes of submental and submandibular lymph nodes.[21]

Lymph node groups are generally palpated systematically with the pads of the index and middle fingers. Although normal lymph nodes cannot be felt, knowledge of their anatomic location is necessary to perform the examination correctly. Lymph nodes in a healthy individual are soft, nonpalpable structures. Lymph nodes that are palpable, swollen, hard, painful, fixed, or nodular indicate possible infection, inflammation, or neoplasm. The cause of abnormal nodes should be determined.[21]

### Intraoral examination

Depending on the chief complaint(s) and the associated history, the patient may be given a cursory or thorough intraoral examination. When appropriate, the examination should include a complete dental and periodontal evaluation, examination of the oral soft tissues, and any necessary diagnostic radiographs. Electric pulp testing and/or thermal testing may be used to help evaluate the condition of the pulp. Percussion and mobility testing may also be helpful.

Soft tissue or superficial pain may arise from lesions of the integument caused by trauma, such as chemical, mechanical, or thermal irritants, as well as from neoplasm. The evaluation for soft tissue sources of orofacial pain requires visual inspection and palpation of suspected sources of pain. The tongue, floor of the mouth, palate, gingival tissue, and buccal mucosa should be carefully inspected. Oral ulcers, infections, and tongue and mucosal ridging should be noted. For superficial pains, diagnostic anesthesia, either topical and/or local, may assist the diagnostic process. An anesthetic challenge may be the most useful diagnostic procedure.

Dental occlusion should be evaluated when indicated, keeping in mind that occlusal findings may be the result of a TMD process rather than its cause. The occlusion is evaluated by analyzing the distribution and stability of the occlusal contacts in the intercuspal position as well as the patterns of wear and any attrition. These baseline studies may be of importance in a progressive disease process.

### Behavioral and psychosocial assessment

Orofacial pain, and chronic pain in general, may be amplified by psychologic and behavioral issues, which may contribute to the

---

**Box 2-5** Checklist of psychologic and behavioral factors

1   Inconsistent, inappropriate, and/or vague reports of pain
2   Symptoms incompatible with the innervation and function of anatomic structures
3   Overdramatization of symptoms
4   Symptoms that vary with life events
5   Significant pain for more than 6 months
6   Repeated failures with conventional therapies
7   Inconsistent response to medications
8   History of other stress-related disorders
9   Major life events, eg, new job, marriage, divorce, death of loved one
10  Evidence of alcohol and drug abuse
11  Clinically significant anxiety or depression
12  Evidence of secondary gain

---

primary etiology, be a factor in the patient's symptoms, and have an influence on effective treatment.

A high percentage of TMD patients show some significant psychologic abnormality that can influence symptom patterns and treatment direction.[22,23] Consequently, it is advised that the history-gathering portion of the comprehensive evaluation include an evaluation of behavioral, social, emotional, and cognitive factors that can sustain or result from the patient's pain complaints (Box 2-5).

Comprehensive psychologic inventories are not necessary for a routine screening or examination of all orofacial pain patients.[24–26] However, before initiating treatment for the pain, the clinician should screen for oral habits, depression, anxiety, stressful life events, lifestyle changes, secondary gain, and overuse of the health care system.[27] In uncomplicated cases, this screening can be accomplished during the initial interview and examination by the clinician. Further assessment or referral is recommended when significant factors are identified.

Anxiety and depression can frequently be identified by simply asking the patient.[28] Other psychologic factors may be identified through pain diaries or self-assessment instruments such as the Holmes and Rahe Scale for life changes.[29] The Interactive Microcomputer Patient Assessment Tool for Health (IMPATH),[30] the TMJ Scale,[31–34] and Screen[35] are screening devices specifically for TMDs. The initial psychosocial assessment may indicate the necessity for a more comprehensive evaluation and further testing by a psychologist or psychiatrist. Instruments that may be used in these cases include the Symptom Checklist-90-Revised (SCL-90-R), Minnesota Multiphasic Personality Inventory (MMPI), Hamilton Depression Scale, West Haven–Yale Multidimensional Pain Inventory, McGill Pain Questionnaire, Multiaxial Assessment of Pain, or the Million Behavioral Questionnaire.[36–44] It is important to interpret the results of these tests within the context of the history and examination.[45]

## Diagnostic tests

The gold standard for diagnosis of TMDs and orofacial pain is a thorough history, examination, and psychosocial assessment. Adjunctive diagnostic tests are not necessary for every patient; however, there are tests and procedures that may be of diagnostic importance. The selection of diagnostic tests should be judged by their scientific merit. Further, a test should be performed only if it adds information necessary for arriving at a diagnosis or if it is estimated that the test result may change the course of treatment.

### Scientific validation of diagnostic tests

For an instrument to become clinically useful, it must first be documented to consistently and reliably identify or measure the specific target sign or symptom that the manufacturer claims it can measure. *Reliability* refers to the degree of consistency in measurements, and *validity* refers to accuracy of measurements. Other measures important in determining the usefulness of certain instruments include sensitivity, specificity, and positive and negative predictive values. *Sensitivity* is a measure of how well a certain test is able to identify a disease when the disease is actually present. *Specificity* is a measure of how well a test identifies those who do not have the disorder. If sensitivity is high without regard to specificity, many patients will be wrongly identified as having the disorder.

For appropriate diagnosis, sensitivity and specificity should be over 70%. Many instruments meet the criteria for validity and reliability[46,47] but demonstrate low sensitivity and specificity, and therefore should not be used to establish a diagnosis.[48-53] Relying on such diagnostic tests could lead to

overtreatment and unnecessary increased medical costs. Finally, the *positive predictive value* is a measure of the probability that a person has the disease, and the *negative predictive value* is the probability that a person does not have the disease. The lack of scientific validation of many diagnostic tests may lead to many false-positive diagnoses and some false-negative diagnoses. There are immediate and implied future health and financial costs related to treating false-positive diagnoses and delayed costs of not treating false-negative diagnoses.

### Diagnostic casts

Since occlusion is not a common cause of TMDs (see chapter 8), diagnostic casts have little value in diagnosis and evaluation. They are helpful in identifying wear patterns and recording a baseline occlusion for comparison during treatment.[54] Occlusal analysis is often not accurate when the joints and muscles are sore. Any in-depth evaluation of the occlusion should be performed only after the pain is under control.[55] Even the most accurate casts will not, by themselves, provide enough information for an accurate diagnosis of joint or muscle pathology.[56]

### Electrodiagnostic testing

There are many electronic devices on the market that claim to aid in the diagnosis and treatment of TMDs, but their reliability, validity, safety, and efficacy have yet to be established.[57] Until well-controlled, double-blind, clinical trials are performed on specific subgroups of orofacial pain patients and are compared with control groups, electrodiagnostic tests should be considered experimental and should not be used in routine clinical practice.[58-62]

## Jaw tracking devices

It is helpful to observe and document mandibular motion in the process of diagnosing TMDs. Jaw tracking devices provide a clear record of these movements and make it easy to visualize specific mandibular movements in different excursions. The meaning of these tracings for diagnostic purposes is still unclear,[48,50,63-67] and the evidence is not adequate to support routine use for diagnosis. A further review of recent literature showed no new articles that support the use of jaw tracking as a diagnostic aid in TMDs, but did show articles on newer methods of jaw tracking.[68-71] These devices are cleared by the Food and Drug Administration but only from a safety standpoint and with a special notation that documentation for efficacy in diagnosis has to be provided for each device.

There are no data to demonstrate that jaw tracking devices are any more useful in measuring mandibular function than a traditional millimeter ruler. With this in mind, cost efficiency should be considered. Therefore, jaw tracking devices are not recommended as part of the orofacial pain evaluation.

## Electromyography

A useful tool for measuring muscle activity and nerve conduction is electromyography (EMG),[47] which has been shown by studies to be reliable.[72-75] However, a thorough review of the evidence-based literature indicates that due to limitations with regard to reliability, validity, sensitivity, and specificity, EMG testing is of limited value in the diagnosis of TMDs[50,59,63,76-79] and that increased EMG activity is not a valid indicator of masticatory muscle pain.[80-82] The current literature shows intraoperator reliability[72-75] and reliability in monitoring the progression of symptoms in particular patients.[53,63,83]

## Thermography

The presence of thermal asymmetries of the skin may reflect painful neurologic and musculoskeletal conditions when comparing normal with abnormal sites. The applicability of thermography for the diagnosis of orofacial pain has been studied, with conflicting results.[84,85] It is suggested that asymptomatic subjects have symmetric thermogram results[86] and that asymmetric thermogram findings suggest the presence of a TMD or other form of orofacial pain.[87] While some studies indicate that TMD patients have increased thermal emission on the symptomatic side,[88] especially over an affected joint,[89] other studies state the opposite. It is expected that TMJ osteoarthritis is characterized by larger thermographic hot zones at the symptomatic joint, low levels of symmetry, elevated absolute temperatures at the TMJ, and large differences between right and left facial zones. However, a study by Finney et al[90] suggests that TMD patients have decreased thermal emission on the symptomatic side. The variability of normal facial surface temperature between sides may be considerable.[91,92]

A comprehensive review of the literature revealed conflicting evidence on the direction of temperature shift over the painful site and high within-patient variability.[53] The results of thermography can also vary greatly according to the technique and instrument positioning. The results of clinical investigations suggest that thermographic "hot spots" in the back are not associated with active trigger points, and that "cold patches" on the face or head are not diagnostic for headache.[93,94] Several studies indicate that thermography may be able to distinguish TMD patients from healthy subjects[95,96] and may be useful in the diagnosis of some orofacial pain disorders.[91,97-104]

However, a more recent review indicated that there is insufficient evidence to support its use in routine clinical practice.[105]

## Sonography

Measurements of joint sounds may be used to diagnose TMDs, but the clinical significance and reproducibility of sounds emanating from the TMJ is not high. Studies evaluating sonography for the diagnosis of disc displacement have found that clinical and sonographic examination had high sensitivity but low specificity compared with magnetic resonance imaging (MRI).[106,107] In short, there is insufficient evidence to justify the use of sonography for detection of joint sounds and internal derangements in lieu of palpation/auscultation.

## Vibration analysis

The vibrations in joint sounds may assist in the diagnosis of a TMD with internal derangements.[108,109] Some studies show that vibration analysis can accurately identify disc displacement in patients.[110] However, sensitivity and specificity have been lower than desired, with many false-negatives and -positives.[11,111,112] No controlled clinical trials investigating the usefulness of joint vibration analysis were found. Hence, there is insufficient evidence to justify the use of vibration analysis versus the use of a stethoscope and palpation in detecting joint sounds.[113,114]

## Diagnostic imaging of the TMJ

There are a number of imaging modalities that may confirm the presence of suspected pathology, screen for unsuspected pathology, or identify staging of a disease. Diagnostic imaging may be used to rule out den-tal or periodontal pathology or to rule out pathology in areas of the head and neck other than the dentition and TMJs. If pathology is suspected that falls outside the scope of dental practice, appropriate medical referral should be made for proper diagnosis.

The type of imaging is indicated based on the relevant clinical findings.[115] While panoramic, transcranial, and tomographic studies are used for evaluating the hard tissues of the TMJs, they do not demonstrate the interarticular disc. Arthrography and MRI can depict the soft tissues of the joint. Because of the invasiveness and the level of technical skills needed, arthrography has been out-favored by MRI.

*Panoramic radiography*, also known as *orthopantography*, is a type of extraoral radiograph in which the maxilla and the mandible are depicted on a single film. After intraoral dental radiographs, it is the most common radiographic study performed in a dental office. The panoramic radiograph is useful for depicting the entire mandible and can demonstrate gross pathology, fractures, arthritic changes, and disparity in symmetry.

*Transcranial radiography* uses standard dental x-ray equipment and normally includes views of each condyle in the open, closed, and "rest" positions. The *rest position* is not a fixed point, but merely a comfortable mid-opening position for visualizing the condyle. Transcranial radiographs provide information concerning contours of bony elements. Some practitioners feel that the position of the condyle in relation to the fossa may also be determined with the transcranial radiograph, but that assumption is not universally shared. This view may be useful in ruling out gross arthritic changes as well as fracture.

*Transpharyngeal radiography* can be useful in screening for gross degenerative changes and evaluating condylar translation.

*Anteroposterior radiography* (transmaxillary or transorbital) may enhance the diagnostic accuracy when assessing degenerative pathology of the condyles.

*Tomography* is another radiographic technique that offers an evaluation of osseous structures, but it is more accurate in that it can focus on "cuts" only several millimeters thick. This study can view a TMJ like a loaf of bread, evaluating one slice at a time. Greater detail of the articular surfaces compared with transcranial views is rendered, and more accurate information on condylar displacement and arthritic changes is also possible to obtain.[116,117]

*Computerized tomography* is a noninvasive technique used to image not only the hard, bony tissues, but soft tissues as well.[118] Through computerized analysis of the radiographic signal, soft tissues such as the TMJ disc may be observed. This procedure has been demonstrated to be fairly accurate in its depiction of disc position, although often lacking in detail.[119] It also exposes the patient to a large amount of radiation.

*Arthrography* is a method of imaging the interarticular disc position. It is performed by injecting radiopaque substance into the inferior, or in some cases the inferior and superior, joint compartments, where it outlines the disc. This procedure, which may be combined with videofluoroscopy, provides a great deal of information. The drawback of this technique is that it can be quite painful for the patient and requires a high degree of clinical expertise. It also exposes the patient to higher levels of radiation.

*MRI* represents the current gold standard of diagnostic imaging for soft tissues.[120] It does not use radiation; rather, it is produced by computer analysis of signals emitted by the oscillation of protons in water molecules within soft tissues. The remarkable detail of soft tissues of the TMJ revealed by MRI is diagnostically useful.[121] In addition, the muscles of mastication can be imaged.[122] The test is noninvasive and provides the maximum amount of information with the smallest risk.

*Radionucleotide imaging*, also know as *scintigraphy*, is used clinically to show increased osteoblastic and/or osteoclastic activity, but its primary use is to identify malignancy and other diseases involving bone.[123] This highly sensitive test can detect areas of increased cellular activity (eg, as in inflammation, growth, or neoplasm), but it is very nonspecific with regard to identifying a specific disease or disorder.[124] A radioactive isotope is introduced intravenously, and the isotope concentrations are imaged using either a scintillation camera or single-photon emission computerized tomography. The former technique produces a plain study, and the latter produces a study similar to a tomographic or radiographic series.

*Ultrasonography* has been studied for the ability to depict internal derangements. Dynamic high-resolution sonography has shown more accurate and reliable results for detecting disc displacement with or without reduction[125,126] but not for detecting condylar erosion. In other studies, three-dimensional sonography has proved useful to exclude osteoarthrosis and disc degeneration,[127] but sensitivity and accuracy with regard to diagnosing disc dislocation compared with MRI were not satisfactory.[128] At this time, there is insufficient evidence for the use of ultrasonography in depicting osteoarthrosis and internal derangements, although the new technologic developments seem promising.

*Cone-beam computerized tomography* is the newest imaging technique for the maxillofacial region. This technique uses less radiation and is less time consuming than conventional tomography. The technology provides transaxial, axial, and panoramic images, which can be reconstructed in two- and three-dimensional layers. In contrast with conventional radiographs, variations in skull position do not lead to distortions in measurements with the cone-beam technology.[129,130] While there are no studies yet demonstrating the value of cone-beam technology in diagnosing internal derangements of the TMJ, it appears that this method may provide an accurate, cost-effective, and dose-effective diagnostic tool for the evaluation of osseous abnormalities of the TMJ.[131]

Of the imaging studies discussed, arthrography, computerized tomography, and MRI might be appropriate options to further study the anatomy of the TMJ. These imaging studies should not be done routinely for every patient or as an initial diagnostic test. While panoramic and transcranial radiographs are considered baseline studies for patients with a recognizable joint disorder, these more sophisticated imaging tests should only be prescribed if the study can provide information that has the potential to alter treatment.

## Diagnostic anesthesia

Neural blockade, somatic and sympathetic nerve blocks, and myoneural (trigger point) injections (Table 2-3) may be used as diagnostic methods. The chief examples of somatic nerve blocks in the head and neck include trigeminal, supraorbital, infraorbital, greater occipital, sphenopalatine ganglion, and cervical plexus nerve blocks. Somatic neural blockade is used not only to determine whether pain is emanating from a particular nerve, but whether the source of pain is proximal or distal to a particular site along the nerve. In addition to its diagnostic potential, somatic neural blockade may be useful in providing pain relief to the affected area by breaking the cycle of pain.

An injection to the TMJ can be achieved by a lateroposterior and slightly inferior intracapsular approach, a posterior meatal intracapsular approach, or an extracapsular block of the auriculotemporal nerve at the posterior aspect of the neck of the condyle.

Lidocaine (1% to 2%, often with epinephrine) is recommended for diagnostic nerve blocks because it produces prompt, long-lasting, and extensive anesthesia. Neural blockade is of particular prognostic value before neurolytic blockade or surgical sympathectomy (neurolysis). When prolonged anesthesia is desired for pain management, bupivacaine (0.25%) can be used.

Primary musculoskeletal pain, that is, pain that is localized to an injured or pathologic muscle or joint, may be arrested by a local or regional anesthetic block. Myofascial pain may be eliminated only if the anesthetic blocks the source or primary site of pain. Procaine is the least myotoxic anesthetic for injecting myofascial trigger points. Since procaine is not available in a dental carpule, many dentists use 2% lidocaine (without epinephrine). Bupivacaine appears to be relatively myotoxic and should be avoided for muscle injections.

Neuropathic pain responds uniquely to diagnostic blockade. If a regional block, such as a mandibular block, eliminates pain distal to the site of injection, the source of pain is confirmed to be located in the region of the anesthetized area. An ineffective diagnostic block suggests that the neuro-

**Table 2-3** Diagnostic anesthesia

| Type of anesthetic block | Type of pain |
| --- | --- |
| Dental block | Odontogenic pain |
| Trigger point injections | Myofascial pain |
| Trigger zone infiltration | Trigeminal neuralgia |
| Auriculotemporal nerve block | Intracapsular TMJ pain |
| Intracapsular block | Intracapsular TMJ pain |
| Greater occipital block | Cervicogenic pain |
| Sphenopalatine block | Neuropathic facial pain<br>Neurovascular pain |
| Stellate ganglion block | Sympathetically maintained pain |

pathic pain is more central and may be due to neuroplastic changes or other central nervous system phenomena.

Autonomic nerve blocks used in patients with orofacial pain most commonly include the stellate ganglion block (sympathetic) and the sphenopalatine block (parasympathetic). They are commonly used for diagnosis and treatment of autonomic-related pains, such as sympathetically mediated pains. Performing a stellate ganglion block requires special training and is usually done in an operating room by a trained anesthesiologist.

## Laboratory testing

A comprehensive assessment may include selective serologic testing, but it should not be a routine part of the orofacial pain examination.[132] Blood chemical analysis can rule out hematologic, rheumatologic, metabolic, or other abnormalities suggestive of systemic disease (Box 2-6). The clinician should know the appropriate serologic studies and be able to collect and interpret the data to establish a differential diagno-

sis. If systemic disease has not been ruled out, referral to a physician is indicated.

## Pretreatment testing and patient monitoring

Specific tests are sometimes necessary before beginning as well as during certain pharmacotherapeutic treatment. For example, the use of antiepileptic drugs such as carbamazepine must be preceded by a baseline complete blood cell count, a blood differential test, and liver function tests. Tricyclic antidepressant drugs should be preceded by a baseline electrocardiogram for assessment of arrhythmia, especially in older patients.

### Renal function

The kidneys are responsible for regulating fluid volume and acid-base balance of the plasma, excreting nitrogenous waste, and synthesizing erythropoietin, hydroxycholecalciferol, and renin. End-stage renal disease occurs when the kidney loses the ability to perform these functions. The early phase of renal disease, which is usually

34. Spiegel EP, Levitt SR. Measuring symptom severity with the TMJ scale. J Clin Orthod 1991;25(1):21–26.

35. de Leeuw JR, Ros WJ, Steenks MH, Lobbezoo-Scholte AM, Bosman F, Winnubst JA. Multidimensional evaluation of craniomandibular dysfunction. II: Pain assessment. J Oral Rehabil 1994;21(5):515–532.

36. Derogatis L. SCL-90-R: Administration, Scoring and Procedures Manual-II. Townson, MD: Clinical Pyschometric Research, 1983.

37. Beck AT, Ward CH, Mendelson M, Mock J, Erbaugh J. An inventory for measuring depression. Arch Gen Psychiatry 1961;4:561–571.

38. Melzack R. The McGill Pain Questionnaire: Major properties and scoring methods. Pain 1975;1(3):277–299.

39. Millon T, Green C, Meagher R. Millon Behavioral Health Inventory Manual. Minneapolis: National Computer Systems, 1982.

40. Speculand B, Goss AN. Psychological factors in temporomandibular joint dysfunction pain. A review. Int J Oral Surg 1985;14(2):131–137.

41. Eversole LR, Machado L. Temporomandibular joint internal derangements and associated neuromuscular disorders. J Am Dent Assoc 1985;110(1):69–79.

42. Kerns RD, Turk DC, Rudy TE. The West Haven–Yale Multidimensional Pain Inventory (WHYMPI). Pain 1985;23(4):345–356.

43. Gerschman JA, Wright JL, Hall WD, Reade PC, Burrows GD, Holwill BJ. Comparisons of psychological and social factors in patients with chronic oro-facial pain and dental phobic disorders. Aust Dent J 1987; 32(5):331–335.

44. Turk DC, Rudy TE. Towards a comprehensive assessment of chronic pain patients. Behav Res Ther 1987; 25(4):237–249.

45. Rugh JD. Association between bruxism and TMD. In: McNeill C (ed). Current Controversies in Temporomandibular Disorders. Chicago: Quintessence, 1992: 29–31.

46. Greene CS, Lund JP, Widmer CG. Clinical diagnosis of orofacial pain: Impact of recent FDA ruling on electronic devices. J Orofac Pain 1995;9(1):7–8.

47. Gallo LM, Gross SS, Palla S. Nocturnal masseter EMG activity of healthy subjects in a natural environment. J Dent Res 1999;78(8):1436–1444.

48. Greene CS. Can technology enhance TM disorder diagnosis? J Calif Dent Assoc 1990;18(3):21–24.

49. Goulet JP, Clark GT. Clinical TMJ examination methods. J Calif Dent Assoc 1990;18(3):25–33.

50. Widmer CG, Lund JP, Feine JS. Evaluation of diagnostic tests for TMD. J Calif Dent Assoc 1990;18(3): 53–60.

51. Mohl ND, McCall WD Jr, Lund JP, Plesh O. Devices for the diagnosis and treatment of temporomandibular disorders. Part I. Introduction, scientific evidence, and jaw tracking. J Prosthet Dent 1990;63(2): 198–201.

52. Mohl ND, Lund JP, Widmer CG, McCall WD Jr. Devices for the diagnosis and treatment of temporomandibular disorders. Part II. Electromyography and sonography. J Prosthet Dent 1990;63(3):332–336.

53. Mohl ND, Ohrbach RK, Crow HC, Gross AJ. Devices for the diagnosis and treatment of temporomandibular disorders. Part III. Thermography, ultrasound, electrical stimulation, and electromyographic biofeedback. J Prosthet Dent 1990;63(4):472–477.

54. Pullinger AG, Seligman DA. The degree to which attrition characterizes differentiated patient groups of temporomandibular disorders. J Orofac Pain 1993; 7(2):196–208.

55. Dyer EH. Importance of a stable maxillomandibular relation. J Prosthet Dent 1973;30(3):241–251.

56. Alexander SR, Moore RN, DuBois LM. Mandibular condyle position: Comparison of articulator mountings and magnetic resonance imaging. Am J Orthod Dentofacial Orthop 1993;104(3):230–239.

57. Lund JP, Widmer CG, Feine JS. Validity of diagnostic and monitoring tests used for temporomandibular disorders. J Dent Res 1995;74(4):1133–1143.

58. Douglass CW, McNeil BJ. Clinical decision analysis methods applied to diagnostic tests in dentistry. J Dent Educ 1983;47(11):708–714.

59. Mohl ND, Crow H. Role of electronic devices in diagnosis of temporomandibular disorders. N Y State Dent J 1993;59(10):57–61.

60. Mohl ND, Dixon DC. Current status of diagnostic procedures for temporomandibular disorders. J Am Dent Assoc 1994;125(1):56–64.

61. Mohl ND. Reliability and validity of diagnostic modalities for temporomandibular disorders. Adv Dent Res 1993;7(2):113–119.

62. Klasser GD, Okeson JP. The clinical usefulness of surface electromyography in the diagnosis and treatment of temporomandibular disorders. J Am Dent Assoc 2006;137(6):763–771.

63. Baba K, Tsukiyama Y, Yamazaki M, Clark GT. A review of temporomandibular disorder diagnostic techniques. J Prosthet Dent 2001;86(2):184–194.

64. Feine JS, Hutchins MO, Lund JP. An evaluation of the criteria used to diagnose mandibular dysfunction with the mandibular kinesiograph. J Prosthet Dent 1988;60(3):374–380.

65. Velasco J, Tasaki T, Gale EN. Study of pantographic tracings of TMD patients and asymptomatic subjects [abstract]. J Dent Res 1991;70(special issue):843.

66. Theusner J, Plesh O, Curtis DA, Hutton JE. Axiographic tracings of temporomandibular joint movements. J Prosthet Dent 1993;69(2):209–215.

67. Tsolka P, Preiskel HW. Kinesiographic and electromyographic assessment of the effects of occlusal adjustment therapy on craniomandibular disorders by a double-blind method. J Prosthet Dent 1993; 69(1):85–92.

68. Kinuta S, Wakabayashi K, Sohmura T, et al. Measurement of masticatory movement by a new jaw tracking system using a home digital camcorder. Dent Mater J 2005;24(4):661–666.

69. Palla S, Gallo LM, Gossi D. Dynamic stereometry of the temporomandibular joint. Orthod Craniofac Res 2003;6(suppl 1):37–47.

70. Hansdottir R, Bakke M. Joint tenderness, jaw opening, chewing velocity, and bite force in patients with temporomandibular joint pain and matched healthy control subjects. J Orofac Pain 2004;18(2):108–113.

71. Sae-Lee D, Wanigaratne K, Whittle T, Peck CC, Murray GM. A method for studying jaw muscle activity during standardized jaw movements under experimental jaw muscle pain. J Neurosci Methods 2006;157(2):285–293.

72. Bowley JF, Marx DB. Masticatory muscle activity assessment and reliability of a portable electromyographic instrument. J Prosthet Dent 2001;85(3):252–260.

73. Cecere F, Ruf S, Pancherz H. Is quantitative electromyography reliable? J Orofac Pain 1996;10(1):38–47.

74. Ferrario VF, Sforza C, D'Addona A, Miani A Jr. Reproducibility of electromyographic measures: A statistical analysis. J Oral Rehabil 1991;18(6):513–521.

75. Levine E, Levine JS. The choice of surface-EMG for muscle functional capacity evaluation. Am J Pain Manage 1999;9:104–108.

76. Rugh JD, Davis SE. Accuracy of diagnosing MPD using electromyography [abstract 1319]. J Dent Res 1990;69:273.

77. Schroeder H, Siegmund H, Santibanez G, Kluge A. Causes and signs of temporomandibular joint pain and dysfunction: An electromyographical investigation. J Oral Rehabil 1991;18(4):301–310.

78. Carlson CR, Okeson JP, Falace DA, Nitz AJ, Curran SL, Anderson D. Comparison of psychologic and physiologic functioning between patients with masticatory muscle pain and matched controls. J Orofac Pain 1993;7(1):15–22.

79. Bosman F, van der Glas HW. Electromyography. Aid in diagnosis, therapy and therapy evaluation in temporomandibular dysfunction [in Dutch]. Ned Tijdschr Tandheelkd 1996;103(7):254–257.

80. Majewski RF, Gale EN. Electromyographic activity of anterior temporal area pain patients and non-pain subjects. J Dent Res 1984;63(10):1228–1231.

81. Lindauer SJ, Gay T, Rendell J. Effect of jaw opening on masticatory muscle EMG-force characteristics. J Dent Res 1993;72(1):51–55.

82. Keefe FJ, Dolan EA. Correlation of pain behavior and muscle activity in patients with myofascial pain-dysfunction syndrome. J Craniomandib Disord 1988;2(4):181–184.

83. Lund JP, Widmer CG. Evaluation of the use of surface electromyography in the diagnosis, documentation, and treatment of dental patients. J Craniomandib Disord 1989;3(3):125–137.

84. Pogrel MA, Yen CK, Taylor RC. Infrared thermography in oral and maxillofacial surgery. Oral Surg Oral Med Oral Pathol 1989;67(2):126–131.

85. Pogrel MA, Erbez G, Taylor RC, Dodson TB. Liquid crystal thermography as a diagnostic aid and objective monitor for TMJ dysfunction and myogenic facial pain. J Craniomandib Disord 1989;3(2):65–70.

86. Feldman F, Nickoloff EL. Normal thermographic standards for the cervical spine and upper extremities. Skeletal Radiol 1984;12(4):235–249.

87. Gratt BM, Sickles EA. Thermographic characterization of the asymptomatic temporomandibular joint. J Orofac Pain 1993;7(1):7–14.

88. Berry DC, Yemm R. Variations in skin temperature of the face in normal subjects and in patients with mandibular dysfunction. Br J Oral Surg 1971;8(3):242–247.

89. Steed PA. The utilization of contact liquid crystal thermography in the evaluation of temporomandibular dysfunction. Cranio 1991;9(2):120–128.

90. Finney JW, Holt CR, Pearce KB. Thermographic diagnosis of temporomandibular joint disease and associated neuromuscular disorders. Paper presented at: the Academy of Neuromuscular Thermography, Dallas, TX, 1986.

91. Gratt BM, Sickles EA, Wexler CE. Thermographic characterization of osteoarthrosis of the temporomandibular joint. J Orofac Pain 1993;7(4):345–353.

92. Johansson A, Kopp S, Haraldson T. Reproducibility and variation of skin surface temperature over the temporomandibular joint and masseter muscle in normal individuals. Acta Odontol Scand 1985;43(5):309–313.

93. Swerdlow B, Dieter JN. The vascular "cold patch" is not a prognostic index for headache. Headache 1989;29(9):562–568.

94. Swerdlow B, Dieter JN. An evaluation of the sensitivity and specificity of medical thermography for the documentation of myofascial trigger points. Pain 1992;48(2):205–213.

95. McBeth SB, Gratt BM. Thermographic assessment of temporomandibular disorders symptomology during orthodontic treatment. Am J Orthod Dentofacial Orthop 1996;109(5):481–488.

96. Canavan D, Gratt BM. Electronic thermography for the assessment of mild and moderate temporomandibular joint dysfunction. Oral Surg Oral Med Oral Pathol Oral Radiol Endod 1995;79(6):778–786.

97. Gratt BM, Pullinger A, Sickles EA, Lee JJ. Electronic thermography of normal facial structures: A pilot study. Oral Surg Oral Med Oral Pathol 1989;68(3):346–351.

45

98. Gratt BM, Sickles EA, Graff-Radford SB, Solberg WK. Electronic thermography in the diagnosis of atypical odontalgia: A pilot study. Oral Surg Oral Med Oral Pathol 1989;68(4):472–481.

99. Gratt BM, Sickles EA, Ross JB, Wexler CE, Gornbein JA. Thermographic assessment of craniomandibular disorders: Diagnostic interpretation versus temperature measurement analysis. J Orofac Pain 1994;8(3):278–288.

100. Gratt BM, Sickles EA, Wexler CE, Ross JB. Thermographic characterization of internal derangement of the temporomandibular joint. J Orofac Pain 1994;8(2):197–206.

101. Gratt BM, Sickles EA, Shetty V. Thermography for the clinical assessment of inferior alveolar nerve deficit: A pilot study. J Orofac Pain 1994;8(4):369–374.

102. Shetty V, Gratt BM, Flack V. Thermographic assessment of reversible inferior alveolar nerve deficit. J Orofac Pain 1994;8(4):375–383.

103. Gratt BM, Graff-Radford SB, Shetty V, Solberg WK, Sickles EA. A 6-year clinical assessment of electronic facial thermography. Dentomaxillofac Radiol 1996;25(5):247–255.

104. Graff-Radford SB, Ketelaer MC, Gratt BM, Solberg WK. Thermographic assessment of neuropathic facial pain. J Orofac Pain 1995;9(2):138–146.

105. Fikackova H, Ekberg E. Can infrared thermography be a diagnostic tool for arthralgia of the temporomandibular joint? Oral Surg Oral Med Oral Pathol Oral Radiol Endod 2004;98(6):643–650.

106. Tanzilli RA, Tallents RH, Katzberg RW, Kyrkanides S, Moss ME. Temporomandibular joint sound evaluation with an electronic device and clinical evaluation. Clin Orthod Res 2001;4(2):72–78.

107. Puri P, Kambylafkas P, Kyrkanides S, Katzberg R, Tallents RH. Comparison of Doppler sonography to magnetic resonance imaging and clinical examination for disc displacement. Angle Orthod 2006;76(5):824–829.

108. Christensen LV. Physics and the sounds produced by the temporomandibular joints. Part II. J Oral Rehabil 1992;19(6):615–627.

109. Paiva G, Paiva PF, de Oliveira ON. Vibrations in the temporomandibular joints in patients examined and treated in a private clinic. Cranio 1993;11(3):202–205.

110. Wabeke KB, Spruijt RJ, van der Weyden KJ, Naeije M. Evaluation of a technique for recording temporomandibular joint sounds. J Prosthet Dent 1992;68(4):676–682.

111. Christensen LV, Donegan SJ, McKay DC. Temporomandibular joint vibration analysis in a sample of non-patients. Cranio 1992;10(1):35-41; discussion 41–42.

112. Ishigaki S, Bessette RW, Maruyama T. Vibration analysis of the temporomandibular joints with meniscal displacement with and without reduction. Cranio 1993;11(3):192–201.

113. Widmer CG. Temporomandibular joint sounds: A critique of techniques for recording and analysis. J Craniomandib Disord 1989;3(4):213–217.

114. Motoyoshi M, Hayashi A, Arimoto M, Ohnuma M, Namura S. Studies of temporomandibular joint sounds. Part 3. The clinical usefulness of TMJ Doppler. J Nihon Univ Sch Dent 1995;37(4):209–213.

115. Brooks SL, Brand JW, Gibbs SJ, et al. Imaging of the temporomandibular joint: A position paper of the American Academy of Oral and Maxillofacial Radiology. Oral Surg Oral Med Oral Pathol Oral Radiol Endod 1997;83(5):609–618.

116. Major PW, Kinniburgh RD, Nebbe B, Prasad NG, Glover KE. Tomographic assessment of temporomandibular joint osseous articular surface contour and spatial relationships associated with disc displacement and disc length. Am J Orthod Dentofacial Orthop 2002;121(2):152–161.

117. Pullinger AG, Seligman DA. Multifactorial analysis of differences in temporomandibular joint hard tissue anatomic relationships between disk displacement with and without reduction in women. J Prosthet Dent 2001;86(4):407–419.

118. Jager L, Rammelsberg P, Reiser M. Diagnostic imaging of the normal anatomy of the temporomandibular joint [in German]. Radiologe 2001;41(9):734–740.

119. Honda K, Larheim TA, Johannessen S, Arai Y, Shinoda K, Westesson PL. Ortho cubic super-high resolution computed tomography: A new radiographic technique with application to the temporomandibular joint. Oral Surg Oral Med Oral Pathol Oral Radiol Endod 2001;91(2):239–243.

120. Emshoff R, Innerhofer K, Rudisch A, Bertram S. Clinical versus magnetic resonance imaging findings with internal derangement of the temporomandibular joint: An evaluation of anterior disc displacement without reduction. J Oral Maxillofac Surg 2002;60(1):36–41; discussion 42–43.

121. Haley DP, Schiffman EL, Lindgren BR, Anderson Q, Andreasen K. The relationship between clinical and MRI findings in patients with unilateral temporomandibular joint pain. J Am Dent Assoc 2001;132(4):476–481.

122. Rudisch A, Innerhofer K, Bertram S, Emshoff R. Magnetic resonance imaging findings of internal derangement and effusion in patients with unilateral temporomandibular joint pain. Oral Surg Oral Med Oral Pathol Oral Radiol Endod 2001;92(5):566–571.

123. Jones BE, Patton DD. Bone scans of the facial bones: Normal anatomy. Am J Surg 1976;132(3):341–345.

124. Okeson JP (ed). Orofacial Pain: Guidelines for Assessment, Diagnosis, and Management. Chicago: Quintessence, 1996.

125. Emshoff R, Jank S, Bertram S, Rudisch A, Bodner G. Disk displacement of the temporomandibular joint: Sonography versus MR imaging. AJR Am J Roentgenol 2002;178(6):1557–1562.

126. Emshoff R, Brandlmaier I, Bodner G, Rudisch A. Condylar erosion and disc displacement: Detection with high-resolution ultrasonography. J Oral Maxillofac Surg 2003;61(8):877–881.

127. Landes CA, Goral W, Mack MG, Sader R. 3-D sonography for diagnosis of osteoarthrosis and disk degeneration of the temporomandibular joint, compared with MRI. Ultrasound Med Biol 2006; 32(5):627–632.

128. Landes CA, Goral WA, Sader R, Mack MG. 3-D sonography for diagnosis of disk dislocation of the temporomandibular joint compared with MRI. Ultrasound Med Biol 2006;32(5):633–639.

129. Ludlow JB, Laster WS, See M, Bailey LJ, Hershey HG. Accuracy of measurements of mandibular anatomy in cone beam computed tomography images. Oral Surg Oral Med Oral Pathol Oral Radiol Endod 2007;103(4):534–542.

130. Pinsky HM, Dyda S, Pinsky RW, Misch KA, Sarment DP. Accuracy of three-dimensional measurements using cone-beam CT. Dentomaxillofac Radiol 2006; 35(6):410–416.

131. Honda K, Larheim TA, Maruhashi K, Matsumoto K, Iwai K. Osseous abnormalities of the mandibular condyle: Diagnostic reliability of cone beam computed tomography compared with helical computed tomography based on an autopsy material. Dentomaxillofac Radiol 2006;35(3):152–157.

132. Wright EF, Des Rosier KF, Clark MK, Bifano SL. Identifying undiagnosed rheumatic disorders among patients with TMD. J Am Dent Assoc 1997;128: 738–744.

133. Little JW, Falace DA, Rhodus NL, Miller CS. Dental Management of the Medically Compromised Patient, ed 5. St Louis: Mosby, 1997.

# Differential Diagnosis of Orofacial Pain

The ability to understand and investigate pathophysiologic processes underlying a disorder depends on a valid, reliable classification system and common terminology to facilitate communication among clinicians, researchers, academicians, and patients. Without a universal system of organization in place, discussion, investigation, and, ultimately, understanding of a disorder is difficult to achieve.

Classification begins by grouping disorders according to common signs and symptoms and dividing further by common pathophysiology and treatment approaches. It is not important to further divide categories when all of the disorders within a given group are managed by the same therapy. After the classification criteria have been developed, the validity and reliability of the criteria must be analyzed. Once the criteria have proven valid and reliable, research efforts can be directed toward gaining better insight into the prevalence, etiology, and natural course of a given disorder, eventually leading to more effective treatment.

Knowledge can only be advanced when agreement is met on specific disorders so that research efforts can be compared between patients and various research groups. At this time it is uncertain whether diagnostic criteria for research purposes are compatible with diagnostic criteria for determining therapy. For example, it is quite reasonable to separate muscle disorders from intracapsular joint disorders for the purpose of studying the natural course of these disorders. However, merely identifying that a patient has one of these types of disorders may not be adequate to effectively manage the condition. The most useful classification schema would provide advantages to both research and clinical diagnosis.

In this chapter, past and present terminology and diagnostic classification systems for temporomandibular disorders (TMDs) and orofacial pain disorders are discussed, and a classification system for orofacial pain disorders based on American Academy of Orofacial Pain (AAOP) guidelines is presented.

# Terminology

Over the years, functional disturbances of the masticatory system have been identified by varying terminology, which has likely led to some confusion. In 1934, James Costen[1] isolated a group of symptoms that centered around the ear and temporomandibular joints (TMJs) and called it *Costen syndrome*. In 1959, Shore[2] used the term *temporomandibular joint dysfunction syndrome* for those symptoms. *Functional temporomandibular joint disturbances* was introduced by Ramfjord and Ash later.[3] Some earlier terms were based on possible etiologic factors related to the symptoms, such as *occlusomandibular disturbance*[4] and *myoarthropathy of the temporomandibular joint*.[5] Other terminology stressed the featured pain symptom, such as in *temporomandibular pain-dysfunction syndrome*[6] and *myofascial pain dysfunction syndrome*.[7]

However, because the symptoms are not restricted to the TMJs, some authors believed that the previously mentioned terms were too limited and that a broader, more collective term should be used, such as *craniomandibular disorders*.[8] Bell[9] suggested the term *temporomandibular disorders*, which has gained wide acceptance and popularity. TMDs are considered musculoskeletal disorders of the masticatory system.

# Diagnostic Classification Schemes

Many classification schemes have been proposed, with varying advantages and disadvantages. Categories of division have included etiologic factors, common signs and symptoms, and tissue origin or functional region of the body.

Perhaps the first classification scheme for TMDs was created by Weinmann and Sicher.[10] In 1951, they classified TMJ problems into (*1*) vitamin deficiencies, (*2*) endocrine disorders, and (*3*) arthritis. Two years later, Schwartz[11] introduced the term *temporomandibular joint pain-dysfunction syndrome* to distinguish organic disturbances of the joint proper from masticatory muscle disorders. In 1960, Bell[12] developed a classification system composed of six groups, recognizing both intracapsular and muscular (extracapsular) disorders. Acknowledging the need for a suitable classification system for functional disorders of the masticatory system, the AAOP published a position paper with a suggested classification scheme.[8] Soon after, the American Dental Association (ADA) organized a national conference in which Bell suggested the term *temporomandibular disorders* and a revised classification of TMDs consisting of five categories. Both the term and classification were accepted by the ADA.[13]

In 1989, Stegenga et al[14] proposed a system of classification emphasizing TMJ articular disorders. They divided their classification into inflammatory and noninflammatory articular disorders, and nonarticular disorders. The subcategories of osteoarthrosis and internal derangements were further divided according to staging over time.

The similarities between TMDs and other medical conditions was apparent to those in the dental profession, and the need for a classification system bridging medicine and dentistry was recognized. In 1986, the International Association for the Study of Pain (IASP)[15] published a classification of pain conditions. Of the 32 categories of pain disorders, category III was designated as *craniofacial pain of musculoskeletal origin*. Within this category were two subcategories: *temporomandibular pain and dysfunc-tion syndrome*, and *osteoarthritis of the TMJ*. This classification failed to recognize any pain disorders arising from the masticatory muscles.

Two years after the IASP classification was published, the International Headache Society (IHS)[16] proposed a classification for headache made up of 13 categories. The 11th category comprised *headache or facial pain attributed to disorder of cranium, neck, eyes, ears, nose, sinuses, teeth, mouth, or other facial or cranial structures*. There were no subcategories for TMDs, however, despite recommendations by the AAOP.[17] The 1996 AAOP Guidelines provided diagnostic criteria and subcategories,[18] although to date there have been no studies to determine the validity and reliability of these criteria.

In 1990, the American Academy of Head, Neck, Facial Pain and TMJ Orthopedics[19] proposed a classification with five TMD categories and two non-TMD categories. The subcategories represented a mixture of both traditional and nontraditional disorders. There were 19 subcategories under myofascial disorders, some of which were separated by the specific muscle or tendon involved. Some of the diagnostic categories, such as bruxism, might have better represented a precipitating or contributing factor of muscle pain rather than a muscle pain disorder itself.

A few more recent classification methods are worthy to mention because they offer certain advantages. Truelove et al[20] proposed a classification scheme that allowed for multiple diagnoses within the same subject group. Required operational criteria were listed for each diagnostic group, allowing the researcher to investigate a sample population and determine the types and severity of disorders present. This concept was further elaborated in the Research Diagnostic Criteria (RDC) offered by Dworkin and LeResche.[21] Their classification not only provided very specific diagnostic criteria for eight TMD subgroups, it also recognized that another level must be considered when evaluating and managing TMD pain: the psychosocial level. For the first time in any classification schema, a dual diagnosis was established that recognized the physical (Axis I) and the psychologic (Axis II) conditions that contribute to the suffering, pain behavior, and disability associated with the patient's pain experience. (This Axis II should not be confused with the designated axis system endorsed by the *Diagnostic and Statistical Manual of Mental Disorders, Fourth Edition*, of the American Psychiatric Association.) This dual-axis classification approach has been incorporated into Bell's classification for all orofacial pain disorders.[22]

Data are being collected to validate the reliability of RDC suggested by Dworkin and LeResche.[21] Although the RDC have proven useful in standardizing research efforts in the field of TMDs, it is questionable whether these criteria help the clinician select appropriate therapy for the patient.

More recently, a much broader approach to classification was suggested. Woda and Pionchon[23] proposed the adoption of a unifying classification for *idiopathic orofacial pain disorders*. Most clinicians who treat orofacial pain disorders recognize that there are certain patients who present with clinical symptoms that do not easily fit into the known and generally well-accepted categories of orofacial pain disorders. These unclassified conditions have been termed *atypical facial pain* and *atypical odontalgia*. Perhaps among these atypical cases are common clinical symptoms associated with common pathophysiologic mechanisms. Yet, until these mechanisms are better understood, grouping them into a large classification will not likely improve treatment selection.

Recently the IHS classification was updated.[24] Some clinicians favor this classification system because it comprises all types of head pains. However, with more than 230 types of headaches listed, it requires extensive knowledge in all orofacial pain disorders to establish a proper diagnosis. In addition, the reliability and validity of the various diagnostic criteria have not yet been established, and the classification does not provide for dual-axis diagnoses. The RDC[21] are more specific for TMDs and offer a dual-axis system, but they do not include all TMD subcategories, nor do they include other orofacial pain conditions. It is therefore concluded that the ideal classification system has not yet been developed.

# Differential Diagnosis

The diagnostic process is a clinical skill in which both art and science are wed. The goals of the process are to determine the primary, secondary, tertiary, etc, physical (Axis I) and/or psychologic (Axis II) diagnoses as well as the contributing factors. Listing conditions that may be responsible for each of the presenting complaints of the patient and including other contributing factors usually facilitate the process. Ruling out specific disorders that can cause similar symptoms should be pursued using inclusive diagnostic criteria until all correct diagnoses are established. It is important to rule out serious, life-threatening intracranial or extracranial disorders or diseases early in the process.

Establishing the correct diagnosis in patients with orofacial pain is particularly difficult, owing to the complex interrelationship of physical and psychologic factors in chronic pain syndromes and the similar signs and symptoms shared by many disorders. If the source of pain is uncertain, the appropriate diagnosis is "pain, cause unknown or undetermined." Further challenges to the process are those complex chronic orofacial disorders, which require a team approach to diagnosis and management, especially when significant Axis II factors are present.[25]

The new AAOP guidelines will use the main classification structure of the IHS,[24] which places TMDs in the 11th category, "Headache or facial pain attributed to disorders of cranium, neck, eyes, ears, nose, sinuses, teeth, mouth, or other facial or cranial structures" (Boxes 3-1 and 3-2), and neuropathic pains in the 13th category, "Cranial neuralgias and central causes of facial pain." As in the past[17,18,26] the AAOP will propose a classification of subcategories of TMDs that offer diagnostic value to both the clinician and researcher and is based on the revised work of Bell.[22] When available, the diagnostic criteria will be included with the assertion that their reliability and validity have not been determined. To better accommodate the variety of orofacial pain types, the AAOP will include some of the category 11 subcategories of the IHS but with different titles or additional elements. For example, subcategory 11.1, "Headache attributed to disorder of cranial bones" will be changed to "Headache or facial pain attributed to disorder of cranial bones" (Box 3-3). Further, whereas headaches or facial pain attributed to the TMJs are recognized as a separate subcategory (IHS 11.7), head-

| **Box 3-1** The International Classification for Headache Disorders according to the IHS[24] | |
|---|---|
| Part 1 | Primary headaches |
| IHS 1 | Migraine headache |
| IHS 2 | Tension-type headache |
| IHS 3 | Cluster headache and other trigeminal autonomic cephalalgias |
| IHS 4 | Other primary headaches |
| Part 2 | Secondary headaches |
| IHS 5 | Headache attributed to head and/or neck trauma |
| IHS 6 | Headache attributed to cranial or cervical vascular disorder |
| IHS 7 | Headache attributed to nonvascular intracranial disorders |
| IHS 8 | Headache attributed to a substance or its withdrawal |
| IHS 9 | Headache attributed to infection |
| IHS 10 | Headache attributed to disorder of homeostasis |
| IHS 11 | Headache or facial pain attributed to disorders of cranium, neck, eyes, ears, nose, sinuses, teeth, mouth, or other facial or cranial structures |
| IHS 12 | Headache attributed to psychiatric disorder |
| Part 3 | Cranial neuralgias, central and primary facial pain, and other headaches |
| IHS 13 | Cranial neuralgias and central causes of facial pain |
| IHS 14 | Other headache, cranial neuralgia, central or primary facial pain |

| **Box 3-2** Recommended diagnostic classification[24] for IHS 11: Headache or facial pain attributed to disorders of cranium, neck, eyes, ears, nose, sinuses, teeth, mouth, or other facial or cranial structures | |
|---|---|
| IHS 11.1 | Headache attributed to disorder of cranial bone |
| IHS 11.2 | Headache attributed to disorder of neck |
| IHS 11.3 | Headache attributed to disorder of eyes |
| IHS 11.4 | Headache attributed to disorder of ears |
| IHS 11.5 | Headache attributed to rhinosinusitis |
| IHS 11.6 | Headache attributed to disorder of teeth, jaws, or related structures |
| IHS 11.7 | Headache or facial pain attributed to TMD |
| IHS 11.8 | Headache attributed to other disorder of cranium, neck, eyes, ears, nose, sinuses, teeth, mouth, or other facial or cervical structures |

aches or facial pain attributed to masticatory muscle disorders are not. Therefore, subcategory 11.7, "Headache or facial pain attributed to temporomandibular joint (TMJ) disorder" will be renamed, "Headache or facial pain attributed to temporomandibular disorder," and a subdivision will be added to distinguish masticatory muscle disorders (11.7.2) from TMJ disorders (11.7.1; Boxes 3-4 and 3-5).

In this chapter, the eight broad diagnostic categories of orofacial pain will be briefly introduced (Box 3-6). A more complete description of each will be elaborated in separate chapters later in this text.

**Box 3-3** Recommended modification of diagnostic classification[18] for IHS 11.1: Headache or facial pain attributed to disorder of cranial bones

| | |
|---|---|
| 11.1.1 | **Congenital and developmental disorders** |
| 11.1.1.1 | Aplasia |
| 11.1.1.2 | Hypoplasia |
| 11.1.1.3 | Hyperplasia |
| 11.1.1.4 | Dysplasia |
| 11.1.2 | **Acquired disorders** |
| 11.1.2.1 | Neoplasia |

**Box 3-4** Recommended modification of diagnostic classification[18] for IHS 11.7.1: Headache or facial pain attributed to TMJ disorder

| | |
|---|---|
| 11.7.1.1 | **Disc derangement disorders** |
| 11.7.1.1.1 | Disc displacement with reduction |
| 11.7.1.1.2 | Disc displacement without reduction |
| 11.7.1.2 | **TMJ dislocation** |
| 11.7.1.3 | **Inflammatory disorders** |
| 11.7.1.3.1 | Synovitis and capsulitis |
| 11.7.1.3.2 | Polyarthritides |
| 11.7.1.4 | **Non-inflammatory disorders** |
| 11.7.1.4.1 | Osteoarthritis: Primary |
| 11.7.1.4.2 | Osteoarthritis: Secondary |
| 11.7.1.5 | **Ankylosis** |
| 11.7.1.6 | **Fracture (condylar process)** |

**Box 3-5** Recommended modification of diagnostic classification[18] for IHS 11.7.2: Headache or facial pain attributed to disorder of masticatory muscles

| | |
|---|---|
| 11.7.2.1 | Local myalgia |
| 11.7.2.2 | Myofascial pain |
| 11.7.2.3 | Centrally mediated myalgia |
| 11.7.2.4 | Myospasm |
| 11.7.2.5 | Myositis |
| 11.7.2.6 | Myofibrotic contracture |
| 11.7.2.7 | Neoplasia |

**Box 3-6** Differential diagnosis of orofacial pain

**Intracranial pain disorders (see chapter 4)**

Neoplasm, aneurysm, abscess, hemorrhage, hematoma, edema

**Primary headache disorders (see chapter 5)**

Migraine, tension-type headache, cluster headache, other trigeminal autonomic cephalalgias

**Secondary headache disorders**

Temporal (giant cell) arteritis, posttraumatic headache, medication overuse, headaches

**Neuropathic pain disorders (see chapter 6)**

Episodic neuralgias: trigeminal, glossopharyngeal, nervus intermedius, superior laryngeal neuralgias

Continuous neuropathic pains: deafferentation pain syndromes, peripheral neuritis, postherpetic neuralgia, posttraumatic and postsurgical neuralgia

Sympathetically maintained pain

**Intraoral pain disorders (see chapter 7)**

Dental pulp, periodontium, mucogingival tissues, tongue pain disorders

**TMDs (see chapter 8)**

TMJ pain, masticatory muscle pain

**Cervical pain disorders (see chapter 9)**

Cervical strain (whiplash), cervical arthritis, cervical disc disorders

**Associated structures (see chapter 10)**

Ears, eyes, nose, paranasal sinuses, throat, lymph nodes, salivary glands

**Axis II mental disorders (see chapter 11)**

Somatoform disorders, factitious disorders, malingering

## Intracranial pain disorders

Disorders of the intracranial structures, such as neoplasm, aneurysm, abscess, hemorrhage or hematoma, and edema, should be considered first in the differential diagnosis because they can be life threatening and require immediate attention. The characteristics of serious intracranial disorders include new or abrupt onset of pain or progressively more severe pain, interruption of sleep by pain, and pain precipitated by exertion or positional change (eg, coughing, sneezing). Other characteristics of intracranial disorders are weight loss, ataxia, weakness, fever, and neurologic signs or symptoms (eg, seizure, paralysis, vertigo, neurologic deficits).[22,25]

## Primary headache disorders

Primary headache disorders include migraine, tension-type headache, cluster headaches, and other trigeminal autonomic ceph-alalgias. These disorders are neurovascular in origin, whereby a neurologic mechanism triggers a vascular response. The character-istics of the headaches vary. Migraine, for example, is described as a disabling throb-bing, pulsating, or beating pain, whereas tension-type headache is characterized as a nondisabling dull, steady, aching pain. The dental profession has become increasingly active in managing some of these pain dis-orders; however, the major burden of man-aging most of these disorders still lies within the medical community.

## Neuropathic pain disorders

Neuropathic pain disorders arise from func-tional abnormalities of the nervous sys-tem.[27-29] There are two main categories of neuropathic pain disorders: episodic and continuous.[29] The episodic conditions are paroxysmal neuralgias characterized by sud-den, shock-like pain that lasts only seconds to minutes; they are named according to the nerve affected, such as trigeminal neu-ralgia, glossopharyngeal neuralgia, nervus intermedius neuralgia, and superior laryn-geal neuralgia. Occipital neuralgia is re-viewed in less detail, because the character-istic pain is located in the back of the cranium above the nuchal line rather than in the orofacial region.

Continuous neuropathic pain disorders can have peripheral and central compo-nents. The peripheral neuropathic pain dis-orders are the result of changes that have occurred in the peripheral neurons such as neuritis, postherpetic neuralgia, and deaf-ferentation pain, which occurs secondary to trauma (ie, postsurgical neuroma). This pain is usually described as unremitting and burning, and patients frequently report abnormal sensations (paresthesias) that are exacerbated by movement or touch.

Centrally mediated neuropathic pain is caused by pathologic changes in the central nervous system. It may be difficult to deter-mine the degree of peripheral and central in-fluence in a particular neuropathic pain condition.[30,31] The condition may be further complicated because of the influence the sympathetic nervous system may have on the pain condition.[32,33]

## Intraoral pain disorders

Intraoral pain is the most common source of orofacial pain. The clinician plays an im-portant role in the diagnosis of intraoral pain because many of these disorders are solely managed by the dental profession. The clinician must be very thorough in rul-ing out intraoral pain disorders involving the dental pulp, periodontium, mucogingi-val tissues, and tongue.

## Temporomandibular disorders

TMDs include disorders involving the masti-catory muscles and/or the TMJ. TMDs have been identified as a major cause of non-dental pain in the orofacial region and is considered to be a subclassification of mus-culoskeletal disorders.[34]

## Cervical pain disorders

Cervical pain disorders represent a very com-mon division of musculoskeletal disorders, and they can greatly influence the orofacial structures. These disorders are subdivided into those that predominantly originate in the muscles and those that predominantly originate in the cervical spine. These struc-tures very commonly refer pain to the face[35,36] and therefore represent a significant diagnostic consideration.

## Extracranial and systemic causes of orofacial pain

There are a variety of associated structures that can cause orofacial pain, such as the ears, eyes, nose, paranasal sinuses, throat, lymph nodes, and salivary glands. Many of these structures produce heterotopic (referred) pain felt in the orofacial region, which is often misinterpreted as dental or TMD pain. Although pain from these structures may not be primarily managed by the dental practitioner, a thorough understanding of their characteristics is necessary in order to establish an accurate diagnosis.

## Psychologic factors

There are many psychologic factors that contribute to a patient's pain experience. Rarely does pain exist without some influence of Axis II conditions, especially as pain becomes more chronic. Even common stressful life events (eg, conflicts in home or work relationships, financial problems, and cultural readjustment) may contribute to illness and chronic pain.[37-40] These stressors may heighten tensions, insecurities, and dysphoric effects that may in turn lead to increased strains on the masticatory system by way of unusual parafunctional behaviors. Once established, these adjustments (often with mixed disturbance of emotions and conduct) lead to an upregulation of the autonomic nervous system, which can further exacerbate the physical condition.[41,42]

Depression, anxiety, and prolonged negative feelings are common among patients with chronic pain and may make the persistent pain more difficult to tolerate or manage. People who unconsciously tend toward somatic expressions of emotions and conflicts are thought to be at higher risk for developing psychogenic somatic symptoms, including TMDs, through increased autonomic nervous system arousal, chronic muscle tension, and neuroendocrinologic activation. Negative cognitive factors, such as counterproductive thoughts or attitudes, can make resolution of the illness more difficult. Confusion and misunderstanding are commonly seen in chronic pain patients, because they have often received many varied opinions, diagnoses, and treatment suggestions. This confusion reduces motivation and increases anger or noncompliance. Also, patients with persistent pain often have unrealistic expectations and may expect complete or immediate pain relief.

It should be emphasized that psychologic disorders and orofacial pain disorders are not mutually exclusive conditions. Individuals with psychiatric disturbances may have bonafide orofacial pain disorders and, conversely, a lack of clear organic findings in patients with persistent orofacial pain is insufficient to suggest a psychogenic origin. The diagnosis of an Axis II psychologic disorder requires the presence of specific signs and symptoms and should never be based on the exclusion of organic disease alone. When psychologic factors are prominent in the patient's presentation, collaboration with a mental health professional should be an integral dimension of assessment and management.

# References

1. Costen JB. Syndrome of ear and sinus symptoms dependent upon functions of the temporomandibular joint. Ann Otol Rhinol Laryngol 1934;3:1–4.
2. Shore NA. Occlusal Equilibration and Temporomandibular Joint Dysfunction. Philadelphia: JB Lippincott, 1959.
3. Ramfjord SP, Ash MM. Occlusion. Philadelphia: WB Saunders, 1971.
4. Gerber A. Temporomandibular joint and dental occlusion [in German]. Dtsch Zahnarztl Z 1971;26:119–141.
5. Graber G. Neurologic and psychosomatic aspects of myoarthropathies of the masticatory apparatus [in German]. ZWR 1971;80:997–1000.
6. Schwartz L. Disorders of the Temporomandibular Joint. Philadelphia: WB Saunders, 1959.
7. Laskin DM. Etiology of the pain-dysfunction syndrome. J Am Dent Assoc 1969;79(1):147–153.
8. McNeill C, Danzig D, Farrar W, et al. Position paper of the American Academy of Craniomandibular Disorders. Craniomandibular (TMJ) disorders—State of the art. J Prosthet Dent 1980;44:434–437.
9. Bell WE. Clinical Management of Temporomandibular Disorders. Chicago: Year Book Medical, 1982.
10. Weinmann JP, Sicher H. Pathology of the temporomandibular joint. In: Sarnat BG (ed). The Temporomandibular Joint. Springfield, IL: Charles C Thomas, 1951:65–81.
11. Schwartz LL. A temporomandibular joint pain-dysfunction syndrome. J Chronic Dis 1956;3:284–293.
12. Bell WE. Temporomandibular Joint Disease. Dallas: Egan, 1960.
13. Report of the president's conference on examination, diagnosis and management of temporomandibular disorders. J Am Dent Assoc 1983;106:75–77.
14. Stegenga B, de Bont L, Boering G. A proposed classification of temporomandibular disorders based on synovial joint pathology. Cranio 1989;7(2):107–118.
15. Merskey H. Classification of chronic pain: Descriptions of chronic pain syndromes and definitions of pain terms. Pain 1986;(suppl 3):S1–S226.
16. Oleson J. Classification and diagnostic criteria for headache disorders, cranial neuralgias and facial pain. Cephalalgia 1988;8(suppl 7):S1–S97.
17. McNeill C. Temporomandibular Disorders: Guidelines for Classification, Assessment, and Management, ed 2. Chicago: Quintessence, 1993.
18. Okeson JP. Orofacial Pain: Guidelines for Classification, Assessment, and Management, ed 3. Chicago: Quintessence, 1996.
19. Talley RL, Murphy GJ, Smith SD, Baylin MA, Haden JL. Standards for the history, examination, diagnosis, and treatment of temporomandibular disorders (TMD): A position paper. J Craniomandib Pract 1990;8:60–77.
20. Truelove EL, Sommers EE, LeResche L, Dworkin SF, Von Korff M. Clinical diagnostic criteria for TMD. New classification permits multiple diagnoses [comments]. J Am Dent Assoc 1992;123(4):47–54.
21. Dworkin SF, LeResche L. Research Diagnostic Criteria of Temporomandibular Disorders: Review, criteria, examinations and specifications, critique. J Craniomandib Disord 1992;6:301–355.
22. Okeson JP. Bell's Orofacial Pains, ed 6. Chicago: Quintessence, 2005.
23. Woda A, Pionchon P. A unified concept of idiopathic orofacial pain: Pathophysiologic features. J Orofac Pain 2000;14(3):196–212.
24. Headache Classification Subcommittee of the International Headache Society. The International Classification of Headache Disorders: 2nd edition. Cephalalgia 2004;24(suppl 1):9–160.
25. Fricton JR, Kroening RF, Hathaway KW. TMJ and Craniofacial Pain: Diagnosis and Management. St Louis: Ishiyaku EuroAmerica, 1988.
26. McNeill C. Craniomandibular Disorders: Guidelines for Evaluation, Diagnosis, and Management. Chicago: Quintessence, 1990.
27. Fields H. Pain. New York: McGraw-Hill, 1987.
28. Wall P, Melzack R. Textbook of Pain, ed 4. Edinburgh: Churchill Livingston, 1999.
29. Okeson JP. Principles of pain diagnosis. In: Okeson JP. Bell's Orofacial Pains, ed 6. Chicago: Quintessence, 2005:141–196.
30. Wasner G, Schattschneider J, Binder A, Baron R. Complex regional pain syndrome—Diagnostic, mechanisms, CNS involvement and therapy. Spinal Cord 2003;41(2):61–75.
31. Raja SN, Grabow TS. Complex regional pain syndrome I (reflex sympathetic dystrophy). Anesthesiology 2002;96(5):1254–1260.
32. Singh B, Moodley J, Shaik AS, Robbs JV. Sympathectomy for complex regional pain syndrome. J Vasc Surg 2003;37(3):508–511.
33. Ochoa JL. Truths, errors, and lies around "reflex sympathetic dystrophy" and "complex regional pain syndrome." J Neurol 1999;246(10):875–879.

34. Okeson JP. Pains of muscle origin. In: Okeson JP. Bell's Orofacial Pains, ed 6. Chicago: Quintessence, 2005:287–328.

35. Piovesan EJ, Kowacs PA, Tatsui CE, Lange MC, Ribas LC, Werneck LC. Referred pain after painful stimulation of the greater occipital nerve in humans: Evidence of convergence of cervical afferences on trigeminal nuclei. Cephalalgia 2001;21(2):107–109.

36. Wright EF. Manual of Temporomandibular Disorders. Ames, IA: Blackwell, 2005.

37. Bertolotti G, Vidotto G, Sanavio E, Frediani F. Psychological and emotional aspects and pain. Neurol Sci 2003;24(suppl 2):S71–S75.

38. Rollman GB, Gillespie JM. The role of psychosocial factors in temporomandibular disorders. Curr Rev Pain 2000;4(1):71–81.

39. Korszun A, Papadopoulos E, Demitrack M, Engleberg C, Crofford L. The relationship between temporomandibular disorders and stress-associated syndromes. Oral Surg Oral Med Oral Pathol Oral Radiol Endod 1998;86(4):416–420.

40. Dworkin SF. Behavioral, emotional, and social aspects of orofacial pain. In: Stohler CS, Carlson DS (eds). Biological and Psychological Aspects of Orofacial Pain. Ann Arbor: Univ of Michigan, 1994.

41. Carlson C, Bertrand P, Ehrlich A, Maxwell A, Burton RG. Physical self-regulation training for the management of temporomandibular disorders. J Orofac Pain 2001;15:47–55.

42. Curran SL, Carlson CR, Okeson JP. Emotional and physiologic responses to laboratory challenges: Patients with temporomandibular disorders versus matched control subjects. J Orofac Pain 1996;10(2):141–150.

# Vascular and Nonvascular Intracranial Disorders

By their very nature, intracranial causes of orofacial pain are difficult to diagnose and do not usually offer pathognomonic features. These disorders may present in a nonspecific fashion with only mild to moderate pain but may cause significant morbidity and, in some cases, mortality. Thus, a careful analysis of the patient's history, with special emphasis on identification of red flags, offers the best chance of accurate diagnosis and appropriate testing and referral.

This chapter reviews intracranial sources of orofacial pain that may be life threatening or may impair a patient's ability to accomplish independent activities of daily living (Box 4-1).

## Preliminary Investigation

Certain tissues are exquisitely nociceptive,[1,2] while others are relatively insensitive to pain (Box 4-2). Because many intracranial structures are insensitive to pain, intracranial pathologic processes must be diagnosed according to concomitant symptoms or historical facts. Signs of extracranial pathology are more specific and correspond better with the location of the pain.

The American Headache Society's mnemonic tool, *SNOOP*, outlines aspects of a patient's signs and symptoms that may indicate a severe or life-threatening disorder (Box 4-3)[3]:

*Systemic symptoms/disease:* Pain in the setting of systemic features such as fever, weight loss, arthralgias, stiff neck, or rash could indicate meningoencephalitis, bacteremia/sepsis, collagen vascular diseases, or neoplastic processes. Preexisting risk factors such as human immunodeficiency virus (HIV), systemic cancer, or long-term treatment with immunotherapy predispose to serious disease. HIV is associated with both intracranial infections and cancer.

*Neurologic signs/symptoms:* Signs or symptoms ranging from mild confusion or sedation to frank neurologic deficits, such as aphasia or hemiparesis, typically herald more than a primary pain disorder. Focal neurologic signs and symptoms (eg, hemiparesis, visual obscuration, imbalance, or numbness) warrant further investigation to rule out stroke, a mass lesion, infiltrating lesions affecting multiple cranial nerves, arteriovenous malformations, thrombotic disease, or focal/systemic infections. However, migraines, for example, can be accompanied

**Box 4-1** Life-threatening secondary causes of intracranial head, neck, and orofacial pain

| Vascular disorders | Nonvascular disorders |
|---|---|
| Ischemic cerebrovascular disease (IHS 6.1) | High cerebrospinal fluid pressure (IHS 7.1) |
| Traumatic intracranial hemorrhage (IHS 5.5) | Low cerebrospinal fluid pressure (IHS 7.2) |
| Nontraumatic intracranial hemorrhage (IHS 6.2) | Intracranial noninfectious inflammation (IHS 7.3) |
| Unruptured vascular malformation (IHS 6.3) | Intracranial neoplasm (IHS 7.4) |
| Arteritis (IHS 6.4) | Intracranial infection (IHS 9.1) |
| Carotid or vertebral artery pain (IHS 6.5) | |
| Venous thrombosis (IHS 6.6) | |

by changes in cognition or hemiparesis. In basilar migraines, signs and symptoms are produced by a focus of pathology in the distribution of the basilar artery and may include imbalance, vertigo, dysarthria, and diplopia, while in familial hemiplegic migraine, patients may present with stroke-like features of hemiparesis, dysarthria, and confusion. Obviously, these "benign" syndromes warrant urgent referral to rule out worrisome causes.

*Onset sudden:* Severe and generalized headache of sudden onset must be considered serious until proven otherwise. The differential diagnosis for life-threatening acute-onset headaches must include subarachnoidal hemorrhage, aneurysm, cerebral venous thrombosis, carotid or vertebral artery dissection, cerebral hematoma or infarction, hypertensive encephalopathy, ischemic and hemorrhagic stroke, and central nervous system infections.[4,5] Headaches precipitated by a cough, sneeze, straining, or exertion warrant imaging of the brain to exclude an intracranial lesion such as a Chiari malformation. Headaches that arouse a patient from sleep need to be investigated further to rule out causes of increased intracranial pressure (eg, tumor, abscess, inflammatory processes). Posttraumatic headache may be manifest without any identifiable

pathology; however, fractures, hematoma, or infections must be excluded. Headache upon standing can be a sign of low cerebrospinal fluid (CSF) pressure due to a CSF leak. Headache upon lying down can be due to increased intracranial pressure related to an intracranial mass. Headaches that occur only in the morning may be associated with obstructive sleep apnea, medication rebound, or oral parafunctional habits.

*Older age:* In patients older than 40 years, new-onset and/or progressive headaches should arouse suspicion. Migraines may begin at any age, but most patients experience onset by the age of 40 years. Contingent upon the entire history and physical, computerized tomography (CT) or magnetic resonance imaging (MRI) of the head and at least an erythrocyte sedimentation rate should be ordered to rule out giant cell arteritis. Progressively worsening headaches at any age need to be carefully assessed.

*Pattern change:* When patients experience the first headache of a certain type or the worst headache they have ever had, or if there is a change in attack frequency, severity, or quality, the clinician should review the case for other red flags and consider further investigation. Chronic, recurrent headaches that have similar features over time are not likely due to a serious disorder.

**Box 4-2** Structure sensitivity to pain

| Sensitive to pain | Insensitive to pain |
|---|---|
| Intracranial: | Intracranial: |
| Dura mater | Brain parenchyma |
| Venous sinuses and their tributaries | Pia mater |
| Intracranial arteries | Arachnoid membrane |
| Neural structures: | Ependyma |
|   Glossopharyngeal nerve | Choroid plexus |
|   Vagus nerve | |
|   Trigeminal nerve | Extracranial: |
|   Upper cervical nerves | Skull/bones |
| Extracranial: | |
| Carotid, vertebral, and basilar arteries | |
| Blood vessels within the scalp and skin | |
| Skin | |
| Mucosa | |
| Muscles | |
| Fascia | |
| Synovium within the temporomandibular joint | |
| Teeth | |
| Periosteum | |

**Box 4-3** SNOOP: Signs and symptoms of concern[3]

| Characteristic | Symptoms |
|---|---|
| Systemic symptoms | Fever, weight loss |
| Systemic disease | HIV, systemic cancer |
| Neurologic signs/symptoms | Confusion, clumsy, weak, aphasic |
| Onset sudden | Thunderclap, progressive, positional |
| Older age | Temporal arteritis, cancer, infection |
| Pattern change | Existing headache now with new pattern, quality, and/or severity |

# Headache Associated with Vascular Disorders (IHS 6)

## Acute ischemic cerebrovascular disease (IHS 6.1)

Headache associated with acute ischemic cerebrovascular disease is usually mild to moderate, but there is nothing pathogno-monic about the quality, severity, or location of the pain. Acute neurologic deficits associated with cerebral ischemia include visual obscurations, weakness, numbness, altered cognition, dysarthria, aphasia, and ataxia. Transient ischemic attacks present with the neurologic deficits that might be seen in an acute ischemic stroke but resolve, by definition, within 24 hours and usually within several minutes.

Signs or symptoms consistent with cerebral ischemia indicate emergent referral to a physician. While it is more likely to occur in older individuals with vascular risk factors (eg, diabetes, hypertension, hypercholesterolemia, and tobacco use), stroke can occur at any age. CT of the head may be sufficient for diagnosis, especially if acute blood accumulation is suspected, but a diffusion-weighted MRI will have a much higher sensitivity and specificity for detection of acute cerebral ischemia. The differential diagnosis for a patient with headache and neurologic symptoms includes migraine.

## Intracranial hemorrhage (IHS 5.5 and 6.2.1)

Headache secondary to traumatic intracranial hematoma may be due to an epidural (IHS 5.5.1) or subdural (IHS 5.5.2) hematoma. Headache secondary to nontraumatic intracranial hematoma may be due to an intracerebral hemorrhage (IHS 6.2.1) or a subarachnoid hemorrhage (ISH 6.2.2). Like pain associated with ischemia, pain stemming from hemorrhage is best diagnosed according to its accompanying symptoms.

An epidural hemorrhage[6] is most often caused by trauma to the middle meningeal artery. Following trauma, there may be a "lucid interval" wherein the patient apparently recovers for the most part, only to become somnolent and then comatose in quick succesion.[7] This lucid interval is more the exception than the rule; more frequently, patients will continue to have severe pain followed by a change in cognition. Rapid drainage of epidural hematomas is necessary to prevent mortality.

A subdural hemorrhage[6] may present acutely, subacutely, or with chronic symptoms. After trauma such as a fall, the sub-dural space fills with blood after the bridging veins coursing through it rupture. Besides pain, symptoms may include gait disturbance, personality change, somnolence, or visual disturbances. Surgical evacuation of the hematoma is the mode of treatment. Older patients are at greater risk, because their bridging veins are not as resistant to trauma, and they are more likely to have gait instability. Patients taking anticoagulants are also at risk even in cases of seemingly minimal head trauma.

Head pain associated with a nontraumatic intracerebral hemorrhage[6] typically presents with acute neurologic deficits. Hemorrhage within the brain parenchyma may be the result of hypertension, neoplasia, arteriovenous malformations, or other condition, and may quickly lead to death depending on the source of trauma and the volume of blood, amount of cerebral tissue damage, mass effect, and herniation.

A very-sudden-onset, "thunderclap headache" that reaches its maximal intensity in less than 1 minute indicates subarachnoid hemorrhage. In the past, medical personnel were taught to ask whether a patient was experiencing "the worst headache of their life," but it is the suddenness, not the intensity, that is the greater red flag. Other presenting signs and symptoms include nausea and vomiting, a stiff neck, and rapid loss of consciousness. A ruptured saccular aneurysm is the most common cause of spontaneous subarachnoid hemorrhage. Treatment consists of maintaining hemodynamic stability, neurosurgical consultation for either aneurysmal clipping or endovascular treatment, and avoidance of vasospasm.[7]

A patient with suspected subarachnoid hemorrhage should be sent to an emergency department, where a detailed neurologic examination can be performed followed by a

**Box 4-4** Differential diagnosis of acute-onset secondary headache[8]

| Vascular | Nonvascular |
|---|---|
| Subarachnoid hemorrhage (IHS 6.2.2) | Acute hypertension (IHS 7.1) |
| Saccular aneurysm (IHS 6.3.1) | Benign intracranial hypertension (IHS 7.1.1) |
| Arteriovenous malformation (IHS 6.3.2) | Intermittent hydrocephalus (IHS 7.1.3) |
| Carotid or vertebral artery dissection (IHS 6.5.1) | Intracranial infection (IHS 9.1) |
| Cerebral venous thrombosis (IHS 6.6) | Pheochromocytoma (IHS 10.3.1) |
| Pituitary apoplexy (IHS 6.7.4) | Acute glaucoma (IHS 11.3.1) |
| | Acute mountain sickness |
| | Acute optic neuritis |

head CT. If the CT result is normal, the patient should undergo a lumbar puncture to examine for xanthochromia as well as to rule out other causes of sudden headache, such as meningitis. The differential diagnosis of a thunderclap headache includes primary headache disorders such as crash migraine, cluster headache, exertional headache, and headache associated with sexual activity, as well as the secondary causes[8] outlined in Box 4-4.

## Unruptured vascular malformation (IHS 6.3)

Saccular aneurysms (IHS 6.3.1), arteriovenous malformations (IHS 6.3.2), dural arteriovenous fistulas (IHS 6.3.3), and cavernous angiomas (IHS 6.3.4) are examples of unruptured vascular malformations.[6] These may present with nonspecific head pains or may mimic migraine or tension-type headaches, even responding to the same therapies. Patients can present at any age, and some may complain of pulsatile tinnitus, although this is not always a sign of ominous pathology. A family history is often positive, prompting an imaging study— preferably magnetic resonance angiography

(MRA) or CT angiography. Since the symptoms are nonspecific, the differential diagnosis remains broad.

## Arteritis (IHS 6.4)

Arteritis typically presents with either systemic symptoms or neurologic deficits, but at times may present with head or facial pain. The pain associated with giant cell (temporal) arteritis (IHS 6.4.1)[6] is fairly distinct from other arteritides. Temporal arteritis may rapidly lead to blindness secondary to granulomatous occlusion of blood vessels. It should be suspected and ruled out in all individuals older than 50 years who present with a new persistent headache centered on one or both temples, worsened with cold temperatures, and associated with jaw claudication. Patients may also complain of pain on combing their hair. Examination may reveal an enlarged, tender temporal artery. Laboratory investigations should include an erythrocyte sedimentation rate and/or C-reactive protein.[6] A temporal artery biopsy may be required for diagnosis, but high doses of corticosteroids should be initiated as soon as possible to avoid permanent vision loss.[9]

Temporal arteritis can usually be distinguished from a temporomandibular disorder by palpation of enlarged, tender temporal arteries with reduced pulsatility, abnormal funduscopic examination findings, and an elevated erythrocyte sedimentation rate.

### Carotid or vertebral artery pain (IHS 6.5)

## Carotid or vertebral artery dissection (IHS 6.5.1)[6]

Patients with carotid or vertebral artery dissection present with ipsilateral, focal pain frequently associated with neurologic symptoms. The pain may be felt in the neck, face, or head and may be associated with painful tinnitus or Horner syndrome[10] (oculosympathetic paresis) due to the intimate association of sympathetic fibers around the internal carotid artery.

This condition is a notable cause of stroke in young people but can happen at any age. Patients may be able to recall a specific activity that may have provoked a traumatic dissection, such as blunt trauma to the neck, riding a roller coaster, vigorous chiropractic manipulation, or any other neck-twisting activity or trauma. Often there is no history of injury; in some cases, it may be caused by arterial damage, such as fibromuscular dysplasia. Blood "dissects" between the medial or subintimal layers of an artery, which may then fill to form a pseudoaneurysm. Ischemia may result, either due to occlusion or embolic debris.

Besides checking for new pupillary asymmetry, audible bruits should be sought, which may indicate the presence of turbulent blood flow. Suspected dissection should be followed up immediately by either a neurologist or neurosurgeon for further investigation using extracranial duplex ultrasound scanning, MRI, and MRA or CT angiography.[10] Treatment typically consists of 3 to 6 months of anticoagulant therapy.[6,10]

### Carotidynia

Idiopathic carotidynia is usually a non–life-threatening cause of focal arterial tenderness. In recent years, this diagnosis has fallen into disfavor due to a lack of specificity, and a critical review of the literature revealed that it is not a valid single pathologic entity.[11] Carotidynia may have a viral origin. Other causes include carotid artery dissection, postcarotid endarterectomy, aneurysm, temporal arteritis, or fibromuscular dysplasia.[12] Therefore, management should include referral to a neurologist.

### Venous thrombosis (IHS 6.6)

Acute, severe pain or subacute to chronic pain characterizes venous thrombosis. Patients may complain of a severe, new headache associated with visual disturbances, signs of increased intracranial pressure (nausea, vomiting, or papilledema), seizures, or frank neurologic deficits.[13] Venous congestion can produce ischemic or hemorrhagic cerebral infarction. Predisposing factors include dehydration, oral contraceptive pills, the postpartum state, prothrombotic blood dyscrasias, neoplastic conditions, mild to moderate head trauma, or local infection.[13] Patients with suspected venous thrombosis should be immediately referred to a neurologist or neurosurgeon for further investigation using MRI with MR venography or CT scan with CT venography. Treatment may consist of modifying the predisposing factors and at least 6 months of anticoagulation therapy.[14]

# Headache Associated with Nonvascular Intracranial Disorders (IHS 7)

## Increased CSF pressure (IHS 7.1)

Increased CSF pressure may yield a nonspecific headache in any region of the head. Patients may have a mass that exerts pressure or a process that impairs the normal circulation and egress of CSF. This headache typically worsens with the Valsalva maneuver or recumbency and may be associated with nausea and vomiting as well as neurologic deficits.[15] Clinicians should watch for extraocular movement abnormalities and papilledema. Idiopathic intracranial hypertension (pseudotumor cerebri) occurs most often in young, obese females.[16] Oral contraceptive pill use is also a risk factor.

Intracranial hypertension typically produces a daily holocephalic headache with intermittent visual disturbances and possibly tinnitus. MRI results should be unremarkable, but papilledema or abducens nerve palsy may be found on physical examination. Increased opening pressure on lumbar puncture usually confirms the diagnosis. Left untreated, the increased pressure may result in blindness.[15] After proper referral, treatment consists of risk factor modification (weight loss) and possibly acetazolamide, which decreases production of CSF. Some patients may require optic nerve sheath fenestration for relief of papilledema or lumboperitoneal shunting of CSF to lower intracranial pressure, reduce headaches, and prevent further vision loss.[15]

## Low CSF pressure (IHS 7.2)

Headaches due to low CSF pressure may be iatrogenic after dural or lumbar punctures (IHS 7.2.1) or spontaneous (IHS 7.2.3). Spontaneous CSF volume depletion may be associated with meningeal diverticula, weakened dura mater, or connective tissue diseases such as Marfan syndrome.[17] The orthostatic component usually becomes less evident as the condition persists. This type of head pain is caused by traction placed on the vasculature and dura mater by the sagging brain. Accompanying neck stiffness, tinnitus, hypacusia, photophobia, or nausea may occur. Gadolinium-enhanced MRI typically reveals pachymeningeal enhancement of the dura and perhaps descent of the cerebellar tonsils. Headaches are usually relieved by recumbency and worsened within a few minutes of standing. They may either resolve spontaneously or within 48 to 72 hours of treatment, which may involve bedrest, mild analgesics, caffeine or theophylline, or an epidural blood patch.[18]

## Intracranial noninfectious inflammatory diseases (IHS 7.3)

Dental practitioners have a limited role in the workup of many inflammatory conditions such as neurosarcoidosis (IHS 7.3.1) and (aseptic) meningitis (IHS 7.3.2).[6] These entities cause various and nonspecific symptoms, whose recognition comes only with vigilant observation and detection of red flags. Investigations necessary for diagnosis include MRI of the head, CSF examination, and blood chemical analysis.

## Intracranial neoplasm (IHS 7.4)

Headaches manifest in approximately 50% of patients with intracranial neoplasia and may be the first presenting symptom in approximately 20% of cases.[19,20] There is nothing specific about the headache produced by an intracranial neoplasm. Headaches may be attributed to increased intracranial pressure or hydrocephalus caused by the neoplasm (IHS 7.4.1), to the neoplasm itself (IHS 7.4.2), or to carcinomatous meningitis (IHS 7.4.3).[6] The time course is most typically subacute to chronic and, usually, there will be other symptoms that make the diagnosis suspect, such as weight loss, personality change, seizures, neurologic deficits (eg, aphasia, weakness, incoordination), or signs of increased intracranial pressure (eg, nausea and vomiting). If a patient presents with a new headache with some of the aforementioned symptoms, an imaging study is warranted. Occasionally, neoplastic processes can occlude normal CSF flow, producing a ball-valve mechanism that manifests as posture-dependent symptoms. Head pain brought on acutely by coughing or the Valsalva maneuver is usually benign but can, in rare cases, be due to a tumor causing increased intracranial pressure.

Many patients with neck, face, or head pain are concerned that their pain may be due to a tumor. Persistent concern can by itself be ample justification to refer the patient to a medical specialist in order to obtain reassurance.

## Intracranial infection (IHS 9.1)

Headaches may be attributed to intracranial infections, including bacterial meningitis (IHS 9.1.1), lymphocytic meningitis (IHS 9.1.2), encephalitis (IHS 9.1.3), brain abscess (IHS 9.1.4), and subdural empyema (IHS 9.1.5).[6] The symptomatic headache is most commonly holocephalic in association with fever, arthralgias, stiff neck, photophobia, nausea and/or vomiting, altered consciousness, and confusion.[21] Symptom onset may occur over minutes to hours, and the patient's condition may deteriorate rapidly. Progression of symptoms over hours may be the most important clue, since fever or meningismus may be absent, especially in the very young, old, or immunocompromised. Patients may die within hours if not properly treated.

Herpes simplex is the most common cause of nonepidemic viral encephalitis, and typically presents with acute headache, fever, cognitive changes, and seizures. Early antiviral therapy greatly reduces permanent neurologic sequelae. Patients with an abscess or subdural empyema present similarly to those with a severe meningitis, with headache, fever, malaise, and possibly signs of increased intracranial pressure.

Infection is diagnosed using procedures such as blood cultures, Gram staining, polymerase chain reaction, and examination of CSF. Imaging techniques include CT and MRI. The clinician should be aware that patients with acquired immune deficiency syndrome (AIDS) may suffer from head, neck, and orofacial pain as a result of numerous possible infections, including any of those discussed above.

## Summary

Intracranial sources of orofacial pain are numerous and may lead to disability or death if not managed expeditiously. Their diagnosis rests primarily on a careful history and an alertness to red flags. The SNOOP acronym is a useful mnemonic device for screening. If red flags disclose features consistent with a life-threatening cause of pain, the patient should be referred to the appropriate medical specialist for further management. Careful application of these general rules can guide appropriate referrals and provide a rationale for reassurance when consultation is not warranted.

# References

1. Ray BS, Wolfe HG. Experimental studies on headache. Pain-sensitive structures of the head and their significance in headache. Arch Surg 1940;41:813–856.
2. Penfield W. A contribution to the mechanism of intracranial pain. Assoc Res Nerv Ment Dis 1935;15:399–416.
3. Dodick D. Clinical clues and clinical rules: Primary vs secondary headache. Adv Stud Med 2003;3:S550–S555.
4. Welch KMA. Headache. In: Loeser JD (ed). Bonica's Management of Pain. Philadelphia: Lippincott Williams &Wilkins, 2001:925–935.
5. Valade D. Headaches in the emergency room. In: Olesen J, Goadsby PJ, Ramadan NM, Tfelt-Hansen P, Welch KMA (eds). The Headaches. Philadelphia: Lippincott Wilkins & Williams, 2006:1133–1138.
6. Headache Classification Subcommittee of the International Headache Society. The International Classification of Headache Disorders: 2nd edition. Cephalalgia 2004;24(suppl 1):9–160.
7. Chung C-S, Caplan LR. Neurovascular disorders. In: Goetz CG (ed). Textbook of Clinical Neurology. Philadelphia: Saunders, 2003:991–1016.
8. Silberstein SD, Lipton RB, Goadsby PJ. Headache in Clinical Practice. Oxford: ISIS Medical Media, 2002.
9. Wall M, Corbett JJ. Arteritis. In: Olesen J, Goadsby PJ, Ramadan NM, Tfelt-Hansen P, Welch KMA (eds). The Headaches. Philadelphia: Lippincott Williams & Wilkins, 2006:901–910.
10. Biousse V, Mitsias P. Carotid or vertebral artery pain. In: Olesen J, Goadsby PJ, Ramadan NM, Tfelt-Hansen P, Welch KMA (eds). The Headaches. Philadelphia: Lippincott Williams & Wilkins, 2006:911–918.
11. Biousse V, Bousser M. The myth of carotidynia. Neurology 1994;44:993–995.
12. Silberstein SD, Young WB. Headache and facial pain. In: Goetz CG (ed). Textbook of Clinical Neurology. Philadelphia: Saunders 2003:1187–1205.
13. Tietjen GE. Cerebral venous thrombosis. In: Olesen J, Goadsby PJ, Ramadan NM, Tfelt-Hansen P, Welch KMA (eds). The Headaches. Philadelphia: Lippincott Williams & Wilkins, 2006:919–924.
14. Bousser MG, Russell RR. Cerebral venous thrombosis. In: Bousser MG, Russell RR (eds). Major Problems in Neurology. London: Saunders, 1997:175.
15. Friedmann DI, Corbett JJ. High cerebrospinal fluid pressure. In: Olesen J, Goadsby PJ, Ramadan NM, Tfelt-Hansen P, Welch KMA (eds). The Headaches. Philadelphia: Lippincott Williams & Wilkins, 2006:925–933.
16. Kesler A, Goldhammer Y, Gadoth N. Do men with pseudomotor cerebri share the same characteristics as women? A retrospective review of 141 cases. J Neuroophthalmol 2001;21:15–17.
17. Mokri B. Headache associated with abnormalities in intracranial structure or function: Low cerebrospinal fluid pressure headache. In: Silberstein SD, Lipton RB, Dalessio DJ (eds). Wolff's Headache and Other Head Pain. Oxford: Oxford Press, 2001:417–433.
18. Vilming ST, Mokri B. Low cerebrospinal fluid pressure. In: Olesen J, Goadsby PJ, Ramadan NM, Tfelt-Hansen P, Welch KMA (eds). The Headaches. Philadelphia: Lippincott Williams & Wilkins, 2006:935–944.
19. Forsyth PA, Posner JB. Headaches in patients with brain tumors: A study of 111 patients. Neurology 1993;43:1678–1683.
20. Jaeckle KA. Causes and management of headaches in cancer patients. Oncology (Williston Park) 1993;7:27–31; discussion 31–32, 34.
21. Weber JR, Sakai F. Headaches attributed to infection. In: Olesen J, Goadsby PJ, Ramadan NM, Tfelt-Hansen P, Welch KMA (eds). The Headaches. Philadelphia: Lippincott Williams & Wilkins, 2006:981–987.

# 5

# Primary Headache Disorders

Primary headaches are disorders unto themselves and are diagnosed by their symptom profile. In contrast, secondary headaches are due to an underlying condition and are classified according to their cause, and they will not be discussed in this chapter. The International Headache Society (IHS)[1] classification breaks the primary headache disorders into four categories:

1. Migraine
2. Tension-type headache (TTH)
3. Cluster headache and other trigeminal autonomic cephalalgias
4. Other primary headaches

The main subcategories of primary headache disorders are listed in Box 5-1. However, it is not within the scope of this chapter to discuss all of these disorders. Those that are more widely prevalent (ie, migraine, TTH, and cluster headache) will be discussed more thoroughly.

## Migraine (IHS 1.x.x; ICD-9 346.10)

### Clinical presentation and diagnosis

Migraine is a disorder of the trigeminal system. A diagnosis of *migraine* may be confirmed when certain IHS criteria are met after organic disease is excluded: *(1)* Patients need to have experienced at least five attacks, each lasting 4 to 72 hours; *(2)* two of the following pain characteristics must be present: unilateral pain, pulsatile quality, moderate-to-severe intensity, and aggravation by routine physical activity; and *(3)* the attack must be accompanied by nausea (and/or vomiting) or photophobia and phonophobia.

Migraines may occur *without aura* (IHS 1.1) or *with aura* (IHS 1.2). *Aura* is the presence of reversible focal neurologic symptoms that gradually develop over 5 to 20 minutes and last for no more than 1 hour

**Box 5-1** Condensed list of primary headaches according to the IHS[1]

| IHS code | Diagnosis |
|----------|-----------|
| 1. | Migraine |
| 1.1 | Migraine without aura |
| 1.2 | Migraine with aura |
| 1.5 | Complications of migraine |
| 1.5.1 | Chronic migraine |
| 1.5.2 | Status migrainosus |
| 1.6 | Probable migraine |
| 2. | Tension-type headache (TTH) |
| 2.1 | Infrequent episodic TTH |
| 2.2 | Frequent episodic TTH |
| 2.3 | Chronic TTH |
| 2.4 | Probable TTH |
| 3. | Cluster headache and other trigeminal autonomic cephalalgias |
| 3.1 | Cluster headache |
| 3.1.1 | Episodic cluster headache |
| 3.1.2 | Chronic cluster headache |
| 3.2 | Paroxysmal hemicrania |
| 3.2.1 | Episodic paroxysmal hemicrania |
| 3.2.2 | Chronic paroxysmal hemicrania (CPH) |
| 3.3 | Short-lasting unilateral neuralgiform headache attacks with conjunctival injection and tearing (SUNCT) |
| 3.4 | Probable trigeminal autonomic cephalalgia |
| 4. | Other primary headaches |
| 4.1 | Primary stabbing headache |
| 4.2 | Primary cough headache |
| 4.3 | Primary exertional headache |
| 4.4 | Primary headache associated with sexual activity |
| 4.4.1 | Preorgasmic headache |
| 4.4.2 | Orgasmic headache |
| 4.5 | Hypnic headache |
| 4.6 | Primary thunderclap headache |
| 4.7 | Hemicrania continua |
| 4.8 | New daily persistent headache (NDPH) |

and a simultaneous reduction in regional cerebral blood flow. Aura may also occur in the absence of a typical migraine headache (IHS 1.2.3). Patients may experience premonitory symptoms hours to a day or two before a migraine attack (with aura or without aura). These include various combinations of fatigue, difficulty concentrating, neck stiffness, sensitivity to light or sound, nausea, blurred vision, yawning, and pallor.

If migraine occurs on more than 15 days per month for at least 3 months in the absence of medication overuse, the migraine is called *chronic* (IHS 1.5.1), and if it lasts for more than 3 days, it is called *status migrainosus* (IHS 1.5.2). Serious complications of migraines are rare and include migrainous stroke (IHS 1.5.4), aura- or migraine-triggered seizures (IHS 1.5.5), and persistent aura (IHS 1.5.3).[2]

## Epidemiology

Estimates of migraine prevalence vary, ranging from 4% to about 20%.[3-8] Before puberty onset, migraine is slightly more common in boys, with the highest incidence between 6 and 10 years of age. In females, the incidence is highest between 14 and 19 years of age. In general, females are more commonly affected than males. The prevalence of migraine in the United States is 17% to 18% for women and 6% for men.[6-8]

The American Migraine Study found that the 1-year prevalence of migraine increased with age among women and men, reaching the maximum at ages 35 to 45 years and declining thereafter.[9] Migraine prevalence is inversely proportional to income, with the low income group having the highest prevalence. Race and geographic region are also influential factors; the prevalence is highest in North America and Western Europe and among those of European descent.[7] Because the condition usually affects people during their most productive years, migraine is a burden to the patient and society. Not only does migraine affect the patient's quality of life by impairing his or her ability to participate in family, social, and recreational activities, it affects society in terms of direct costs (eg, medical care) and indirect costs (eg, absenteeism and reduced effectiveness at work). The American Migraine Study estimates that 23 million US residents have

severe migraines. Twenty-five percent of women experience four or more severe attacks per month; 35% experience one to three severe attacks per month; and 40% experience one or less than one severe attack per month.

## Pathogenesis

Many mechanisms and theories explaining the causes of migraine have been proposed, although the full picture is still elusive. A strong familial association and the early onset of the disorder suggest a genetic component, which has led some to question whether it is a channelopathy. The trigeminal vascular model by Moskowitz[10] explains that trigeminal activation resulting in the release of neuropeptides produces neurogenic inflammation, increased vascular permeability, and dilation of blood vessels. Other pathophysiologic mechanisms behind migraine have been proposed, such as serotonin, calcitonin gene-related peptide, nitric oxide, dopamine, norepinephrine, glutamate, and other substances,[11,12] as well as mitochondrial dysfunction.[13] It has recently been recognized that central sensitization producing allodynia and hyperalgesia is an important clinical manifestation of migraine.[14]

## Treatment

Pharmacologic treatment of migraine may be abortive/symptomatic or prophylactic. Patients who experience frequent severe migraines often require both approaches. The choice of treatment should be guided by the frequency of the attacks. Infrequent attacks (two or fewer per week) may be treated with abortive medications,[15] and more frequent attacks should be treated with prophylactic medications. If there is a concurrent illness,

---

**Box 5-2** Common medications used to abort a migraine[15]

| Specific | Nonspecific |
|---|---|
| Selective serotonin agonists (triptans) | Acetaminophen, aspirin, and caffeine |
| Dihydroergotamine | Aspirin |
| | Butorphanol |
| | Ibuprofen |
| | Naproxen sodium |

---

**Box 5-3** Common medications used for the prevention of migraine[15,17,18]

| Most effective | Moderately effective |
|---|---|
| Amitriptyline | Gabapentin |
| Divalproex sodium/sodium valproate | Nimodipine |
| Topiramate | Verapamil |
| Propranolol | Ketoprofen |
| Timolol | Naproxen |
| Metoprolol | |

---

a single agent should be used to treat both when possible, and agents that might aggravate a comorbid illness should be avoided. Nonpharmacologic methods such as biofeedback, relaxation techniques, acupuncture, and other behavioral interventions can be used as adjunctive therapy.[16] Patient preferences should also be considered.

Several medications have been used for acute migraine treatment, including selective 5-HT$_{1B/D}$ (serotonin) agonists, analgesics, nonsteroidal anti-inflammatory drugs, antiemetics, anxiolytics, ergot alkaloids, steroids, neuroleptics, and narcotics. Drugs with proven statistical and clinical benefit according to the American Academy of Neurology are listed in Box 5-2 and should be given as first-line treatment.[15]

When migraine becomes more frequent and the use of acute medications exceeds two to three times per week, preventive medications are used. Preventive treatments include a broad range of medications, most notably antidepressants, anticonvulsants, and beta-blockers (Box 5-3).[15,17,18] Serotonin antagonists, nonsteroidal anti-inflammatory drugs, and calcium-channel blockers appear to be less effective.[15] These medications are started at low doses and titrated to the desired effect to minimize side effects and arrive at the minimal dose needed. In more refractory cases, polypharmacy may be necessary. Botulinum toxin type A is an alternative that continues to be studied.[19-21]

Patients can help themselves, too, by learning to identify and avoid headache triggers. Important triggers are environmental factors, including light, noise, allergens, and barometric changes; behavioral factors, such as missing meals or getting too much or too little sleep; and food/beverage items, such as cured meats, cheese, chocolate, and those containing aspartame, monosodium glutamate, and nitrites.

# Tension-Type Headache (IHS 2.x.x; *ICD-9* 307.81)

## Clinical presentation and diagnosis

TTHs are divided into *infrequent episodic* (IHS 2.1), *frequent episodic* (IHS 2.2), *chronic* (IHS 2.3), and *probable* (IHS 2.4) (see Box 5-1). The categories are typically subdivided according to the presence or absence of pericranial tenderness as assessed by manual palpation.

TTH is described as a dull ache or a nonpulsating pain of mild-to-moderate intensity often manifesting as tightness, pressure, or soreness in a "band-like" distribution as if the patient were wearing a hat. The pain location is not specific, though it is often bilateral and may extend into the neck. Temporalis and masseter muscle involvement may be present, and mastication may be affected in some patients. TTH is not accompanied by nausea or vomiting, nor is it aggravated by routine physical activity, but it may be associated with sensitivity to light or noises.

The headaches may last from 30 minutes to 7 days. They are classified as *infrequent* if they occur on less than 1 day per month (less than 12 per year) and as *frequent* if they occur on more than 1 day per month but less than 15 days per month for at least 3 months. Chronic TTH evolves from episodic TTH and is diagnosed when headaches occur daily or more often than 15 days per month for at least 3 months. In contrast, if a new-onset daily or unremitting headache with tension-type characteristics develops, the headache is classified as *new daily persistent headache* (IHS 4.8). Sensitivity to light and/or noises and mild nausea may be present with these headaches. It may be difficult to distinguish between chronic migraine and chronic TTH, and these disorders may be present simultaneously.

## Epidemiology

TTH is the most common of all primary headaches. For example, in a cross-sectional population study of 740 adult subjects, 74% had experienced TTH within the previous year, while 31% of the same population had experienced TTH for more than 14 days during the previous year.[22] In another study, a 1-year prevalence rate for TTH in males was 63% and in females, 86%.[23] The onset of the headaches is usually between 20 and 40 years of age.

## Pathogenesis

For many years, TTH was thought to be directly related to muscle tension and was referred to as a *muscle contraction* or *muscle tension* headache. Muscle tenderness may be present in some individuals; however, increased levels of electromyographic activity are not always associated with the condition.[24] Some studies[25,26] report that electromyography revealed increased activity in response to emotional stressors in patients compared with controls. It has been suggested, however, that this increase in electromyographic-detected activity may not be the cause of the pain but, rather, a response to the pain. Emotional stress, anxiety, and depression seem to have causal relationships with TTHs.[27]

A very controversial boundary exists between migraine and TTH. Some experts see these disorders as distinct entities, while others see them at opposite ends of a continuum, varying in severity and features but having a common pathogenesis.[28–30] At this time, the pathophysiology of TTH remains unclear. The latest theories include peripheral and central sensitization concepts, with a possible role for nitric oxide.[31-33]

### Treatment

Patients with TTH tend to self medicate with over-the-counter analgesics, anti-histamines, caffeine, and other medications. Rarely do they consult their physician for relief unless the frequency or severity of these headaches increases. Treatment of TTH may include relaxation techniques, pharmacotherapy, and physical therapy.

Since emotional stress plays an important role in TTH, the patient should be assessed for any significant stressors; when significant stressors are identified, corrective behaviors or, when possible, avoidance should be encouraged. Stress management skills, relaxation training, and biofeedback techniques can be important therapies for TTH,[34] but patients must be willing to take time to work with these therapies. If a major depression disorder or anxiety disorder is present, however, these conditions need to be managed by the proper health care professional.

Pharmacotherapy may be needed, but the patient should be aware of the potential complications. Nonsteroidal anti-inflammatory inhibitors are often effective. Tricyclic antidepressants, such as amitriptyline or nortriptyline, can be helpful in managing frequently occurring TTH but should be taken at bedtime because of their sedative effects.

When TTH is present in association with a masticatory muscle disorder, efforts should be first directed to treating the disorder. A nighttime occlusal appliance for nocturnal bruxism may help a headache that occurs upon awaking. During the day, the patient should practice techniques in cognitive awareness, habit reversal, and self-relaxation to reduce or eliminate tension and clenching or grinding of the teeth.

Often TTH is a heterotopic pain originating in the cervical muscles. When a cervical myofascial pain disorder is present, treatment should be oriented toward resolving this disorder. If myofascial trigger points are the source of headache, the use of postural, stretching, and strengthening exercise programs combined with the use of a vapocoolant spray and/or trigger point injections may be effective.[35]

## Cluster Headache (IHS 3.x.x; ICD-9 346.20)

### Clinical presentation and diagnosis

Cluster headache is a throbbing, sharp, or boring pain of severe intensity usually localized to the orbital, supraorbital, and/or temporal region. These headaches are typically side fixed, remaining on the same side of the head for the patient's lifetime. Only 15% of patients will experience a side shift between cluster periods. To confirm the diagnosis, patients should have experienced at least five attacks of severe, unilateral, orbital, supraorbital, and/or temporal pain lasting from 15 to 180 minutes if left untreated.[1] The headache also needs to be associated with at least one of the following signs or symptoms: lacrimation, conjunctival injection, rhinorrhea, nasal congestion, forehead and facial sweating, miosis, ptosis, or eyelid edema.

During a cluster headache, patients cannot and do not want to remain still. They typically pace the floor or even bang their heads against the wall to try to alleviate the pain. Cluster headaches are short in duration compared with some of the other primary headache disorders, usually lasting an average of 45 minutes to 1 hour, and patients will frequently have between one and three attacks per day. The headaches have a predilection for the first REM sleep phase, so the patient will awaken with a severe headache 60 to 90 minutes after falling asleep. This is an important distinguishing characteristic, as very few other pain problems are known to wake a person from sleep.

Cluster headaches can be of an *episodic* (greater than 1 month of headache-free days per year; ISH 3.1.1) or *chronic* (occurring for more than 1 year without remission or with remissions lasting less than 1 month; IHS 3.1.2) subtype. Between 80% and 90% of cluster patients have the episodic variety. Cluster periods, or the time when patients are experiencing daily cluster headache attacks, usually last between 2 and 12 weeks, and patients can have 1 to 2 cluster periods per year. It is common for a patient to experience a cluster period at the same time each year. This circadian periodicity suggests a hypothalamic generator for cluster headaches.[36]

## Epidemiology

Cluster headache was thought to affect primarily men; however, more recent studies have determined the ratio of men to women to be approximately 4:1.[37,38] Prevalence estimates vary between 0.09% and 0.32%.[39,40] In a recent population-based sample in Germany, the 1-year prevalence of cluster headache was estimated to be 119/100,000.[41] The mean age of onset for cluster headache is nearly 10 years later than that of migraine, at approximately 27 to 31 years of age.[42]

## Pathogenesis

The primary mechanism associated with cluster headache is unknown, but it is believed to be central. The three defining aspects of cluster headache are the trigeminal distribution, periodicity of attacks, and unilaterality. The rhythmic periodicity and the predilection for attacks to occur during sleep has implicated circadian and circannual rhythms, which indicate hypothalamic involvement.[36,43]

Studies have shown a close relationship between cluster headaches and sleep-disordered breathing and sleep apnea.[44,45] Kudrow[46] postulated that altered hypothalamic influence of the brainstem centers controlling respiration and vasomotor function diminishes carotid chemoreceptor activity. This factor may explain the positive response of cluster headaches to oxygen, as well as the relationship between cluster headaches and altitude and sleep apnea.[46]

## Treatment

The treatment of cluster headache is essentially pharmacologic, with the goal of shortening and alleviating the cluster headache attacks and shortening the cycle of attacks; therefore, like migraine therapy, it can be divided into symptomatic/abortive and prophylactic regimens (Box 5-4). Due to the nature of cluster headaches, symptomatic treatment is rapid-acting. Agents used are oxygen, serotonin receptor agonists (triptans), and dihydroergotamine. Individual attacks will usually respond to oxygen delivered at 7 L per minute for approximately 15 minutes. Due to the frequency of headaches, the use of ergotamine preparations is largely limited because of the hypertensive effects of the ergot alkaloid. Also, because

---

**Box 5-4** Common medications used to treat cluster headache[47–49]

| Abortive | Prophylactic |
|---|---|
| Oxygen inhalation | Verapamil |
| Selective serotonin agonists (triptans) | Corticosteroids (short-term) |
| Dihydroergotamine | Lithium |
| | Divalproex sodium |
| | Topiramate |

---

of the rapid onset of pain and relatively short duration, oral narcotic analgesics should be limited.

Prophylactic therapies should be initiated as soon as the cycle begins. Verapamil may be used as first-line treatment.[47,48] Corticosteroids are also very effective but should be used only as initiation therapy for a short period of time.[48] Others, such as lithium carbonate, divalproex sodium, and topiramate, have shown superiority over placebo in several trials.[48,49] There is insufficient evidence for the use of gabapentin at this time. More controlled trials are needed to establish the appropriate protocol for prophylactic treatment of cluster headaches. The preventive medications are usually continued for 1 month after the last cluster attack and then discontinued until the next cycle begins.

Surgical intervention has been limited to cases of intractable cluster headache. Limited information from small case series is available and indicate varying degrees of success. The procedures included sphenopalatine ganglion blockade,[50] trigeminal rhizotomy,[51,52] microvascular decompression of the trigeminal nerve,[53] and gamma knife radiation.[54] More recently, occipital nerve stimulation and deep brain stimulation of the hypothalamic area in patients with intractable chronic cluster headaches has

been studied,[55–58] and these small case series have yielded promising results. Surgical interventions are reserved for extreme unremitting cases of cluster headache when all medications have failed to provide relief.

## Paroxysmal Hemicrania (IHS 3.2.x; *ICD-9* 346.20)

Paroxysmal hemicrania is a headache with clinical characteristics similar to those of cluster headache, but the headache attacks are shorter lasting (2 to 30 minutes), more frequent, and occur more commonly in women.[1] The attacks are also strictly unilateral, predominantly in the periorbital region. Like cluster headache, the diagnosis is confirmed when the headache is accompanied by at least one of the following signs or symptoms: lacrimation, conjunctival injection, rhinorrhea, nasal congestion, forehead and facial sweating, miosis, ptosis, and eyelid edema. Attacks occurring in periods lasting 7 days to 1 year separated by pain-free periods lasting 1 month or more are classified as *episodic* (IHS 3.2.2), and attacks occurring for more than 1 year without remission or with remissions lasting less than 1 month are classified as *chronic* (IHS 3.2.2).

Unlike with cluster headache, very little is known about the pathophysiologic mechanisms behind paroxysmal hemicrania, but it is thought that disturbances in the hypothalamus play a central role in this entity as well.[59]

The disorder is peculiar in that it is 100% responsive to indomethacin.[48,60] Contrasting reports are available about the efficacy of sumatriptan.[61,62] Topiramate appears to be promising.[63]

# References

1. Headache Classification Subcommittee of the International Headache Society. The International Classification of Headache Disorders, ed 2. Cephalalgia 2004;24(suppl 1):9–160.

2. Agostoni E, Aliprandi A. The complications of migraine with aura. Neurol Sci 2006;27(suppl 2):S91–S95.

3. Diamond S, Bigal ME, Silberstein S, Loder E, Reed M, Lipton RB. Patterns of diagnosis and acute and preventive treatment for migraine in the United States: Results from the American Migraine Prevalence and Prevention study. Headache 2007;47: 355–363.

4. MacGregor EA, Brandes J, Eikermann A. Migraine prevalence and treatment patterns: The global Migraine and Zolmitriptan Evaluation survey. Headache 2003;43:19–26.

5. Stewart WF, Lipton RB, Liberman J. Variation in migraine prevalence by race. Neurology 1996;47:52–59.

6. Lipton RB, Bigal ME, Diamond M, Freitag F, Reed ML, Stewart WF. Migraine prevalence, disease burden, and the need for preventive therapy. Neurology 2007;68:343–349.

7. Stewart WF, Lipton RB, Celentano DD, Reed ML. Prevalence of migraine headache in the United States. Relation to age, income, race, and other sociodemographic factors. JAMA 1992;267:64–69.

8. Lipton RB, Diamond S, Reed M, Diamond ML, Stewart WF. Migraine diagnosis and treatment: Results from the American Migraine Study II. Headache 2001;41:638–645.

9. Lipton RB, Stewart WF, Simon D. Medical consultation for migraine: Results from the American Migraine Study. Headache 1998;38:87–96.

10. Moskowitz MA. Basic mechanisms in vascular headache. Neurol Clin 1990;8:801–815.

11. Longoni M, Ferrarese C. Inflammation and excitotoxicity: Role in migraine pathogenesis. Neurol Sci 2006;27(suppl 2):S107–S110.

12. Peroutka SJ. Migraine: A chronic sympathetic nervous system disorder. Headache 2004;44(1):53–64.

13. Sparaco M, Feleppa M, Lipton RB, Rapoport AM, Bigal ME. Mitochondrial dysfunction and migraine: Evidence and hypotheses. Cephalalgia 2006;26(4):361–372.

14. Dodick D, Silberstein S. Central sensitization theory of migraine: Clinical implications. Headache 2006;46 [Suppl 4]:S182–S191.

15. Silberstein SD. Practice parameter: Evidence-based guidelines for migraine headache (an evidence-based review): Report of the Quality Standards Subcommittee of the American Academy of Neurology. Neurology 2000;55(6):754–762.

16. Holroyd KA, Drew JB. Behavioral approaches to the treatment of migraine. Semin Neurol 2006;26(2):199–207.

17. Ramadan NM. Current trends in migraine prophylaxis. Headache 2007;47(suppl 1):S52–S57.

18. Chronicle E, Mulleners W. Anticonvulsant drugs for migraine prophylaxis. Cochrane Database Syst Rev 2004;(3):CD003226.

19. Conway S, Delplanche C, Crowder J, Rothrock J. Botox therapy for refractory chronic migraine. Headache 2005;45:355–357.

20. Binder WJ, Brin MF, Blitzer A, Pogoda JM. Botulinum toxin type A (BOTOX) for treatment of migraine. Dis Mon 2002;48:323–335.

21. Silberstein S, Mathew N, Saper J, Jenkins S. Botulinum toxin type A as a migraine preventive treatment. For the BOTOX Migraine Clinical Research Group. Headache 2000;40:445–450.

22. Rasmussen BK, Jensen R, Olesen J. A population-based analysis of the diagnostic criteria of the International Headache Society. Cephalalgia 1991;11:129–134.

23. Rasmussen BK, Jensen R, Schroll M, Olesen J. Epidemiology of headache in a general population—A prevalence study. J Clin Epidemiol 1991;44:1147–1157.

24. Pikoff H. Is the muscular model of headache still viable? A review of conflicting data. Headache 1984;24:186–198.

25. Schoenen J, Gerard P, De Pasqua V, Juprelle M. EMG activity in pericranial muscles during postural variation and mental activity in healthy volunteers and patients with chronic tension type headache. Headache 1991;31:321–324.

26. Feuerstein M, Bush C, Corbisiero R. Stress and chronic headache: A psychophysiological analysis of mechanisms. J Psychosom Res 1982;26:167–182.

27. Olesen J. Clinical and pathophysiological observations in migraine and tension-type headache explained by integration of vascular, supraspinal and myofascial inputs. Pain 1991;46(2):125–132.

28. Jensen R. Mechanisms of tension-type headache. Cephalalgia 2001;21:786–789.

29. Lipton RB, Stewart WF, Cady R, et al. 2000 Wolfe Award. Sumatriptan for the range of headaches in migraine sufferers: Results of the Spectrum Study. Headache 2000;40(10):783–791.

30. Rasmussen BK, Jensen R, Schroll M, Olesen J. Interrelations between migraine and tension-type headache in the general population. Arch Neurol 1992; 49(9):914–918.

31. Bendtsen L. Central and peripheral sensitization in tension-type headache. Curr Pain Headache Rep 2003;7(6):460–465.

32. Ashina S, Bendtsen L, Ashina M. Pathophysiology of tension-type headache. Curr Pain Headache Rep 2005;9(6):415–422.

33. Jensen R. Peripheral and central mechanisms in tension-type headache: An update. Cephalalgia 2003;23 (suppl 1):49–52.

34. Penzien DB, Rains JC, Lipchik GL, Creer TL. Behavioral interventions for tension-type headache: Overview of current therapies and recommendation for a self-management model for chronic headache. Curr Pain Headache Rep 2004;8:489–499.

35. Graff-Radford SB, Reeves JL, Jaeger B. Management of chronic head and neck pain: Effectiveness of altering factors perpetuating myofascial pain. Headache 1987;27:186–190.

36. May A, Bahra A, Buchel C, Frackowiak RS, Goadsby PJ. Hypothalamic activation in cluster headache attacks. Lancet 1998;352:275–278.

37. Manzoni GC. Gender ratio of cluster headache over the years: A possible role of changes in lifestyle. Cephalalgia 1998;18(3):138–142.

38. Bahra A, May A, Goadsby PJ. Cluster headache: A prospective clinical study with diagnostic implications. Neurology 2002;58(3):354–361.

39. Ekbom K, Ahlborg B, Schele R. Prevalence of migraine and cluster headache in Swedish men of 18. Headache 1978;18(1):9–19.

40. Torelli P, Castellini P, Cucurachi L, Devetak M, Lambru G, Manzoni GC. Cluster headache prevalence: Methodological considerations. A review of the literature. Acta Biomed 2006;77(1):4–9.

41. Katsarava Z, Obermann M, Yoon MS, et al. Prevalence of cluster headache in a population-based sample in Germany. Cephalalgia 2007;27:1014–1019.

42. Manzoni GC, Terzano MG, Bono G, Micieli G, Martucci N, Nappi G. Cluster headache—Clinical findings in 180 patients. Cephalalgia 1983;3:21–30.

43. Leone M, Bussone G. A review of hormonal findings in cluster headache. Evidence for hypothalamic involvement. Cephalalgia 1993;13:309–317.

44. Chervin RD, Zallek SN, Lin X, Hall JM, Sharma N, Hedger KM. Sleep disordered breathing in patients with cluster headache. Neurology 2000;54:2302–2306.

45. Graff-Radford SB, Newman A. Obstructive sleep apnea and cluster headache. Headache 2004;44:607–610.

46. Kudrow L. A possible role of the carotid body in the pathogenesis of cluster headache. Cephalalgia 1983; 3:241–247.

47. Capobianco DJ, Dodick DW. Diagnosis and treatment of cluster headache. Semin Neurol 2006;26: 242–259.

48. May A, Leone M, Afra J, et al. EFNS guidelines on the treatment of cluster headache and other trigeminal-autonomic cephalalgias. Eur J Neurol 2006;13:1066–1077.

49. Pascual J, Lainez MJ, Dodick D, Hering-Hanit R. Antiepileptic drugs for the treatment of chronic and episodic cluster headache: A review. Headache 2007; 47:81–89.

50. Felisati G, Arnone F, Lozza P, Leone M, Curone M, Bussone G. Sphenopalatine endoscopic ganglion block: A revision of a traditional technique for cluster headache. Laryngoscope 2006;116:1447–1450.

51. Pieper DR, Dickerson J, Hassenbusch SJ. Percutaneous retrogasserian glycerol rhizolysis for treatment of chronic intractable cluster headaches: Long-term results. Neurosurgery 2000;46:363–368; discussion 368-70.

52. Taha JM, Tew JM Jr. Long-term results of radiofrequency rhizotomy in the treatment of cluster headache. Headache 1995;35:193–196.

53. Lovely TJ, Kotsiakis X, Jannetta PJ. The surgical management of chronic cluster headache. Headache 1998; 38:590–594.

54. McClelland S 3rd, Barnett GH, Neyman G, Suh JH. Repeat trigeminal nerve radiosurgery for refractory cluster headache fails to provide long-term pain relief. Headache. 2007;47:298–300.

55. Starr PA, Barbaro NM, Raskin NH, Ostrem JL. Chronic stimulation of the posterior hypothalamic region for cluster headache: Technique and 1-year results in four patients. J Neurosurg 2007;106:999–1005.

56. Burns B, Watkins L, Goadsby PJ. Treatment of medically intractable cluster headache by occipital nerve stimulation: Long-term follow-up of eight patients. Lancet 2007;369:1099–1106.

57. McClelland S III, Tendulkar RD, Barnett GH, Neyman G, Suh JH. Long-term results of radiosurgery for refractory cluster headache. Neurosurgery 2006;59: 1258–1262; discussion 62–63.

58. Leone M, Franzini A, Broggi G, Bussone G. Hypo-thalamic stimulation for intractable cluster headache: Long-term experience. Neurology 2006;67:150–152.

59. Matharu MS, Goadsby PJ. Functional brain imaging in hemicrania continua: Implications for nosology and pathophysiology. Curr Pain Headache Rep 2005; 9:281–288.

60. Antonaci F, Pareja JA, Caminero AB, Sjaastad O. Chronic paroxysmal hemicrania and hemicrania continua. Parenteral indomethacin: The 'indotest'. Headache 1998;38:122–128.

61. Pascual J, Quijano J. A case of chronic paroxysmal hemicrania responding to subcutaneous sumatriptan. J Neurol Neurosurg Psychiatry 1998;65:407.

62. Antonaci F, Pareja JA, Caminero AB, Sjaastad O. Chronic paroxysmal hemicrania and hemicrania continua: Lack of efficacy of sumatriptan. Headache 1998;38:197–200.

63. Cohen AS, Goadsby PJ. Paroxysmal hemicrania responding to topiramate. J Neurol Neurosurg Psychiatry 2007;78:96–97.

# Episodic and Continuous Neuropathic Pain

*Neuropathic pain* is defined as pain that arises from injury, disease, or dysfunction of the peripheral or central nervous system[1] as compared with *somatic pain*, which occurs in response to noxious stimulation of normal neural receptors. It is generally classified according to the agent of insult and anatomic distribution of the pain. Neuropathic pain can be episodic or continuous and can be peripherally generated or centrally mediated. Oftentimes, both central and peripheral sensitization play a role in sustaining the condition.

## Episodic Neuropathic Pain

Head and neck pain are mediated by afferent fibers in the trigeminal nerve, nervus intermedius, glossopharyngeal and vagus nerves, and the upper cervical roots via the occipital nerves. Neuralgia results when these nerves are stimulated by compression, distortion, exposure to cold, or other forms of irritation, or a lesion in the central pathways. The aggravating stimulus may be mild and innocuous. The pain is characterized by a paroxysmal stabbing or electric shock–like quality felt in the area innervated by the involved nerve. Neuralgia is named according to the nerve involved, and the most common type of episodic neuropathic pain is trigeminal neuralgia.

### Trigeminal neuralgia (IHS 13.1; ICD-9 350.1)

*Trigeminal neuralgia* (tic douloureux) affects the face unilaterally in a distribution of one or more divisions of the trigeminal nerve. The second and/or third divisions of the trigeminal nerve are most commonly affected; the first division is affected in only 1% to 2% of patients. The pain does not cross the midline of the face, although the condition may affect the face bilaterally in as many as 3% to 5% of patients. The condition is characterized by brief (paroxysmal) electric shock–like or lancinating pains that are typically precipitated by nonpainful stimuli, such as washing or lightly touching the face, shaving, smoking, talking, and brushing the teeth. The pain may also occur without an obvious stimulus. The paroxysms of pain are usually severe and short-lived, with a duration of seconds or less.

There is often a refractory period in which an outburst cannot be provoked. Sometimes several paroxysms will occur in succession and "fuse," effecting a longer duration of pain. Some patients who have frequent attacks of pain will describe a longer-lasting burning sensation in the same distribution. Trigeminal neuralgia is marked by remission periods lasting days to years, but the pain-free intervals usually become shorter and the exacerbations intensify as the neuralgia progresses.[2–4]

The neurologic examination results are normal in these patients.[5] The average age of onset is approximately 50 years, and the prevalence has been estimated to be 107.5 males/million and 200.2 females/million.[6]

## Pathogenesis

The pathogenesis of trigeminal neuralgia is not completely understood. Trigeminal neuralgia has been investigated as a problem related to demyelination of the nerve fibers caused by compression of the trigeminal nerve root close to its entry into the pons by overlying blood vessel(s).[7] This compression and resultant deformation of the trigeminal nerve root and some of its myelin is thought to allow for spontaneous nerve firing and ephaptic stimulation of adjacent fibers.[8] This theory may explain how stimulation of light touch sensory nerve fibers by innocuous stimuli can cause a cross stimulation of C-fibers, resulting in perception of pain.

Other possible causes for demyelinating compression of the trigeminal nerve include tumors.[9] This compression can be caused by invasion of the tumor itself or by the trigeminal nerve being trapped between the tumor and an adjacent structure or blood vessel. Occasionally, saccular aneurysm, arteriovenous malformation, or other vascular anomalies can cause compression and resultant demyelination.[8] Rarely is trigeminal nerve compression caused by a bony malformation or disease process. Tumors, usually carcinoma, can cause infiltration of the trigeminal nerve root or ganglion, as well as any other part of the trigeminal nerve, but are rarely the cause of typical trigeminal neuralgia.

Primary demyelinating disorders such as multiple sclerosis may also be associated with the symptoms of trigeminal neuralgia. A minority of patients with multiple sclerosis show vascular compression of the trigeminal nerve root. Decompression procedures on these patients often relieve the neuralgia-like symptoms.[10]

Nondemyelinating lesions, such as those associated with an infarction of the brainstem or angioma can also cause trigeminal neuralgia.[11] Some researchers have described familial trigeminal neuralgia, implicating autosomal dominant genetic traits.[12] Charcot-Marie-Tooth disease is an autosomal dominant sensory motor type I neuropathy associated with peripheral demyelination and hence could produce trigeminal neuralgia–like symptoms.[13]

Although there appears to be a clear connection between demyelination and trigeminal neuralgia, demyelination theories alone do not account for many of the characteristics of this particular neuropathy. Devor and coworkers[14] proposed the *ignition hypothesis*, which seems to take the demyelination theories further. The ignition hypothesis attempts to explain the phenomena of:

- *Triggering,* or how a trigger stimulus such as light touch can cause severe pain that long outlasts the stimulus.
- *Amplification,* or how the innocuous stimulus results in a spreading response far beyond

the innervated area by the originally stimulated nerve fibers.

• *Stop mechanism,* or how the pain response is sustained for a period and then stops itself.[14]

Earlier, Rappaport and Devor[15] explained 13 of 14 key features of trigeminal neuralgia based on neuronal abnormalities related to nerve injury. In most cases, this injury is related to nerve root compression, but other forms of injury may apply. Nerves that are injured become hyperexcitable and therefore may fire with little or no stimulus. These so-called ectopic pacemaker sites may actually be at points of demyelination or at the ends of severed nerves.[14] Some sites may fire continuously at a low level, producing a dull background burning pain, and others may require only the slightest stimulation to produce a long-lasting burst of impulses that results in severe pain lasting long beyond the initial stimulus.[16]

Nerve fibers may recruit other adjacent fibers and so on, causing short-lasting shooting pain from one point to another.[14] Once ignited, there can be further amplification of the pain by *ephapsis* or electrical cross talk between nerve fibers at a site of injury or compression, whereby the adjacent nerve fibers have lost the myelin sheaths, hence allowing direct "short circuit" stimulation.[17]

The stop mechanism and refractory period can be explained by hyperpolarization of the neuron, which stops the burst until the ionic imbalance returns to its prestimulation levels. During this time the nerve fiber can no longer be stimulated.[14]

In most patients who have undergone surgical treatment of trigeminal neuralgia, microvascular compression of the trigeminal nerve root and sometimes, the trigeminal ganglion,[18] has been found.

If no pathologic factor other than vascular compression is identifiable, the neuralgia is termed *classical trigeminal neuralgia* (IHS 13.1.1). If the neuralgia is caused by a verifiable lesion, such as a tumor, epidermoid cyst (eg, acoustic neurilemoma or meningioma), cholesteatoma, osteoma, aneurysms, and vascular malformations,[19] it is termed *symptomatic trigeminal neuralgia* (IHS 13.1.2). Trigeminal neuralgia must be differentiated from other causes of face pain, including local dental disorders, sinus disease, head and neck neoplasms and infections, atypical postherpetic neuralgia, persistent idiopathic facial pain, and headache or facial pain associated with a temporomandibular disorder (IHS 11.7). Additionally, two other pain conditions that have to be considered in the differential diagnosis are SUNCT syndrome (short-lasting, unilateral, neuralgiform pain with conjunctival injection and tearing; IHS 3.3) and primary stabbing headache, previously called the *jabs and jolts syndrome* (IHS 4.1). As part of identifying other causes of the pain, imaging studies of the head/brain may be indicated.

## Treatment

The treatment of classical trigeminal neuralgia can be divided into two modalities, medical and surgical.

### Medical management

Carbamazepine is the most effective medication for trigeminal neuralgia. The starting dose is 100 mg/day and is increased, as tolerated or as needed, by 100 mg every 2 days to a maximum of 1,200 mg/day in a divided-dose regimen. A beneficial effect is often apparent within hours to a couple of days after starting this medication. The most common side effects include drowsiness, dizziness, unsteadiness, nausea, and anorexia. These are often transient and can be reduced by starting with a low dose and increasing the dose slowly. Aplastic anemia is a rare side effect; patients taking this drug need to have their blood levels watched carefully for this complication. Sustained-release preparations of carbamazepine (eg, Tegretol XR [Novartis], Carbatrol [Shire]) have improved compliance and reduced the medication's sedating side effects. The most recent Cochrane Database systematic review of the efficacy of carbamazepine for the treatment of trigeminal neuralgia revealed only four placebo and three active randomized controlled trials (RCTs). The populations in these studies were small but showed that there is evidence that carbamazepine is effective in the treatment of trigeminal neuralgia.[20]

Phenytoin has also been prescribed for the treatment of trigeminal neuralgia. However, long-term success was achieved in only 25% of the cases when used alone. The combination of phenytoin and baclofen seems to be more effective.[21,22] Common side effects are drowsiness, dizziness, asthenia, and gastrointestinal discomfort.

Gabapentin may be a useful alternative first-line treatment. Compared with carbamazepine and phenytoin, gabapentin has minimal side effects and is better tolerated by older patients.[23,24] However, there are no RCTs specifically investigating the efficacy of phenytoin or gabapentin for trigeminal neuralgia.[25,26]

Of the newer anticonvulsants, oxcarbazepine, a keto-analog of carbamazepine that has no known potential for bone marrow or hepatic toxicity, has also shown efficacy in the treatment of trigeminal neuralgia.[27,28] Oxcarbazepine is started at 150 mg twice daily and increased as tolerated to 300 to 600 mg twice daily. Side effects are similar to those of carbamazepine except that hyponatremia occurs more frequently. There are no controlled clinical trials studying the efficacy of oxcarbazepine for the treatment of trigeminal neuralgia.

One small double-blind placebo-controlled study showed that lamotrigine was superior to placebo in treating trigeminal neuralgia.[27] It has recently been validated for refractory cases, especially in trigeminal neuralgia due to multiple sclerosis, with doses between 100 and 400 mg daily.[29] Side effects may include diplopia, ataxia, dizziness, headache, and gastrointestinal discomfort. Lamotrigine should be promptly discontinued at the first sign of any rash, as serious rashes, including Stevens-Johnson syndrome, have occurred in approximately 0.1% of patients and usually appear within 2 to 9 weeks of starting treatment.[30]

Topiramate has shown initial promise in one very small randomized placebo-controlled pilot study.[31,32] Topiramate is started at 25 mg twice daily and increased slowly by 100 mg/day every 1 to 2 weeks, aiming for a daily dose of 100 to 400 mg divided twice daily. Side effects can include anorexia, weight loss, somnolence, anxiety, fatigue, psychomotor slowing, urolithiasis, and glaucoma. For all of the newer anticonvulsants, including gabapentin and oxcarbazepine, larger RCTs are needed to more precisely estimate their effectiveness.

A Cochrane Database systematic review concluded that there is insufficient evidence from RCTs to advocate the use of non-seizure medications, including baclofen, tizanidine, tocainide, proparacaine, pimozide, clomipramine, and amitriptyline for the treatment of trigeminal neuralgia, and side effects were common.[33]

## Surgical management

Several peripheral and central surgical procedures have been recommended to treat trigeminal neuralgia. Peripheral procedures include neurectomy, cryotherapy, and alcohol injection. Procedures aimed at traumatizing or destroying nerve tissue in or near the gasserian ganglion include radiofrequency thermocoagulation, percutaneous glycerol rhizotomy, and percutaneous balloon microcompression. The central surgical procedures include microvascular decompression surgery and stereotactic radiosurgery, also called *gamma knife surgery.*

*Neurectomy* is a peripheral ablative procedure in which the offending trigeminal nerve branch is avulsed under local or general anesthesia. Hypo- and paresthesias are common side effects,[34,35] and recurrence of pain is frequent. *Cryotherapy* is a peripheral ablative procedure in which the offending trigeminal branch is frozen under general or local anesthesia. A recently designed probe allows the procedure to be performed without surgical exposure of the nerve.[36] Generally, the effects of cryotherapy are short-lasting (6 to 12 months),[36,37] although longer pain relief has been reported.[38] Side effects may include atypical face pain and sensory deficits. *Alcohol injections* are administered under local anesthesia. After the affected branch of the trigeminal nerve is anesthetized, a small amount of absolute alcohol is injected. Compared with neurectomy and radiofrequency thermocoagulation, alcohol blocks have fewer side effects but a higher percentage of recurrence.[34] Side effects typically include hypo-, par-, and dysesthesia. Duration of pain relief is generally less than 1 year.[39] However, the proce-

dure can be repeated without affecting the extent or duration of pain relief.[39]

Three types of gasserian ganglion procedures are available for trigeminal neuralgia. *Percutaneous radiofrequency thermocoagulation* and *percutaneous glycerol rhizotomy* are neurosurgical procedures in which a needle, guided by radiographic fluoroscopy, is placed into the foramen ovale of the sedated patient. After careful manipulation and feedback from the patient, the selected nerve fibers are destroyed by thermal lesioning[40] or by injection of anhydrous glycerol.[41,42] Corneal numbness and masseter weakness are the most common complications of radiofrequency thermocoagulation (10% to 12%).[43] Corneal numbness and dysesthesia are the most common complications of percutaneous glycerol rhizotomy (8% each).[43] *Percutaneous balloon microcompression* is a neurosurgical procedure in which the trigeminal nerve is compressed by inflating a tiny balloon in the area of the involved nerve fibers.[44,45] The needle placement is similar to that of the other two procedures. Recent reports show high rates of immediate pain relief with balloon compression (91% to 100%),[46-48] whereas the recurrence rates at 12 to 18 months were low (2.5% to 5%).[46,48] A retrospective study with an average follow-up of almost 11 years reported 19% recurrence within a 5-year period and 32% recurrence within a 20-year period.[49] Side effects of this procedure include numbness and dysesthesia, the severity of which may be related to the amount of compression applied.[46] Transient masseter weakness is a common side effect. Other complications include arterial and cranial nerve injuries.

An alternative to rhizotomy is microvascular decompression of the trigeminal ganglion and dorsal root, first described in

1952 by Taarnhoj[50] in Denmark and by Love[51] in the United States. Jannetta[52] refined and popularized this procedure, which involves a craniotomy, in which the posterior fossa is opened and explored and the cortex is carefully lifted to expose the root entry zone of the trigeminal nerve and the compressing vessel or lesion. If the compressor is the superior cerebellar artery, which is the most common offender, it is carefully dissected from the trigeminal nerve, and a sponge is placed between the structures. Remarkable immediate success has been reported with this procedure.

Although microvascular decompression appears to have great long-term success, such a major surgical procedure carries risks of morbidity and mortality. Patient selection is therefore extremely important. Relatively young, healthy patients are obviously the best candidates.

The newest minimally invasive method of treating trigeminal neuralgia is *stereotactic neurosurgery* (gamma knife surgery). Precisely focused radiation of 40 to 90 Gy emitted from 201 photon beams is applied to the trigeminal root entry zone. Compared with other procedures, pain relief is delayed.[53] Reports of pain relief vary from 61% to 92%,[53-56] while recurrence rates vary from 10% to 27%.[54-57] Dysesthesia is the most prominent side effect (9%).[43]

There are no RCTs comparing different types of surgeries or surgeries with medications for trigeminal neuralgia. A recent thorough systematic review of only high-quality studies with actuarial data evaluated the treatment efficacy of radiofrequency thermocoagulation, percutaneous glycerol rhizotomy, percutaneous balloon compression, and stereotactic radiosurgery.[43] This review revealed that whereas radiofrequency

thermocoagulation showed the longest pain relief, the complications, though transient, were also most frequent. Radiofrequency thermocoagulation and percutaneous glycerol rhizotomy yielded higher percentages of complete pain relief at 6, 12, and 24 months than stereotactic radiosurgery. However, after 2 years, the pain-relieving effects of glycerol rhizotomy rapidly declined. A recent study showed that microvascular decompression and balloon compression offered the best prospects of improving the quality of life. Percutaneous glycerol rhizotomy and radiofrequency thermocoagulation also yielded favorable results, whereas medications were the least likely to improve quality of life.[57]

### Pretrigeminal neuralgia (ICD-9 350.9)

Pretrigeminal neuralgia was first described by Sir Charles Symonds.[58] Fromm and co-workers[59] reported on 16 patients who initially complained of a dull, continuous toothache in the maxilla or mandible that changed to classical trigeminal neuralgia. Trigeminal neuralgia can be accompanied by a dull, continuous pain in between attacks. A retrospective record review revealed that 35 of 83 patients with trigeminal neuralgia also reported continuous, dull pain in the same area. Of these patients, the 14% who reported dull pain preceding trigeminal neuralgia may have had pretrigeminal neuralgia.[60] No reports on the prevalence of pretrigeminal neuralgia are available. The diagnosis is based on the description of a dull ache, normal neurologic and dental examination results, and normal results on computerized tomography (CT) or magnetic resonance imaging (MRI) of the head.

Pretrigeminal neuralgia has been treated successfully with medications traditionally used for trigeminal neuralgia.[61]

## Glossopharyngeal neuralgia (IHS 13.2.x; ICD-9 352.1)

*Classical glossopharyngeal neuralgia* (IHS 13.2.1) is similar in character to trigeminal neuralgia but is present in the distribution of the glossopharyngeal nerve and may be present in the distribution of the auricular and pharyngeal branches of the vagus nerve. The pain is typically severe, transient, stabbing or burning, and located in the ear, base of the tongue, tonsillar fossa, or beneath the angle of the mandible. The pain is unilateral, although 1% to 2% of patients may experience nonsimultaneous bilateral pain. The paroxysms of pain usually last seconds to 2 minutes and are provoked by swallowing, chewing, talking, or yawning. It may relapse and remit like trigeminal neuralgias. The neurologic examination results in these patients are normal. The incidence of glossopharyngeal neuralgia is estimated to be 50 to100 times less than trigeminal neuralgia,[62] and the pathophysiology is thought to be similar to that of idiopathic trigeminal neuralgia.

The evaluation of a patient with glossopharyngeal neuralgia should include an MRI with contrast to exclude *symptomatic glossopharyngeal neuralgia* (IHS 13.2.2), which may arise because of posterior fossa tumor, fusiform (dolichoectatic) vertebral or basilar arterial pathology, and vascular anomalies. In addition, local causes of the pain, such as infection and nasopharyngeal tumor, need to be excluded.

Effective treatment can often be accomplished with the same anticonvulsant medications used for the treatment of trigeminal neuralgia, such as carbamazepine, oxcarbazepine, baclofen, phenytoin, or lamotrigine either alone or in combination.[27,63] Surgical procedures include intracranial sectioning of the glossopharyngeal nerve and the upper rootlets of the vagus nerve and microvascular decompression of the glossopharyngeal nerve.[64]

## Nervus intermedius neuralgia (IHS 13.3; ICD-9 351.9)

*Nervus intermedius neuralgia* is a rare condition characterized by unilateral paroxysms of pain felt in the depth of the ear and lasting seconds or minutes. There is often a trigger zone in the posterior wall of the auditory canal. Disorders of lacrimation, salivation, and taste are sometimes present. Local ear disorders need to be ruled out. This type of neuralgia is frequently associated with herpes zoster.[5,65-67] Medications used for trigeminal neuralgia, or surgical section of the nervus intermedius or chorda tympani, may relieve the pain.

## Superior laryngeal neuralgia (IHS 13.4; ICD-9 352.3)

*Superior laryngeal neuralgia* is a rare condition with severe paroxysmal pain felt in the throat, submandibular region, or under the ear, and it can last minutes to hours. Episodes of pain are precipitated by swallowing, straining the voice, or head turning, and a trigger zone is located on the lateral aspect of the throat overlying the hypothyroid membrane through which the internal branch of the superior laryngeal nerve enters the laryngeal structures.[68] The differential diagnosis includes neoplasms, bursitis lateralis, neuritis, and neuritis laryngei cranialis (seen during influenza epidemics). Medications traditionally used for trigeminal neuralgia may be effective. Repeated nerve blocks with high doses (5% to10%) of lidocaine have shown lasting effects.[69]

## Herpes zoster (IHS 13.15.1; ICD-9 053.x)

Acute herpes zoster infection affects 125 of 100,000 people in the older population. The trigeminal ganglion is involved in 10% to15% of cases, and the ophthalmic (first) division is involved in approximately 80% of cases.[70] *Herpes zoster* is characterized by pain followed by a herpetic eruption in the distribution of the trigeminal nerve within 1 week of onset. The disorder is due to reactivation of the varicella virus, which has been latent in the trigeminal ganglion. Inflammation, necrosis, and hemorrhage with intranuclear inclusion bodies occur in the ganglion.[71]

Ophthalmic herpes zoster may be associated with palsies affecting the third, fourth, and sixth cranial nerves. The facial nerve can also be affected, manifested by a vesicular eruption in the auditory meatus, facial weakness, and sometimes hearing loss, tinnitus, and vertigo. Involvement of C2 or C3 may cause pain and eruption over the posterior region of the head. The most common complication of herpes zoster is the development of intractable pain called *postherpetic neuralgia*.

Antivirals such as valacyclovir, famciclovir, and acyclovir can treat all aspects of herpes zoster infection related to healing, new lesions, and acute pain in immunocompetent[72,73] as well as immunocompromised patients.[74] Valacyclovir may be dosed at 1.5 g twice or three times per day with similar treatment efficacy, and 750 mg of famciclovir taken once per day has a similar treatment efficacy as the multiple daily dosing regimens of valacyclovir or 200 mg of acyclovir taken five times daily. Corticosteroids have been shown to shorten the duration of acute pain in elderly patients.[75,76] In most cases, sufficient pain relief cannot be achieved by antivirals and corticosteroids alone or in combination, and therapy may need to be supplemented with analgesics.

Although numerous interventions ranging from topical anesthetics and local subcutaneous injections to sympathetic and epidural blocks have been proposed and tried, prevention of postherpetic neuralgia with these methods has proven difficult.[76,77] In addition, there is currently no clear evidence that administration of antivirals will prevent the development of postherpetic neuralgia.[78]

## Painful ophthalmoplegia (IHS 13.16; ICD-9 378.9)

*Painful ophthalmoplegia* is characterized by episodes of orbital pain that are accompanied by paralysis of one or more of cranial nerves III, IV, or VI. Lesions of these nerves caused by vascular, neurologic, inflammatory, infiltrative, or space-occupying processes may underlie the symptoms. Such lesions may be demonstrated on CT or MR carotid angiography. Episodes are said to last 8 weeks in untreated patients, but pain relief can be achieved within 72 hours after initiation of corticosteroid therapy. The differential diagnosis includes pseudotumor of the orbit, temporal arteritis, vascular lesions, and ophthalmoplegic migraine.[79]

# Continuous Neuropathic Pain

## Idiopathic (trigeminal) neuropathic pain (ICD-9 350.9)

This category has historically been referred to as *atypical facial pain*, and in the recent IHS classification is referred to as *persistent idiopathic facial pain* (IHS 13.18.4). Because both of these terms may be regarded as "catch all" terms, it is preferred to refer to this category as *idiopathic continuous neuropathic pain* to contrast this pain with the neuralgias, which typically are episodic (with the exception of postherpetic neuralgia), but to reflect the neuropathic origin. The diagnosis of continuous neuropathic pain is made by ruling out all other possible conditions. Prior to the diagnosis, all other local or systemic causes, whether dental, oral, facial, sinus, musculoskeletal, or intracranial (eg, intracranial mass lesions) must be excluded. To do so may require additional assessment by an otorhinolaryngologist and/or neurologist.

Neuronal hyperexcitability is the key to the development of chronic pain.[80] The most likely mechanism behind neuropathic pain is partial or complete deafferentation. The clinician should remember that removal of pulpal tissue and extraction of teeth represent deafferentation procedures. Tooth pulp removal in cats has resulted in neuronal hyperexcitability and changes in the somatosensory pathways to the brain.[81] Other animal studies of lesions to the trigeminal nerve have also shown abnormal neural activity and neuroplastic changes.[82-84] Although deafferentation usually results in anesthesia and paresthesias, pain may ensue on occasion. Jensen and Baron[80] divided symptoms into negative and positive symptoms. *Negative symptoms* indicate sensory loss and present as reduced response to touch, pinprick, temperature, and vibration, whereas *positive symptoms* may reflect processes of regeneration and disinhibition, including paresthesia, dysesthesia, hyperalgesia, and deep pain.[80]

Continuous neuropathic pain may be peripherally generated or centrally mediated. Peripheral and central sensitization most likely both play a role in the maintenance of neuropathic pain. The extent that each contributes to the pain experience varies most likely in each patient depending on the underlying disease and genetic factors.[85] In addition, alterations in the function of the descending inhibitory pathways may contribute to increased pain perception.

When the pain is localized to a tooth or area that previously contained a tooth, the condition may be referred to as *atypical odontalgia*. By definition, atypical odontalgia means toothache of unknown cause[86] and has been considered synonymous with the term *phantom tooth pain*.[87] The prevalence of atypical odontalgia is not known; however, studies suggest that between 3% and 5% of endodontically treated patients may experience persistent pain.[88,89] More females than males appear to be afflicted with this condition,[90] and the maxilla seems to be more often involved than the mandible.[90] The patient can usually locate the exact tooth or area that is felt to be responsible for the pain. The pain is described as dull, aching, and persistent. Often the toothache has been present for months or even years, with no significant change in clinical characteristics. It may increase and decrease in intensity but rarely resolves. Most patients with atypical odontalgia have had multiple dental procedures performed in an attempt to remedy the pain before the diagnosis is established. The reason for these unnecessary and unsuccessful procedures is because the patient is often totally convinced that the pain is coming from a tooth. When the treatment fails, the patient will often encourage or sometimes even demand that the dentist continue with additional therapy. Although the pain is felt in the tooth or alveolar process, there is no local pathology present to explain the pain. Local provocation of the tooth or surrounding tissues does not alter the pain.

It is extremely important to differentiate atypical odontalgia from toothache of pulpal source.[91] The following characteristics are common to atypical odontalgia and not to pulpal toothache[92]:

1. There is constant pain in the tooth with no obvious source of local pathology.
2. Local provocation of the tooth does not consistently alter the pain. Hot, cold, or loading stimulation does not reliably affect the pain.
3. The toothache is unchanging over weeks or months. Pulpal pain tends to worsen or improve with time.
4. Repeated dental therapies fail to resolve the pain.
5. Response to local anesthesia is equivocal.

Additional criteria for the diagnosis of atypical odontalgia include the presence of pain for more than 4 months and the absence of referred pain.[93] Often there is a history of trauma or deafferentation.[90] Recent studies indicate that the pain from atypical odontalgia may be only partially generated peripherally.[94,95]

Because there are no RCTs including large samples of patients with continuous trigeminal neuropathic pain, treatment typically relies on therapies proven successful in studies on peripheral neuropathies of different origins. There is support for the effi-cacy of tricyclic antidepressants, gabapentin, pregabalin, tramadol, and topical lidocaine, and limited support for the use of paroxetine, citalopram, venlafaxine, bupropion, and lamotrigine.[96,97] Motor cortex stimulation has been shown to be successful in several patients with refractory neuropathic facial pain.[98-100]

## Postherpetic (trigeminal) neuralgia (IHS 13.15.2; ICD-9 053.12)

Most people heal completely from a bout of herpes zoster within 3 to 4 weeks without any persisting sequelae. However, some people may have irreversible damage to the skin and sensory disturbances. Whereas persisting or recurrent pain is infrequent in the general population, postherpetic neuralgia may affect 50% to 75% of the older population.[101] The IHS describes chronic postherpetic neuralgia as pain developing during the acute phase of herpes zoster and recurring or persisting for more than 3 months after the onset of the herpetic eruption.[5] The pain may be described as *burning*, sometimes accompanied by brief stabbing pain. Postherpetic neuralgia may be accompanied by hyperalgesia and allodynia or by profound sensory loss and anesthesia dolorosa.[101] Risk factors for developing postherpetic neuralgia include female sex, older age, experience of a prodrome, severity of the rash, and the severity of pain.[102]

The pathophysiology of postherpetic neuralgia is still largely unknown, but peripheral and central mechanisms have been suggested. Cell destruction at the level of the dorsal horn and loss of cutaneous nerve endings have been implicated.[103,104] Baron[101] proposed three different types of postherpetic neuralgias, one based on peripheral and central sensitization, one based on predominant degeneration of nociceptive neurons, and one based on mainly skin deafferentation. Depending on the underlying mechanism, different symptoms may prevail and different treatment modalities might be more successful.

According to recent Cochrane Database systematic reviews, the anticonvulsants gabapentin (in very high doses) and carbamazepine (in combination with clomipramine) show satisfactory pain relief,[25] as do the antidepressants amitriptyline, clomipramine, and desipramine.[105] Tramadol may also be helpful.[105] Recent RCTs showed that pregabalin reduced pain more effectively than placebo.[106,107] However, there are no active controlled trials to show whether this new drug is better than previously recommended medications. Topical lidocaine has been advocated for treatment of postherpetic neuralgia. Evidence of its efficacy as first-line treatment, however, is insufficient.[108] To date, there are not enough data to support the use of the newer antidepressants, but if the conventional medications fail or produce too many side effects, a trial of these medications may be indicated. Surgical intervention may be considered in severe, intractable cases.[109]

## Anesthesia dolorosa (IHS 13.18.1)

One of the most feared complications following neurosurgery for trigeminal neuralgia is anesthesia dolorosa. This pain condition is caused by damage to the trigeminal nerve, ganglion, and, less commonly, the trigeminal nuclear complex. *Anesthesia dolorosa* is characterized by severe pain in an area of anesthesia or dysesthesia. In addition to the characteristic pain, a feature of this condition is decreased sensibility to pain and temperature in one or more divisions of the trigeminal nerve. Accordingly, central pain results from lesions that affect the trigeminothalamic pathways.

A recent review revealed a low incidence rate of anesthesia dolorosa (less than 2%) after radiofrequency thermocoagulation and glycerol injections.[43] Balloon microcompression,[47,110] microvascular decompression,[111] and gamma knife surgery[54,112] have not typically been associated with the development of anesthesia dolorosa.

Very few studies are available with regard to the treatment of anesthesia dolorosa. Therefore, treatment remains anecdotal and usually consists of tricyclic antidepressants and anticonvulsants. Microsurgical repair has been shown to be effective in only one of seven patients.[113] In addition, dorsal entry zone lesioning has shown some promise,[114] as has sensory thalamic neurostimulation.[115]

## Central poststroke pain (IHS 13.18.2; ICD-9 338.0)

*Central poststroke pain* is characterized by pain, dysesthesia, and impaired sensation to pinprick and temperature stimulation. This pain condition is due to a lesion somewhere along the spinothalamic pathway and most commonly is the result of a vascular lesion, for example, ischemic or hemorrhagic infarction. The pain is not limited to the facial area; similar symptoms are usually experienced in the entire half of the body contralateral to the infarction. Similar pain can be produced by lesions that involve the ascending pain pathways elsewhere in the central nervous system; thus the term *central pain* is used to indicate such involvement.

Among those underlying processes implicated in the production of central pain of the face are vascular lesions (infarcts and hemorrhages), multiple sclerosis, syringobulbia, trauma, neurosurgical lesions, vascular malformations, tumor, and a variety of inflammatory disorders.

Few RCTs investigating treatment modalities for central poststroke pain have been performed. A recent systematic review identified amitriptyline and lamotrigine as the most effective medications, followed by mexiletine and phenytoin.[116] Carbamazepine did not seem to be effective, whereas gabapentin, although promising, was not studied sufficiently. This review also indicated that intravenous ketamine, propofol, and lidocaine might be helpful for short-term treatment. Invasive procedures may have a place when pharmacologic management fails. The available data are mostly anecdotal but suggest that deep brain stimulation and cortical stimulation may be helpful.[117]

## Complex regional pain syndrome

Complex regional pain syndrome (CRPS) I and II have been proposed to replace, respectively, reflex sympathetic dystrophy (ICD-9 337.20) and causalgia, also described as mononeuritis (ICD-9 355.9). The new terms have not been widely accepted, and the older terms are still frequently used.

According to the International Association for the Study of Pain (IASP),[66] CRPS is characterized by persistent, often burning pain accompanied by allodynia and hyperalgesia and at some point by swelling, changes in blood flow, and/or abnormal sudomotor activity. In CRPS I, the symptoms occur after a mild injury and are disproportionate to the initiating event, and in CRPS II, nerve damage seems to be the preceding factor. A revision to the IASP criteria has recently been proposed.[118] The diagnostic criteria include four symptom categories comprising sensory, vasomotor, sudomotor/edema, and motor/trophic changes, of which at least three must reported and at least two must be present at the time of evaluation. A third CRPS diagnosis, "CRPS not otherwise specified," was added for patients who do not fully meet the criteria.

The pathophysiology of CRPS remains unclear. It may be peripherally or centrally mediated, and its origin may be neuropathic, inflammatory, or immunologic.[119] Estimates of the incidence of CRPS range between 5 and 26 cases per 100,000 persons,[120,121] and women are about three times more often afflicted than men.[121] CRPS is typically found in the extremities, with the upper extremities more often involved, and is not generally described as occurring in the head and neck. A recent review of the lierature between 1947 and 2000 identified only 13 cases with head and neck involvement.[122] The typical features, such as loss of function and skin atrophy, were rarely seen, and, therefore, the diagnoses in most of these cases were debatable.

In some cases of CRPS, the peripheral nociceptors become sensitive to adrenergic stimulation, and any increase in activity of the sympathetic nervous system is likely to increase the pain. Increased levels of emotional stress and even visual or auditory stimuli can markedly increase the pain intensity. Typically, this pain is responsive to sympathetic blockade and, in such cases, the term sympathetically maintained pain is appropriate. Studies trying to resolve which features (eg, mechanical allodynia, cold allodynia) might predict a favorable response to sympathetic blockade have shown contrasting results.[123–125] High anxiety levels, litigation, and disability may be related to poor treatment response to a sympathetic blockade.[125]

Treatment of CRPS generally includes physical rehabilitation, psychologic interventions, and pharmacologic management.[119] Few RCTs with decent sample sizes are available with regard to the treatment of CRPS, and no particular pharmacologic or intervention strategy stands out. Therefore, at this time, pharmacologic treatment should follow the treatment paradigms for neuropathic pain. In the case of sympathetically maintained pain, a series of sympathetic blocks is indicated.

# References

1. Jensen TS. Mechanisms of neuropathic pain. In: Campbell JN (ed). Pain 1996: An Updated Review. Seattle: IASP Press, 1996:77–86.

2. Fromm GH. Pathophysiology of trigeminal neuralgia. In: Fromm GH, Sessle BJ (eds). Trigeminal Neuralgia: Current Concepts Regarding Pathogenesis and Treatment. Boston: Butterworth-Heinemann, 1991:105–130.

3. Cheshire WP. Trigeminal neuralgia: Diagnosis and treatment. Curr Neurol Neurosci Rep 2005;5(2):79–85.

4. Truini A, Galeotti F, Cruccu G. New insight into trigeminal neuralgia. J Headache Pain 2005;6(4):237–239.

5. Headache Classification Committee of the International Headache Society. The International Classification of Headache Disorders: 2nd edition. Cephalalgia 2004;24(suppl):1–151.

6. Penman J. Trigeminal neuralgia. In: Vinken PJ, Bruyn GW (eds). Handbook of Clinical Neurology. Amsterdam: Elsevier, 1968:296–322.

7. Jannetta PJ. Arterial compression of the trigeminal nerve at the pons in patients with trigeminal neuralgia. J Neurosurg 1967;26(1)(suppl):159–162.

8. Love S, Coakham HB. Trigeminal neuralgia pathology and pathogenesis [review]. Brain 2001;124(pt 12):2347–2360 [erratum 2002;125(pt 3):687].

9. Barker FG II, Jannetta PJ, Babu RP, Pomonis S, Bissonette DJ, Jho HD. Long-term outcome after operation for trigeminal neuralgia in patients with posterior fossa tumors. J Neurosurg 1996;84(5):818–825.

10. Broggi G, Ferroli P, Franzini A, Servello D, Dones I. Microvascular decompression for trigeminal neuralgia: Comments on a series of 250 cases, including 10 patients with multiple sclerosis. J Neurol Neurosurg Psychiatry 2000;68(1):59–64.

11. Golby AJ, Norbash A, Silverberg GD. Trigeminal neuralgia resulting from infarction of the root entry zone of the trigeminal nerve: Case report. Neurosurgery 1998;43(3):620–622; discussion 22–23.

12. Smyth P, Greenough G, Stommel E. Familial trigeminal neuralgia: Case reports and review of the literature. Headache 2003;43:910–915.

13. Coffey RJ, Fromm GH. Familial trigeminal neuralgia and Charcot-Marie-Tooth neuropathy. Report of two families and review. Surg Neurol 1991;35(1):49–53.

14. Devor M, Amir R, Rappaport ZH. Pathophysiology of trigeminal neuralgia: The ignition hypothesis. Clin J Pain 2002;18(1):4–13.

15. Rappaport ZH, Devor M. Trigeminal neuralgia: The role of self-sustaining discharge in the trigeminal ganglion. Pain 1994;56(2):127–138.

16. Lisney SJ, Devor M. Afterdischarge and interactions among fibers in damaged peripheral nerve in the rat. Brain Res 1987;415(1):122–136.

17. Devor M, Seltzer Z. Pathophysiology of damaged nerves in relation to chronic pain. In: Wall PD, Melzack R (eds). Textbook of Pain, ed 4. Edinburgh: Churchill Livingstone, 1999:129–164.

18. Beaver DL. Electron microscopy of the gasserian ganglion in trigeminal neuralgia. J Neurosurg 1967;26(1)(suppl):138–150.

19. Fromm GH. Etiology and pathogenesis of trigeminal neuralgia. In: Fromm GH (ed). The Medical and Surgical Management of Trigeminal Neuralgia. Mount Kisco, NY: Futura, 1987:31–41.

20. Wiffen PJ, McQuay HJ, Moore RA. Carbamazepine for acute and chronic pain. Cochrane Database Syst Rev 2005;(3):CD005451.

21. Masdeau JC. Medical treatment and clinical pharmacology. In: Rovit RL, Murali R, Jannetta PJ (eds). Trigeminal Neuralgia. Baltimore: Williams & Wilkins, 1990:79–93.

22. Fromm GH, Terrence CF, Chattha AS. Baclofen in the treatment of trigeminal neuralgia: Double-blind study and long-term follow-up. Ann Neurol 1984;15(3):240–244.

23. Rozen TD, Capobianco DJ, Dalessio DJ. Cranial neuralgias and atypical facial pain. In: Silberstein SD, Lipton RB, Dalessio DJ (eds). Wolff's Headache and Other Head Pain. New York: Oxford Univ Press, 2001:509–524.

24. Cheshire WP. Defining the role for gabapentin in the treatment of trigeminal neuralgia: A retrospective study. J Pain 2002;3(2):137–142.

25. Wiffen P, Collins S, McQuay H, Carroll D, Jadad A, Moore A. Anticonvulsant drugs for acute and chronic pain. Cochrane Database Syst Rev 2005;(3): CD001133.

26. Wiffen PJ, McQuay HJ, Edwards JE, Moore RA. Gabapentin for acute and chronic pain. Cochrane Database Syst Rev 2005;(3):CD005452.

27. Zakrzewska JM, Patsalos PN. Oxcarbazepine: A new drug in the management of intractable trigeminal neuralgia. J Neurol Neurosurg Psychiatry 1989;52(4): 472–476.

28. Royal M, Wienecke G, Movva V, et al. Open label trial of oxcarbazepine in neuropathic pain. Pain Med 2001;2:250–251.

29. Leandri M, Lunardi G, Inglese M, et al. Lamotrigine in trigeminal neuralgia secondary to multiple sclerosis. J Neurol 2000;247(7):556–558.

30. Zakrzewska JM, Chaudhry A, Nurmikko TJ, Patton DW, Mullens EL. Lamotrigine (Lamictal) in refractory trigeminal neuralgia: Results from a double-blind placebo controlled crossover trial. Pain 1997;73(2): 223–230.

31. Gilron I, Booher SL, Rowan JS, Max MB. Topiramate in trigeminal neuralgia: A randomized, placebo-controlled multiple crossover pilot study. Clin Neuropharmacol 2001;24(2):109–112.

32. Solaro C, Uccelli MM, Brichetto G, et al. Topiramate relieves idiopathic and symptomatic trigeminal neuralgia. J Pain Symptom Manage 2001;21(5):367–368.

33. He L, Wu B, Zhou M. Non-antiepileptic drugs for trigeminal neuralgia [review]. Cochrane Database Syst Rev 2006;3:CD004029.

34. Oturai AB, Jensen K, Ericksen J, et al. Neurosurgery for trigeminal neuralgia: Comparison of alcohol block, neurectomy and radiofrequency coagulation. Clin J Pain 1996;12(3):311–315.

35. Murali R, Rovit RL. Are peripheral neurectomies of value in the treatment of trigeminal neuralgia? An analysis of new cases and cases involving previous radiofrequency gasserian thermocoagulation. J Neurosurg 1996;85(3):435–437.

36. Pradel W, Hlawitschka M, Eckelt U, Herzog R, Koch K. Cryosurgical treatment of genuine trigeminal neuralgia. Br J Oral Maxillofac Surg 2002;40(3):244–247.

37. Zakrzewska JM, Thomas DG. Patient's assessment of outcome after three surgical procedures for the management of trigeminal neuralgia. Acta Neurochir (Wien) 1993;122(3–4):225–230.

38. De Coster D, Bossuyt M, Fossion E. The value of cryotherapy in the management of trigeminal neuralgia. Acta Stomatol Belg 1993;90(2):87–93.

39. McLeod NM, Patton DW. Peripheral alcohol injections in the management of trigeminal neuralgia. Oral Surg Oral Med Oral Pathol Oral Radiol Endod 2007;104(1):12–17.

40. Sweet WH, Wepsic JG. Controlled thermocoagulation of trigeminal ganglion and rootlets for differential destruction of pain fibers. I. Trigeminal neuralgia. J Neurosurg 1974;40:143–156.

41. Hakanson S. Trigeminal neuralgia treated by the injection of glycerol into the trigeminal cistern. Neurosurgery 1981;9(6):638–646.

42. Young RF. Glycerol rhizolysis for treatment of trigeminal neuralgia. J Neurosurg 1988;69(1):39–45.

43. Lopez BC, Hamlyn PJ, Zakrzewska JM. Systematic review of ablative neurosurgical techniques for the treatment of trigeminal neuralgia. Neurosurgery 2004;54(4):973–982; discussion 82–83.

44. Mullan S, Lichtor T. Percutaneous microcompression of the trigeminal ganglion for trigeminal neuralgia. J Neurosurg 1983;59(6):1007–1012.

45. Meglio M, Cioni G. Percutaneous procedures for trigeminal neuralgia: Microcompression versus radiofrequency thermocoagulation (personal experience). Pain 1989;38(1):9–16.

46. Lee ST, Chen JF. Percutaneous trigeminal ganglion balloon compression for treatment of trigeminal neuralgia. Part II. Results related to compression duration. Surg Neurol 2003;60(2):149–153; discussion 53–54.

47. Brown JA, Pilitsis JG. Percutaneous balloon compression for the treatment of trigeminal neuralgia: Results in 56 patients based on balloon compression pressure monitoring. Neurosurg Focus [serial online] 2005;18 (5):E10. Available at: http://www.aans.org/education/ journal/neurosurgical/may05/18-5-10.pdf. Accessed November 1, 2007.

48. Liu HB, Ma Y, Zou JJ, Li XG. Percutaneous microballoon compression for trigeminal neuralgia. Chin Med J (Engl) 2007;120(3):228–230.

49. Skirving DJ, Dan NG. A 20 year review of percutaneous balloon compression of the trigeminal ganglion. J Neurosurg 2001;94(6):49–54.

50. Taarnhoj P. Decompression of the trigeminal root and the posterior part of the ganglion as treatment in trigeminal neuralgia; Preliminary communication. J Neurosurg 1952;9(3):288–90.

51. Love JG. Decompression of the gasserian ganglion and its posterior root; A new treatment for trigeminal neuralgia; Preliminary report. Proc Staff Meet Mayo Clin 1952;27(14):257–258.

52. Jannetta PJ. Treatment of trigeminal neuralgia by suboccipital and transtentorial cranial operations. Clin Neurosurg 1977;24:538–549.

53. Henson CF, Goldman HW, Rosenwasser RH, et al. Glycerol rhizotomy versus gamma knife radiosurgery for the treatment of trigeminal neuralgia: An analysis of patients treated at one institution. Int J Radiat Oncol Biol Phys 2005;63(1):82–90.

54. Kondziolka D, Perez B, Flickinger JC, Habeck M, Lunsford LD. Gamma knife radiosurgery for trigeminal neuralgia: Results and expectations. Arch Neurol 1998;55(12):1524–1529.

55. McNatt SA, Yu C, Giannotta SL, Zee CS, Apuzzo ML, Petrovich Z. Gamma knife radiosurgery for trigeminal neuralgia. Neurosurgery 2005;56(6):1295–1301; discussion 1301–1303.

56. Sheehan J, Pan HC, Stroila M, Steiner L. Gamma knife surgery for trigeminal neuralgia: Outcomes and prognostic factors. J Neurosurg 2005;102(3):434–441.

57. Spatz AL, Zakrzewska JM, Kay EJ. Decision analysis of medical and surgical treatments for trigeminal neuralgia: How patient evaluations of benefits and risks affect the utility of treatment decisions. Pain 2007;131(3):302–310.

58. Symonds C. Facial pain. Ann R Coll Surg Engl 1949; 4:206.

59. Fromm GH, Terrence CF, Graff-Radford SB. Can trigeminal neuralgia have a prodrome? Neurology 1990;40:1493–1495.

60. Juniper RP, Glynn CJ. Association between paroxysmal trigeminal neuralgia and atypical facial pain. Br J Oral Maxillofac Surg 1999;37(6):444–447.

61. Fromm GH, Graff-Radford SB, Terrence CF, Sweet WH. Pre-trigeminal neuralgia. Neurology 1990; 40(10):1493–1495.

62. Rushton JG, Stevens JC, Miller RH. Glossopharyngeal (vagoglossopharyngeal) neuralgia. Arch Neurol 1981; 38(4):201–205.

63. Rozen TD. Trigeminal neuralgia and glossopharyngeal neuralgia. Neurol Clin North Am 2004;22:185–206.

64. Kondo A. Follow-up results of using microvascular decompression for treatment of glossopharyngeal neuralgia. J Neurosurg 1998;88(2):221–225.

65. Loeser JD. Cranial neuralgias. In: Loeser JD (ed). Bonica's Management of Pain. Philadelphia: Lippincott Williams & Wilkins, 2001:855–866.

66. Merskey H, Bogduk N (eds). Classification of Chronic Pain, ed 2. Seattle: IASP Press, 1994.

67. Aguggia M. Typical facial neuralgias. Neurol Sci 2005; 26(suppl 2):S68–S70.

68. Bruyn GW. Superior laryngeal neuralgia. Cephalalgia 1983;3:235–240.

69. Takahashi Sato K, Suzuki M, Izuha A, Hayashi S, Isosu T, Murakawa M. Two cases of idiopathic superior laryngeal neuralgia treated by superior laryngeal nerve block with a high concentration of lidocaine. J Clin Anesth 2007;19(3):237–238.

70. Ragozzino MW, Melton LJ 3rd, Kurland LT, Chu CP, Perry HO. Population-based study of herpes zoster and its sequelae. Medicine (Baltimore) 1982;61:310–316.

71. Portenoy RK, Duma C, Foley KM. Acute herpetic and postherpetic neuralgia: Clinical review and current management. Ann Neurol 1986;20(6):651–664.

72. Shafran SD, Tyring SK, Ashton R, et al. Once, twice, or three times daily famciclovir compared with aciclovir for the oral treatment of herpes zoster in immunocompetent adults: A randomized, multicenter, double-blind clinical trial. J Clin Virol 2004;29(4): 248–253.

73. Madkan VK, Arora A, Babb-Tarbox M, Aboutlabeti S, Tyring S. Open-label study of valacyclovir 1.5 g twice daily for the treatment of uncomplicated herpes zoster in immunocompetent patients 18 years of age or older. J Cutan Med Surg 2007;11(3):89–98.

74. Tyring S, Belanger R, Bezwoda W, Ljungman P, Boon R, Saltzman RL. A randomized, double-blind trial of famciclovir versus acyclovir for the treatment of localized dermatomal herpes zoster in immunocompromised patients. Cancer Invest 2001;19(1):13–22.

75. Eaglestein WH, Katz R, Brown JA. The effects of early corticosteroid therapy in the skin eruption and pain of herpes zoster. J Am Med Assoc 1970;211:1681–1683.

76. van Wijck AJ, Opstelten W, Moons KG, et al. The PINE study of epidural steroids and local anaesthetics to prevent postherpetic neuralgia: A randomised controlled trial. Lancet 2006;367(9506):219–224.

77. Opstelten W, van Wijck AJ, Stolker RJ. Interventions to prevent postherpetic neuralgia: Cutaneous and percutaneous techniques. Pain 2004;107(3):202–206.

78. Alper BS, Lewis PR. Does treatment of acute herpes zoster prevent or shorten postherpetic neuralgia? J Fam Pract 2000;49(3):255–264.

79. Bogduk N. Pain of cranial nerve and cervical nerve origin other than primary neuralgias. In: Olesen J, Tfelt-Hansen P, Welch KMA (eds). The Headaches, ed 2. Philadelphia: Lippincott Williams & Wilkins, 2000: 921–922.

80. Jensen TS, Baron R. Translation of symptoms and signs into mechanisms in neuropathic pain. Pain 2003;102(1–2):1–8.

81. Hu JW, Sessle BJ. Effects of tooth pulp deafferentation on nociceptive and nonnociceptive neurons of the feline trigeminal subnucleus caudalis (medullary dorsal horn). J Neurophysiol 1989;61(6):1197–1206.

82. Vos BP, Strassman AM, Maciewicz RJ. Behavioral evidence of trigeminal neuropathic pain following chronic constriction injury to the rat's infraorbital nerve. J Neurosci 1994;14(5 pt 1):2708–2723.

83. Bongenhielm U, Robinson PP. Spontaneous and mechanically evoked afferent activity originating from myelinated fibres in ferret inferior alveolar nerve neuromas. Pain 1996;67(2–3):399–406.

84. Yates JM, Smith KG, Robinson PP. Ectopic neural activity from myelinated afferent fibres in the lingual nerve of the ferret following three types of injury. Brain Res 2000;874(1):37–47.

85. Meyer RA, Ringkamp M, Campbell JN, Raja SN. Peripheral mechanisms of cutaneous nociception. In: McMahon SB, Koltzenburg M (eds). Wall and Melzack's Textbook of Pain, ed 5. London: Churchill Livingstone, 2006:3–34.

86. Rees RT, Harris M. Atypical odontalgia: Differential diagnosis and treatment. Br J Oral Maxillofac Surg 1978;16:212–218.

87. Marbach JJ. Phantom tooth pain. J Endod 1978;4: 362–372.

88. Marbach JJ, Hulbrock J, Hohn C, Segal AG. Incidence of phantom tooth pain: An atypical facial neuralgia. Oral Surg Oral Med Oral Pathol 1982;53(2):190–193.

89. Campbell RL, Parks KW, Dodds RN. Chronic facial pain associated with endodontic neuropathy. Oral Surg Oral Med Oral Pathol 1990;69(3):287–290.

90. List T, Leijon G, Helkimo M, Oster A, Dworkin SF, Svensson P. Clinical findings and psychosocial factors in patients with atypical odontalgia: A case-control study. J Orofac Pain 2007;21(2):89–98.

91. Falace DA, Cailleteau JG. Diagnosis of dental and orofacial pain. In: Falace DA (ed). Emergency Dental Care: Diagnosis and Management of Urgent Dental Problems. Baltimore: Williams & Wilkins, 1995:1–24.

92. Okeson JP. Bell's Orofacial Pains, ed 6. Chicago: Quintessence, 2005.

93. Graff-Radford SB, Solberg WK. Criteria for the Classification of Orofacial Pain and Dysfunction in Clinical Practice. Los Angeles: UCLA School of Dentistry, 1992.

94. List T, Leijon G, Helkimo M, Oster A, Svensson P. Effect of local anesthesia on atypical odontalgia—A randomized controlled trial. Pain 2006;122(3):306–314.

95. Baad-Hansen L, Juhl GI, Jensen TS, Brandsborg B, Svensson P. Differential effect of intravenous S-ketamine and fentanyl on atypical odontalgia and capsaicin-evoked pain. Pain 2007;129(1–2):46–54.

96. Beniczky S, Tajti J, Timea Varga E, Vecsei L. Evidence-based pharmacological treatment of neuropathic pain syndromes. J Neural Transm 2005;112(6):735–749.

97. Sindrup SH, Otto M, Finnerup NB, Jensen TS. Antidepressants in the treatment of neuropathic pain. Basic Clin Pharmacol Toxicol 2005;96(6):399–409.

98. Nguyen JP, Lefaucher JP, Le Guerinel C, et al. Motor cortex stimulation in the treatment of central and neuropathic pain. Arch Med Res 2000;31(3):263–265.

99. Rainov NG, Heidecke V. Motor cortex stimulation for neuropathic facial pain. Neurol Res 2003;25(2): 157–161.

100. Rasche D, Ruppolt M, Stippich C, Unterberg A, Tronnier VM. Motor cortex stimulation for long-term relief of chronic neuropathic pain: A 10 year experience. Pain 2006;121(1–2):43–52.

101. Baron R. Postherpetic neuralgia and other neurologic complications. In: Gross G, Doerr HW (eds). Herpes Zoster: Recent Aspects of Diagnosis and Control. Basel: Karger, 2006.

102. Jung BF, Johnson RW, Griffin DR, Dworkin RH. Risk factors for postherpetic neuralgia in patients with herpes zoster. Neurology 2004;62(9):1545–1551.

103. Oaklander AL. The density of remaining nerve endings in human skin with and without postherpetic neuralgia after shingles. Pain 2001;92(1–2):139–145.

104. Wree A, Schmitt O, Usunoff KG. Neuroanatomy of pain and neuropathology of herpes zoster and postherpetic neuralgia. In: Gross G, Doerr HW (eds). Herpes Zoster: Recent Aspects of Diagnosis and Control. Basel: Karger, 2006.

105. Saarto T, Wiffen PJ. Antidepressants for neuropathic pain. Cochrane Database Syst Rev 2005;(3): CD005454.

106. Dworkin RH, Corbin AE, Young JP Jr, et al. Pregabalin for the treatment of postherpetic neuralgia: A randomized, placebo-controlled trial. Neurology 2003;60(8):1274–1283.

107. Freynhagen R, Strojek K, Griesing T, Whalen E, Balkenohl M. Efficacy of pregabalin in neuropathic pain evaluated in a 12-week, randomised, double-blind, multicentre, placebo-controlled trial of flexible- and fixed-dose regimens. Pain 2005;115(3): 254–263.

108. Khaliq W, Alam S, Puri N. Topical lidocaine for the treatment of postherpetic neuralgia. Cochrane Database Syst Rev 2007;(2):CD004846.

109. Schvarcz JR. Craniofacial postherpetic neuralgia managed by stereotactic spinal trigeminal nucleotomy. Acta Neurochir Suppl 1989;46:62–64.

110. Brown JA, McDaniel MD, Weaver MT. Percutaneous trigeminal nerve compression for treatment of trigeminal neuralgia: Results in 50 patients. Neurosurgery 1993;32(4):570–573.

111. Chang JW, Chang JH, Park YG, Chung SS. Microvascular decompression in trigeminal neuralgia: A correlation of three-dimensional time-of-flight magnetic resonance angiography and surgical findings. Stereotact Funct Neurosurg 2000;74(3–4): 167–174.

112. Gorgulho A, De Salles AA, McArthur D, et al. Brainstem and trigeminal nerve changes after radiosurgery for trigeminal pain. Surg Neurol 2006;66(2): 127–135; discussion 135.

113. Gregg JM. Studies of traumatic neuralgia in the maxillofacial region: Symptom complexes and response to microsurgery. J Oral Maxillofac Surg 1990;48(2):135–140; discussion 141.

114. Nashold BS, El-Naggar A, Mawaffak AW, et al. Trigeminal nucleus caudalis root entry zone: A new surgical approach. Stereotact Funct Neurosurg 1992;59(1–4):45–51.

115. Siegfried J. Sensory thalamic neurostimulation for chronic pain. Pacing Clin Electrophysiol 1987;10(1 pt 2):209–212.

116. Frese A, Husstedt IW, Ringelstein EB, Evers S. Pharmacologic treatment of central post-stroke pain. Clin J Pain 2006;22(3):252–260.

117. Nicholson BD. Evaluation and treatment of central pain syndromes. Neurology 2004;62(5 suppl 2): S30–S36.

118. Harden RN, Bruehl S, Stanton-Hicks M, Wilson PR. Proposed new diagnostic criteria for complex regional pain syndrome. Pain Med 2007;8(4):326–331.

119. Stanton-Hicks MD, Burton AW, Bruehl SP, et al. An updated interdisciplinary clinical pathway for CRPS: Report of an expert panel. Pain Pract 2002;2(1):1–16.

120. Sandroni P, Benrud-Larson LM, McClelland RL, Low PA. Complex regional pain syndrome type I: Incidence and prevalence in Olmsted county, a population-based study. Pain 2003;103:199–207.

121. de Mos M, de Bruijn AG, Huygen FJ, Dieleman JP, Stricker BH, Sturkenboom MC. The incidence of complex regional pain syndrome: A population-based study. Pain 2007;129(1–2):12–20.

122. Melis M, Zawawi K, Al-Badawi E, Lobo Lobo S, Mehta N. Complex regional pain syndrome in the head and neck: A review of the literature. J Orofac Pain 2002;16(2):93–104.

123. Dellemijn PL, Fields HL, Allen RR, McKay WR, Rowbotham MC. The interpretation of pain relief and sensory changes following sympathetic blockade. Brain 1994;117(pt 6):1475–1487.

124. Rommel O, Malin JP, Zenz M, Janig W. Quantitative sensory testing, neurophysiological and psychological examination in patients with complex regional pain syndrome and hemisensory deficits. Pain 2001;93(3):279–293.

125. Hartrick CT, Kovan JP, Naismith P. Outcome prediction following sympathetic block for complex regional pain syndrome. Pain Pract 2004;4(3):222–228.

# Intraoral Pain Disorders

The most prevalent sources of orofacial pain originate from the structures located in the oral cavity. This chapter will review common orofacial pain disorders associated with the teeth and periodontium, the mucogingiva, and the tongue.

## Odontogenic Pain

Toothache is a symptom that commonly confounds the clinician. Establishing a diagnosis is challenging because teeth often refer pain to other teeth as well as to distant locations around the head, neck, and jaws, which may mimic the symptoms of other types of orofacial pain disorders. To further complicate matters, other orofacial pain disorders may refer pain to teeth, mimicking the symptoms of toothache. In order to render effective treatment, the clinician must first determine whether the pain is *odontogenic* in origin and, if so whether the source of the pain is pulpal or periodontal. In some instances, toothache may not actually originate from pulpal or periodontal tissues. These toothaches are generally called *nonodontogenic* toothaches.

### *Pulpal pain*

Classification of pulpal pain

The dental pulp is a visceral organ. Thus, pulpal pain, like visceral pain in general, is a deep, dull, aching pain that is of a threshold nature and is often difficult to localize.[1] This pain can arise from vital or nonvital pulp.

**Vital pulp**
Pain in vital pulp can result from either reversible or irreversible inflammation. *Reversible pulpitis* is characterized by a quick, sharp pain and hypersensitive response that subsides soon after the stimulus is removed. Any irritant, such as food, drink, or caries, may cause this focal pulpal inflammation.[2] Reversible pulpitis is a symptom—not a disease process. If the irritant is removed and the inflamed pulp is palliated, it will return to normal. If the irritant remains, however, the symptoms will persist or become more widespread, leading to an irreversible condition.

*Irreversible pulpitis* is characterized by prolonged pain that may be provoked by a stimulant or occur spontaneously. The pain may be intermittent or continuous, moderate or severe, sharp or dull, affected by the time of day or body position, and localized or diffuse. The intensity of the pain may vary considerably over time and may go through asymptomatic periods. The inflammation is more severe and more widespread in irreversible pulpitis[2] and may lead to pulpal necrosis.

### Nonvital pulp

Untreated irreversible pulpitis, traumatic injury, or any event that causes long-term interruption of the blood supply to the pulp will inevitably lead to partial or total pulpal necrosis. Partial necrosis may present some of the symptoms associated with irreversible pulpitis and is more common in multi-rooted teeth. Total necrosis is asymptomatic before it affects the periodontal ligament.[2] If pulpal disease extends into the periapical tissue, the pain becomes spontaneous and continuous and can be exacerbated by percussion but not by temperature.

## Etiology of pulpal pain

Dentinal sensitivity is caused by exposure of the dentinal tubules to the environment of the oral cavity[3] through attrition, abrasion, erosion, or dental caries. Gingival recession, toothbrush trauma, periodontal diseases, and periodontal surgery are factors that may expose the radicular dentin. The etiologic factors involved in acute pulpal pain can be grouped into three general categories: bacterial, traumatic, and iatrogenic.

### Bacterial

Bacteria are introduced into the pulp as a result of dental caries,[4] fractures,[5-7] and anomalous tracts[8] from the periodontium[9] and the systemic blood supply.[10]

### Traumatic

Direct trauma to a tooth can cause pulpitis, acute pulpalgia, incomplete fracture of a tooth,[6] or complete fracture with exposure of the pulp.[5,6] Trauma may partially or completely avulse a tooth through disruption of the apical blood supply and subsequent pulpitis or necrosis.[11] Repeated direct microtrauma, such as chronic bruxism, may also cause pulpal inflammation followed by necrosis.

### Iatrogenic

The operative procedures involved in tooth restoration may cause pulpitis and acute pulpalgia. The adverse effects from heat and vibrations from the high-speed handpiece, depth of preparation, dehydration of dentin, insertion of pin-retained restorations, and accidental pulp exposure are well documented. Pulpal changes have also been reported in response to impression techniques in which bacteria were forced through the dentinal tubules into the pulp. Many materials and chemicals used to restore teeth may also injure the pulp and cause pulpitis and acute pulpal pain.

## Pathophysiology of pulpal pain

Myelinated (Aδ) and unmyelinated (C) afferent nerve fibers mediate the innervation of dentinal pulp. The Aδ fibers enter the apex of the root and extensively arborize, especially in the coronal part of the tooth. Just below the odontoblastic cell layer, the Aδ fibers lose their myelin sheath and form a network of nerves called the *plexus of Raschkow*.[12] This plexus sends free nerve endings onto and through the odontoblastic cell layer where they synapse with the odontoblastic dendritic processes, whose cell bodies are located at the pulpal end of the odontoblastic tubule.[13] This intimate association of Aδ fibers with the odontoblastic cell layer and dentin is referred to as the *pulpodentinal complex*.[14]

A disturbance in the pulpodentinal complex initially affects the low-threshold Aδ fibers. However, not all stimuli will reach the excitation threshold and generate a painful response. Mild irritants such as incipient dental caries and mild periodontal disease are usually not painful but can stimulate the defensive formation of sclerotic or reparative dentin. If the cellular or fluid contents of the dentinal tubules are sufficiently disturbed to involve the odontoblastic cell layer, the Aδ fibers become excited, and fluid movement in the dentinal tubules is translated into electric signals by sensory receptors located within the tubules or the subjacent odontoblast cell layer.[15-17] These nociceptive signals are immediately perceived as a quick, sharp (bright), momentary pain. On removal of the exciting stimulus (eg, cold liquid), the sensation dissipates quickly.[14] If an external irritant, such as dental caries, is of significant magnitude to injure the pulp, the resulting tissue inflammation and associated vascular response can lead to an increase in tissue pressure. The pulp, however, is surrounded by calcified dentin, which prevents any significant volume change and thus compromises the pulp's compensatory mechanisms to reduce the pressure. The damaged tissue degenerates, and the inflammatory process spreads circumferentially and incrementally from this site to involve adjacent structures, perpetuating the destructive cycle.[18]

An injured tooth with localized inflammation can also emit symptoms of Aδ fiber pain on provocation. Inflammatory mediators, such as bradykinin, 5-hydroxytryptamine, and prostaglandin E$_2$, can sensitize the Aδ fibers by lowering their pain threshold. When the exaggerated Aδ fiber pain subsides, a dull, throbbing ache remains. This second pain symptom signifies the inflammatory involvement of nociceptive C-fibers.[14] C-fibers make up small, unmyelinated nerves that are found in the central portion of the pulp and run subjacent to the Aδ fibers.

When C-fiber pain dominates Aδ fiber pain, the pain is more diffuse and not easily localized. C-fiber pain indicates that irreversible local tissue damage has occurred. Inflammatory mediators, vascular changes in blood volume and blood flow, and increases in tissue pressure modulate the pain response. As the spread of inflammation increases, C-fiber pain becomes the only pain feature. Pain that may start as a short, lingering discomfort can escalate to an intense, prolonged episode or a constant, throbbing pain. The pain becomes more diffuse and can be referred to a distant site or to other teeth.[14]

When the caries lesion penetrates the dentin and contacts the pulp, the nature of the inflammatory response changes from a collection of mostly mononuclear leukocytes to a localized collection of polymorphonuclear leukocytes, which form microabscesses within the lesion.[19,20] It is at this stage that reversible pulpitis becomes irreversible.[21] Eventually, one area of microabscesses leads to numerous other microabscesses. When they are large enough to coalesce, the pulp undergoes liquefaction necrosis and/or dry necrosis. Complete necrosis of the pulp may occur rapidly or may take years to develop, and it may or may not be associated with pain.

## Clinical characteristics of pulpal pain

The hallmark of acute pulpal pain, as with all types of visceral pain, is its diffuseness and variability.[22] Over the dull, aching pain, there may be superimposed sensations of pulsing and throbbing or sharp, burning, and lancinating paroxysms of pain. In these cases, the superimposed sensations are due to the intensification of pulpal pain rather than to vascular or neuropathic mechanisms.

The onset of pulpal pain occurs only when the stimulus achieves a threshold level of intensity, and the threshold level varies according to the provoking stimulus and other factors. Clinical symptoms correlate poorly with the health or histologic status of the pulp.[23-25] Early histopathologic changes in the pulp can cause agonizing pain, while a necrotic tooth may be painless. Therefore, the clinician should not rely on symptoms alone to determine the condition of the pulp.

Pulpal pain can be modified by many factors, including heat and cold, pressure from occlusal contact, head position, and the intensity of the offending stimulus. The preexisting condition of the pulp may modify the inflammatory process and therefore the pain. In addition, emotionally mediated central nervous system activity may increase or decrease the degree of pain.

Acute pulpal pain commonly results in central excitatory effects.[22] When the pain is referred, it tends to follow a laminated segmental pattern within the trigeminal system. Investigators have graphed the probable sites of pain referral from individual teeth. According to these studies,[26,27] maxillary teeth refer pain to maxillary and mandibular teeth on the same side and to cutaneous locations on the face superior to the maxillary teeth, and mandibular teeth refer pain to maxillary and mandibular teeth on the same side. Anterior teeth have been shown to refer pain to both sides of the face,[28] with a cutaneous referral pattern traveling from the ear to locations on the face inferior to the ear.

## Differential diagnosis of pulpal pain

A tooth causing odontogenic pain is identified by the presence of pathology that explains the pain (eg, caries, a failing restoration, radiographic findings).[22] When a suspicious tooth is located, an attempt to induce or increase the pain by noxious stimulation of that tooth by chemical, thermal, mechanical, or electric irritants should be made. If pain can be influenced by local irritation, the tooth should be locally anesthetized to see whether pain is completely arrested even with further stimulation. If local anesthesia has no effect on the pain level, the pain is originating from another pain source, such as a different tooth or a nonodontogenic source. If anesthesia decreases the pain, the pain source is confirmed; however, there may be an additional nonanesthetized contributor to the pain. The next step is to determine whether the pain is pulpal or periodontal in origin.

Pain of pulpal origin tends to respond to a stimulus at a given threshold and may be difficult to localize precisely. Teeth that have only pulpal involvement are not sensitive to percussion. Teeth that have periodontal and/ or periapical involvement respond to a stimulus on a graduated basis, are generally easy to localize, and are sensitive to percussion.[22]

*Reversible pulpitis* is characterized by stimulated pain of brief duration that ceases soon after removal of the stimulus. Cold and electric stimulation provoke a brief response, but there is no sensitivity to percussion.[29] *Irreversible pulpitis* is characterized by stimulated pain of prolonged duration or by spontaneous pain. Cold and electric stimulation yield a prolonged response, but there is usually no sensitivity to percussion unless the inflammatory process in the radicular pulp has begun to involve the periapex.[29]

Necrotic pulp can be extremely painful or asymptomatic. The tooth may be extremely sensitive to percussion if the periapex is inflamed, but neither temperature nor electric stimulation elicits a response.[29]

## Management of pulpal pain

Treatment is directed toward reducing the functional diameter of the dentinal tubules so as to limit fluid movement. There are several treatment options available[30–32]: (1) formation of a smear layer on the sensitive dentin by burnishing the exposed root surface; (2) application of agents such as oxalate compounds that form insoluble precipitates within the tubules; (3) impregnation of the tubules with plastic resins; and (4) application of dentin-bonding agents to seal off the tubules.

Treatment of reversible pulpitis targets removal of the pain-causing stimulus, such as an incipient caries lesion; removal of the lesion and restoration of lost tooth structure will alleviate the pain. Treatment of irreversible pulpitis or necrotic pulp involves extirpation of the offending pulp with a root canal treatment or extraction of the tooth.

## Periodontal pain

The periodontium (periodontal ligament and alveolar bone) is classified as a musculoskeletal organ; therefore, acute periodontal pain is more localized in comparison with pulpal pain. The discriminative capability is so acute that patients can often pinpoint the source of the pain as coming from the apical as opposed to the coronal periodontal ligament. The improved ability to localize the source of pain is attributed to the proprioceptive and mechanoreceptive sensibility of the periodontium.[33] The intensity of the pain is proportionate to the stimulus.[1] At minimal levels of stimulation, the patient may describe a sensation as innocuous such as itching, and at severe levels, unrelenting, throbbing pain is felt. Inflammatory fluid accumulation may cause displacement of the tooth in its socket, with a resulting acute malocclusion and pain. Pain may thus be associated with biting or chewing.

Periodontal pain can be modified. Factors that may increase periodontal pain are pressure from occlusal contact, head position, and the intensity of the stimulus. In addition, central modulation as a result of the patient's emotional state may increase or decrease the degree of pain.

Like pulpal pain, periodontal pain may stimulate secondary central excitatory effects, resulting in regional pain referral to any location around the head and neck. Referred pain to muscles may lead to the development of myofascial trigger points and autonomic nervous system effects such as congested sinuses, conjunctival hyperemia, and puffy eyelids. In addition, areas that have had previous experience with pain are more likely to be sites of referred pain.

Periodontal pain may originate from local factors only; however, systemic factors can modulate the patient's ability to resist the effects of the local factors.

## Periodontal pain caused by local factors only

Periodontal pain localized to a single tooth or area is usually associated with abscesses of the periodontium and combined periodontal-endodontic lesions. Abscesses of the periodontium are categorized by location and include four types: gingival, periodontal, periradicular, and pericoronal.[34]

### Gingival abscess
#### Clinical characteristics
Abscess of the gingiva is relatively uncommon. It usually arises as the result of trauma to a previously healthy gingival unit. The clinical presentation consists of a painful, fluctuant swelling with a smooth and shiny surface, and spontaneous drainage via fistula is common. The differential diagnosis includes periodontal abscess, which occurs in a setting of periodontal attachment loss and pocket formation.[35] The gingival abscess is distinguished from the periodontal abscess by its confinement to the marginal or interdental gingival tissue.

#### Etiology
As noted above, the gingival abscess occurs in a previously healthy site. The precipitating cause is usually traumatic implantation of a foreign body or material.

#### Pathophysiology
The abscess consists of a purulent focus in the connective tissue, surrounded by diffuse infiltration of polymorphonuclear leukocytes, edematous tissue, and vascular engorgement. The surface epithelium presents varying degrees of intra- and extracellular edema, invasion of leukocytes, and ulceration.

#### Management considerations
The goal of therapy is to eliminate the acute signs and symptoms of infection and mitigate the pain. This is accomplished by incision of the fluctuant area to permit drainage and removal of the causative agent. Treatment of the lesion may require irrigation and debridement. Since this lesion, by definition, occurs in a previously healthy site, aggressive root debridement is not usually indicated. The patient is then dismissed for 24 hours with instructions to rinse with a glass of warm salt water every 2 hours. When the patient returns, the lesion is usually reduced in size and symptom free.

### Periodontal abscess
#### Clinical characteristics
The term *periodontal abscess* refers to acute or recurrent inflammatory swellings that occur in periodontally diseased sites. The typical abscess is a localized swelling of the gingiva that may also involve the alveolar mucosa. These lesions often have a violaceous or cyanotic appearance and are usually fluctuant.[36,37] The degree of pain can range from a deep ache of low intensity to severe discomfort. In general, the lesions are somewhat less painful than acute apical periodontal abscesses of endodontic origin, and the pain is often exacerbated by mastication and percussion. The affected tooth is often mobile and slightly extruded, and suppuration may be noted from the pocket orifice. The swelling occurs more coronally than in combined periodontal-endodontic lesions. The tooth pulp is usually vital. In more severe cases, cellulitis, fever, and malaise may occur.[38] The periodontal abscess must be distinguished from lesions of apical periodontitis, which are due to pulpal necrosis or similar conditions.[38]

## Etiology

Bacterial infection is usually the causal factor. Recent studies have found that the abscess microflora is composed mainly of periodontal pathogens, specifically *Porphyromonas gingivalis*, *Prevotella intermedia*, *Fusobacterium nucleatum*, *Peptostreptococcus micros*, and *Bacterioides forsythus*.[39–41] The periodontal abscess may also form when food lacerates the gingiva or when inflammatory exudate from chronic periodontitis cannot drain into the periodontal pocket because of impacted food particles.[42] Trauma or extension of pulpal inflammation into the periapical tissues can also lead to periodontal abscess.[29] Other sources include over-instrumentation in root canal treatment or mechanical trauma from endodontic filling materials.

## Pathophysiology

A periodontal abscess is usually an exacerbation of a preexisting chronic periodontal infection. More than 300 species of microorganisms have been isolated from periodontal pockets, but only a small number are considered capable of causing disease.[43] These microorganisms possess bacterial virulence factors that are constituents or metabolites capable of either disrupting homeostatic or protective host mechanisms or causing the progression or initiation of disease. Most of the tissue destruction in established periodontal lesions is a result of the mobilization of the host tissues via activation of monocytes, lymphocytes, fibroblasts, and other host cells. Engagement of these cellular elements by bacterial factors, in particular bacterial lipopolysaccharide, is thought to stimulate production of both catabolic cytokines and inflammatory mediators, including arachidonic acid metabolites such as prostaglandin $E_2$. Cytokines stimulate inflammatory responses that cause tissue destruction via mobilization of tissue metalloproteinases, a major pathway for connective tissue attachment loss and bone loss in most forms of periodontitis.[44,45]

## Management considerations

Treatment of the abscess consists of drainage (usually through the pocket orifice) and debridement of the root surface under local anesthesia, often accompanied by copious irrigation. Debridement can be performed with hand instruments or ultrasonic lavage. Occlusal adjustment is sometimes indicated but is not a primary component of therapy. Periodontal abscess formation is common in furcation lesions, but debridement of these areas is difficult. Unless the tooth is obviously beyond salvage, it is usually prudent to resolve the symptoms and then reassess the periodontal situation.

## Periradicular abscess

### Clinical characteristics

The onset of periradicular abscess is rapid, with spontaneous pain, pain to percussion, pus formation, and swelling.[2] It must be distinguished from the periodontal abscess, although both processes may be operant in a combined periodontal-endodontic lesion. The periodontal abscess always occurs, by definition, in a setting of periodontal attachment loss and pocket formation. If attachment loss or pocket formation is not present in the site, a periodontal etiology is not likely.

Although the pulp is necrotic and not sensitive to thermal testing, the initial pain is typically intense as long as the abscess is confined to bone. However, extension into the soft tissues reduces the pressure and hence the pain. If there is no pathway for drainage when the infection exits the cortical bone, the abscess may spread along fascial planes to distant locations, which can result in serious space infections. Bacteremia from such lesions rarely causes infections in distant organs or tissues. If the infection does localize, it changes from a hard swelling on the surface into a soft, pus-filled swelling that eventually drains. Increased body temperature and regional lymphadenopathy are usually present.

### Etiology
A periradicular abscess usually develops from a pulp that undergoes rapid degeneration from pulpitis to necrosis with spread of the infection into the periradicular tissues.[14] Occasionally, it may develop from an exacerbation of a *phoenix abscess* (chronic periodontitis located at the periapex).

### Pathophysiology
The periradicular abscess is initiated by a quick infiltration of numerous, virulent bacteria into the apical periodontal ligament from an infection in the pulp, causing an acute inflammatory reaction in four stages. Chemical mediators of inflammation orchestrate these events. The first stage is injury and cell death, followed by microvascular phenomena, such as vascular dilation, stasis, and increased vascular permeability, allowing for release of plasma and inflammatory cells. The third stage mobilizes more polymorphonuclear leukocytes into the lesion, increasing destruction of bacteria and host tissue and forming more pus. If the body contains the pus, it may be absorbed and the lesion will heal. If not, the pus will dissect its way through the marrow spaces in the alveolar bone, perforate the cortical plate, and either drain or spread into soft tissue spaces. The fourth stage is healing.

### Management considerations
Management of the periapical abscess involves draining the abscess by tooth extraction or root canal therapy.

## Pericoronal abscess (pericoronitis)
### Clinical characteristics
This localized purulent infection occurs in tissue that surrounds the crown of a partially erupted tooth, most frequently in the mandibular third molar area. Clinical features may include a markedly red, swollen, edematous, suppurating gingival lesion that is exquisitely tender, with radiating pains to the ear, throat, and floor of the mouth. Patients also report a foul taste and an inability to close the jaws. Frequently, an indentation of the opposing tooth can be seen imprinted on the inflamed gingival flap. Swelling of the cheek in the region of the angle of the jaw and lymphadenitis are common findings. The patient may also present systemic complications such as fever, leukocytosis, and malaise.[36,38]

### Etiology
The space between the crown of the tooth and the overlying gingival flap in the third molar area is an ideal site for the accumulation of food debris and bacterial growth, which is a common foundation for pericoronal abscess formation.

### Pathophysiology
*Cellulitis* occurs as a result of an influx of inflammatory fluid and cellular exudate in the area of the gingival flap due to infection by microorganisms that produce significant amounts of hyaluronidase and fibrinolysins, which act to break down and dissolve, respectively, hyaluronic acid and fibrin. Streptococci are particularly potent producers of

hyaluronidase and are therefore a common causative organism. Cellulitis may stay localized or it may spread posteriorly into the oropharyngeal area and medially to the base of the tongue, making it difficult for the patient to swallow. Depending on the severity and extent of the infection, there may be lymph node involvement of the submandibular, posterior cervical, deep cervical, and retropharyngeal lymph nodes.[46,47]

### Management considerations

An irrigating syringe should be used to perform lavage of the cavity under the flap. As this condition is virtually always associated with partially erupted mandibular third molars, removal of the tooth is generally indicated as soon as the acute episode has resolved. Removal of the operculum is sometimes advocated in lieu of extraction. However, soft tissue management in this area is often difficult and the postoperative result unsatisfying, so extraction is usually the treatment of choice to prevent recurrence. Pericoronal infections can sometimes extend along fascial planes to involve other anatomic spaces. Such space infections should be treated aggressively, owing to the potential for morbidity and, rarely, mortality. Abscess formation is not uncommon and calls for prompt surgical drainage and appropriate antibiotic therapy. Patients with trismus, fever greater than 101°F, and facial swelling should be referred to an oral and maxillofacial surgeon.[48]

## Combined periodontal-endodontic abscess

Combined lesions are of primary periodontal origin, and may begin as marginal periodontitis, which may later cause a "retrograde" endodontic infection by gaining access to the pulp through the apical fora-

mina or accessory canals. It has been suggested that such lesions are uncommon.[4] Alternatively, endodontic infections may drain through the apical or accessory foramina and periodontal ligament, thereby causing "retrograde" periodontitis.[9]

This condition may occur in a patient with preexisting periodontitis or in a setting of normal periodontal health. In most cases, the distinction between primary periodontal and primary endodontic lesions is artificial. The one exception may be the combined lesion that is endodontic in origin and occurs in a patient without significant periodontal involvement. Occasionally, periodontal lesions (ie, involving attachment loss and deep, narrow probing depths) may resolve following endodontic treatment, but only if the lesion is of recent onset.

### Clinical characteristics

Patients present with pain, tenderness to pressure and percussion, increased tooth mobility, increased probing depth/attachment loss, and swelling of the marginal gingiva, simulating a periodontal abscess. The suppurative process may cause the formation of a narrow, deep pocket that can sometimes be traced to the apex with a gutta-percha cone or a periodontal probe. Pulp testing reveals a necrotic pulp or, in the case of a multirooted tooth, an abnormal response.[50] All of these signs are variable, as is the radiographic appearance.

### Pathophysiology

The pathophysiologic processes are detailed in the preceding sections on periodontal and periradicular abscesses.

### Management considerations

The periodontal component of the combined lesion may resolve subsequent to con-

## Management considerations

Early detection of cracked teeth is essential before the crack progresses into the pulp and down the root, resulting in the need for endodontic therapy or even nonrestorability.[59–62] The specific therapy depends on the severity of symptoms and location of the crack. Temporary stabilization can be achieved with an orthodontic stainless steel band or a temporary crown until an overlay or full crown can be fabricated.[57] Endodontic treatment with or without stabilization has been advocated.[58,61,63] In case of extensive cracks, extraction may be the only feasible solution.[2]

# Nonodontogenic Toothache

The clinician should never automatically assume that all toothaches are caused by pulpal or periodontal disease. There are numerous nonodontogenic sources that may be responsible for pain felt in the teeth.[1,22] Since dental pain is so commonly treated in the dental office, nonodontogenic toothaches are often inappropriately treated with dental therapy before being properly diagnosed. Often, only after multiple treatment failures and even tooth extractions does the diagnosis of nonodontogenic toothache become apparent.

The most important step toward proper identification and management is the suspicion that the origin of the toothache is not in the pulp or supporting dental structures. Key identifiers of nonodontogenic toothache include[1,64]:

• Spontaneous multiple toothaches
• Inadequate local dental cause for the pain
• Stimulating, burning, nonpulsatile toothaches
• Constant, unremitting, nonvariable toothaches
• Persistent, recurrent toothaches
• Failure of anesthesia to significantly reduce the pain
• Failure of the toothache to respond to reasonable dental therapy

Nonodontogenic toothache can often be differentiated from odontogenic toothache by local provocation. Pulpal and periodontal pains are increased by stimuli such as percussion, thermal, or biting forces. When toothache is not increased by provocation, the clinician should suspect a nonodontogenic source of pain. Local anesthetic can be helpful in differentiating true dental pain from pain referred to the teeth.[1,65,66] When administered to the site of the nonodontogenic toothache, local anesthetic often will not reduce the pain, since the reported site of pain is not the true source of pain.

Multiple structures may refer pain to the teeth[22,64]; one of the most common of these structures is muscle. Myofascial trigger points in the masseter (most common muscle source), temporalis, medial pterygoid, lateral pterygoid, and anterior digastric muscles are possible sources of referred pain.[27,67,68] Another source of nonodontogenic toothache is the maxillary sinus, which is a common source of maxillary tooth pain.[69] Nonodontogenic toothache may also result from continuous neuropathic pain (eg, neuritis, neuroma, deafferentation, or atypical odontalgia), episodic neuropathic pain (eg, neuralgias), or neurovascular disorders.[66,70–73] Even cardiac pain may be felt as toothache,[74] and, in some instances, psychogenic disorders may present as tooth pain. Knowing the pain characteristics and referral patterns for each of these sources is essential for a good differential diagnosis. A complete review of each of these disorders can be found in other texts.[1,22,64,73]

# Mucogingival and Glossal Pain Disorders

Localized mucogingival or glossal pain is usually associated with a detectable erosive or ulcerative lesion, and diffuse pain may be associated with a widespread infection, a systemic disease due to underlying deficiency, or other unknown factors.

Localized pain associated with a detectable lesion may result from trauma (physical, chemical, or thermal), viral infection, immune dysfunction, or may be of unknown origin. Pain characteristics include a bright, stimulating quality; anatomically accurate, subjective localization; a pain site coincident with its source; a provocation response faithful in incidence, intensity, and location; and a temporary response to topical anesthetic at the pain site.[1,38]

Generalized diffuse pain in the oral mucosa usually has a burning quality and may be accompanied by a change in taste, predominantly of a bitter metallic nature.[38] This pain may result from a direct insult to the tissues due to bacterial, viral, or fungal infection, which can be identified by the characteristic appearance of the oral mucosa. Radiation therapy to the head and neck may result in acute mucositis with severe generalized mucosal pain. A burning sensation of the oral mucosa, particularly the tongue, may also result from traumatic trigeminal neuralgia or some systemic deficiency disease.

## Local mucogingival and glossal pains

### Acute necrotizing ulcerative gingivitis

Necrotizing periodontal conditions are characterized by severe pain, necrotic lesions of the interdental gingiva (ie, "punched-out papillae"), and gingival hemorrhage on slight provocation. The somewhat arbitrary terms *necrotizing ulcerative gingivitis* (NUG) and *necrotizing ulcerative periodontitis* (NUP) have been used to distinguish necrotizing conditions that present with or without attachment loss. The American Academy of Periodontology has recommended that both diseases be considered *necrotizing periodontal diseases* since distinctions between NUG and NUP are somewhat arbitrary.[75] For the sake of simplicity, both diseases will be referred to by the acronym *NUG* in this review. As a historical aside, the term *acute necrotizing ulcerative gingivitis* was formerly used to describe these conditions. However, clinical observation has revealed that acute episodes may often resolve spontaneously into a subacute, indolent infection characterized by episodic recurrences.

**Clinical characteristics**

NUG is associated with painful, hyperemic, fiery red gingiva and punched-out erosion of the interdental papilla. The lesions bleed easily and are often covered with a gray necrotic pseudomembrane. The patient may complain of an inability to eat due to the severity of the pain. Occasionally, systemic symptoms are seen, such as malaise and a low-grade fever. Fetid breath is another common, though not invariable, finding. The lesions may occasionally spread to other areas of the oral mucosa as *necrotizing* ulcerative stomatitis.[76] *Noma* (also known as *gangrenous stomatitis* and *cancrum oris*) is the diagnostic term used when these lesions extend to the facial tissues.[77,78]

In the developed world, necrotizing ulcerative stomatitis is usually seen in debilitated or immunocompromised adults. In the developing world, these diseases also occur in malnourished infants. When the condition occurs in immunocompetent adults, the patient is often a young adult with poor hygiene who is a heavy smoker. Patients who do not fit this profile (eg, a middle-aged nonsmoker with good hygiene) should be evaluated for predisposing immunosuppressive conditions.

### Etiology

Although the precise causative agents are unknown, emotional stress, tobacco use, poor oral hygiene, local trauma, fatigue, and impaired immunity predispose the individual to NUG.[76]

### Pathophysiology

NUG was originally referred to as a *fusospirochetal* disease, since light microscopic and darkfield examination revealed the presence of spirochetes and fusiform bacteria in scrapings from lesions. More recently, *P intermedia* has been implicated, along with various *Treponema*, *Fusobacterium*, and *Selenomona* species.[79]

### Management considerations

Treatment consists of mechanical debridement, antibiotic therapy with metronidazole, tetracycline, or doxycycline, and a 0.12% chlorhexidine mouthrinse. Management of the underlying periodontal disease must follow the acute phase.[76,80]

## Recurrent aphthous stomatitis

Recurrent aphthous stomatitis (RAS), also known as *aphthous ulcers* or *canker sores*, is said to be the most common oral mucosal disease affecting the general population. RAS appears in three clinical forms: minor, major, and herpetiform. The most prevalent form of the disease is RAS minor, with a frequency rate of 17.7% in the general population and 80% in RAS patients.[81,82] The prevalence of RAS major ranges from 7% to 20%,[83] while 7% to 10% of all cases of RAS are of the herpetiform type.[83–85]

### Clinical characteristics

RAS minor appears as discrete, painful, shallow, recurrent ulcers, covered by a yellow-gray pseudomembrane surrounded by an erythematous halo. Ulcers number one to five at any given time, and each measures less than 10 mm in diameter.[82,86] They are almost always painful, and usually heal within 10 to 14 days without scar formation.[87]

RAS major produces coalescent ulcers that are usually larger than 1 cm in diameter and persist for weeks or months.[85,86] They present as very painful, large, deep-based ulcers containing a yellow-gray necrotic center with raised, rolled, indurated walls that have a predilection for the lips, soft palate, and fauces. The lesions may heal with scarring.

Herpetiform RAS occurs in crops of 10 to 100 at a time,[86] usually in the posterior part of the mouth. The ulcers appear in clusters of 1 to 3 mm in diameter that sometimes coalesce, resembling a herpetic infection.

Regardless of the type of RAS, ulcers are confined to the nonkeratinized mucosa of the mouth: the labial mucosa, buccal mucosa, maxillary and mandibular sulci, non-attached gingiva, floor of the mouth, ventral surface of the tongue, soft palate, and tonsillar fauces. The keratinized dorsum of the tongue, attached gingiva, and the hard palate mucosa are spared. While patients often demonstrate submandibular lymphadenopathy, fever is rare.[88]

## Etiology

Factors that play a modifying or triggering role in the development of RAS include hormonal changes, trauma, stress, and food allergies.[89,90] Foods associated with triggering RAS include bovine milk protein, glutens, chocolate, nuts, cinnamon, spices, and preservatives.[88] A number of medications are known to cause RAS. The most common medications reported to cause intraoral aphthous-like lesions are the nonsteroidal anti-inflammatory drugs (NSAIDs).[91] Deficiencies of ferritin and vitamin $B_{12}$ have also been associated with RAS.[92]

## Pathophysiology

No causative microorganisms have been identified. Rather, the disease is considered to result from immune system dysfunction. Studies of peripheral blood from otherwise healthy persons with RAS have found various immune system abnormalities, such as depressed or reversed CD4:CD8 cell ratios (especially in persons with severe RAS)[85,87,93-95] and increased T-cell receptor-$\gamma\delta^+$ cells in patients with active RAS compared with controls. [96]

## Management considerations

Treatment for RAS is palliative and symptomatic. Every effort should be made to eliminate predisposing allergens from the patient's diet. Therapeutic agents such as topical steroids and amlexanox 5% oral paste[97-99] have been effective in decreasing the symptoms and healing time, but nothing has been effective in decreasing the recurrence rate unless a trigger or serum deficiency can be identified. Other types of treatment for RAS minor include topical anesthetics, topical mouthrinses, caustic agents, and laser ablation.[85,88,100] In RAS major, where the healing process may be prolonged and topical corticosteroids may not be effective, therapy may range from intralesional injections of triamcinolone acetonide to the use of thalidomide.[85,88] Other drugs that have been advocated include lysine, dapsone, azathioprine, and etanercept.[87,101]

## Herpes simplex virus infection

Herpes simplex virus (HSV) causes an acute viral infection that may occur in the oral cavity in either a primary or recurrent form and may be from one of two distinct strains of herpes virus hominis, HSV-1 or HSV-2.[102]

### Primary herpetic gingivostomatitis

Primary herpetic gingivostomatitis occurs in individuals with no previous exposure to the virus; therefore, it occurs primarily in children and adolescents.

### Clinical characteristics

The clinical manifestations include systemic involvement as well as oral lesions. The initial presentation is a rapid onset of generalized prodromal signs and symptoms, such as fever, malaise, headache, irritability, and regional lymphadenopathy. The systemic symptoms are followed by the development of oral lesions initially manifested as a severe generalized gingival inflammation. After several days, oral vesicles can appear on any area of the mouth, although the lips, gingiva, tongue, and palate are most often affected. The vesicles rupture very rapidly, forming shallow, ragged, extremely painful ulcerations with a yellowish center and erythematous borders. The lesions begin as numerous punctate ulcerations that coalesce to form large irregular ulcerations, which usually heal within 10 to 14 days. In some cases, extraoral lesions occur on the upper and lower lips, with severe pain, oozing, and crusting. Severe pain, foul odor, and increased salivation usually accompany the oral lesions.[76,100,102,103]

Diagnosis is most often based on the history and clinical presentation. Laboratory diagnosis is not commonly necessary except in a setting of immunosuppression or atypical presentation.[100]

### Secondary herpetic gingivostomatitis

The prevalence of secondary or recurrent herpes simplex virus infection in the general population has been estimated at 20% to 40% worldwide and 35% to 38% in the United States.[104] Recurrent infections can present as either recurrent herpes labialis or recurrent intraoral herpes. Both conditions are commonly due to reinactivation of the virus, which has existed in the trigeminal ganglion in a latent or quiescent state.

#### Clinical characteristics

Recurrent herpes labialis infection is characterized by unilateral vesicular eruptions surrounded by erythema, followed by crusting and healing. The eruptions are sometimes preceded by a prodromal tingling sensation. Oral mucosal lesions are rare, not associated with fever, and usually restricted to small clusters of microvesicles (1 to 3 mm) that rupture, leaving behind punctate ulcers, typically on the palatal gingiva uni-

laterally. The lesions are self-limited, resolving within 1 to 4 days.[103] Because of the acquired immunity during the primary infection, the subjective complaints are usually mild, and constitutional symptoms are usually absent. Extraoral lesions may appear on the skin, genitalia, anal and perianal areas, eyes (eg, keratitis, keratoconjunctivitis), and nervous system (eg, encephalitis, meningitis).[105,106]

### Etiology

The typical route of HSV inoculation is physical contact with an infected individual by someone who has not been previously exposed to the virus or possibly by someone with a low titer of protective antibody to HSV. During the primary infection, only a small percentage of individuals show clinical signs and symptoms, while most experience only subclinical symptoms. This latter group is seropositive and can be identified through laboratory evaluation of circulating antibodies to HSV.[107]

### Pathophysiology

The incubation period ranges from several days to 2 weeks after exposure. A vesiculo-ulcerative eruption then occurs in the oral and perioral tissues at the primary site of inoculation. Following resolution of primary herpetic gingivostomatitis, the virus migrates, through some unknown mechanism, along the periaxonal sheath of the trigeminal nerve to the trigeminal ganglion, where it remains in a latent or quiescent state. Reactivation of the virus may follow exposure to cold, trauma, or stress. Viral particles then travel by way of the trigeminal nerve to the original epithelial surface where replication occurs, resulting in a focal vesiculo-ulcerative eruption. Since the humoral and cell-mediated arms of the immune system have been sensitized to the HSV antigens, the extent of the lesions is limited, and systemic symptoms usually do not occur. As the secondary lesion resolves, the virus returns to the trigeminal ganglion, and evidence of viral particles can no longer be found within the epithelium.[107]

**Management considerations**

Treatment of primary herpetic gingivostomatitis is usually supportive, with fluids and nutrition, to prevent dehydration and electrolyte imbalance. Systemic analgesics such as acetaminophen with or without codeine are useful to control pain. Aspirin and NSAIDs should be avoided in acute viral infections. Systemic antiviral agents such as acyclovir are not routinely indicated for primary herpetic gingivostomatitis except in severely immunocompromised patients or when there is ocular involvement.

Treatment of recurrent herpetic gingivostomatitis consists of local palliative measures and antiviral therapy with acyclovir or one of its congeners (eg, famciclovir, valacyclovir).[108] Topical penciclovir reduces the severity and duration of the viral outbreak by 1 to 2 days.[109,110] Some investigators have reported success with lysine tablets, but this therapy has not been subjected to rigorous trials.[101] A number of agents have been used to prevent or reduce recurrence of mucocutaneous herpetic infections, the most widely used of which are famciclovir and valacyclovir.[108]

Active herpetic lesions should be considered infectious. Patients should be warned of the possibility of transmission to others, especially to infants and the immunocompromised. Auto-inoculation of the virus into other receptive mucosal sites (eg, the eye) is also possible.[103]

## Oral candidiasis

*Oral candidiasis* is a term that encompasses a group of mucosal and cutaneous conditions most commonly caused by the yeast *Candida albicans*. Other members of the *Candida* genus, such as *C tropicalis*, *C krusel*, *C parapsilosis*, and *C guilliermondi* may also be found intraorally, but they rarely cause disease. More recently, oral candidiasis has been associated with *C dubliniensis* in HIV-infected individuals.[111]

*C albicans* can exist in several forms. The *yeast* form is commensal and relatively harmless, while the *hyphal* form is invasive, pathogenic, and the cause of clinical candidiasis. Studies indicate that when the yeast forms grow hyphae, they spread across, attach to, and burrow between and into epithelial cells. This process is commonly seen in more serious tissue invasion and in immunocompromised hosts.[112]

An opportunistic pathogen, *C albicans* normally requires a host and/or site that is somehow compromised. Immunosuppressed patients such as those with AIDS or poorly controlled diabetes are among those most commonly affected.[113] Mucocutaneous candidiasis also may occur as a consequence of antibiotic or glucocorticoid therapy. Local factors or ecologic niches, such as dental prostheses, may also predispose to infection or serve as candidal reservoirs.

**Acute pseudomembranous candidiasis**

This form of candidiasis is the most common, and the two groups frequently affected are infants and elderly persons. The lesions are superficial, curd-like, white plaques that wipe off, leaving an erythematous, eroded, or ulcerated surface. The plaques are composed of fungal organisms, keratotic debris, inflammatory cells, desquamated epithelial cells, bacteria, and fibrin. The lesions may develop at any location, but favor the buccal mucosa and mucobuccal folds, the oropharynx, and the lateral aspects of the dorsal tongue. If the pseudomembrane has not been disturbed, the associated symptoms are minimal. In severe examples, patients may complain of tenderness, burning, and dysphagia. Predisposing factors include a history of broad-spectrum antibiotics, steroids, nutritional deficiency, diabetes, malignancy, chemotherapy, radiation therapy, and cell-mediated immunity dysfunction, including HIV infection.[111,113,114]

### Acute atrophic candidiasis

The persistence of acute pseudomembranous candidiasis may eventually result in loss of the pseudomembrane, which causes red lesions of various sizes surrounded by inflamed tissue. Atrophic lesions are most often seen on the tongue and the palate. The lesions are much more painful than in other forms of candidiasis, and are associated with tenderness, oral burning, and dysphagia. Predisposing factors include broad-spectrum antibiotics and corticosteroid aerosols such as those used by patients with asthma.[111,113]

### Chronic atrophic candidiasis

The lesions in chronic atrophic candidiasis are erythematous and edematous, characterized by a slight velvety/pebbly surface. Small erosions may also be seen. The lesions are located on the palate and maxillary and mandibular edentulous ridges, and are frequently encountered under dentures. Predisposing factors include ill-fitting or poorly cleaned dentures, as well as those factors described for the other forms of candidiasis.[111,113]

### Chronic hypertrophic/hyperplastic candidiasis

Chronic candidal infections are also capable of producing a hyperplastic tissue response. The resulting lesions are hard, nodular lesions that appear white, cream colored, or red, and are not associated with pain. They are located most often on the surface of the tongue, buccal mucosa, palate, denture-bearing areas (eg, papillary hyperplasia), central dorsum of the tongue (eg, median rhomboid glossitis), and in areas of epithelial hyperplasia. Predisposing factors include cellular hyperplasia, oral precancerous lesions, smoking, and denture wearing.

The diagnosis of candidiasis can often be made from the patient history and the clinical appearance and distribution of the mucosal lesions. When necessary, especially in an immunocompromised patient, identification of the organism is made in a culture of the lesion on a selective medium, from a cytologic smear with periodic acid–Schiff staining, or on a wet smear macerated with 10% potassium hydroxide.[100,114]

Oral candidiasis is most often treated with topical antifungal agents such as nystatin ointment, clotrimazole troches, or amphotericin oral suspensions. Oral preparations in the form of troches provide the advantage of prolonged contact with the lesions, and they are safe to use because of their poor systemic absorption.[100] In refractory candidiasis, chronic mucocutaneous candidiasis, or oral candidiasis associated with immunosuppression or HIV, systemic administration of ketoconazole, fluconazole, or itraconazole is indicated, but in the case of azole-resistant candidiasis, amphotericin is used.[113,114]

## Angular cheilitis

The clinical manifestation of angular cheilitis is similar to intraoral chronic atrophic candidiasis but in a different location. The lesions are localized to the corners of the mouth. These deep fissures allow pooling of saliva and are subsequently colonized by yeast organisms. The lesions are moderately painful, eroded, and encrusted. Predisposing factors include ill-fitting dentures with overclosure, drooling at the corners of the mouth, lip-licking habits, and thumb/digit-sucking habits.[111,113]

*Angular cheilitis* is a mixed infection of *C albicans* and the salivary species of streptococci. These lesions respond well to combination therapy containing an antifungal and a topical steroid such as clotrimazole with betamethasone dipropionate or nystatin with triamcinolone acetonide.

## Trauma

Trauma is the most common cause of irritation or ulceration of the oral mucous membranes. Traumatic oral lesions may be either factitial or iatrogenic in their origin and may result from physical, chemical, or thermal insults to the tissue.[115] Traumatic ulcers may be caused by common physical injuries to the oral cavity, such as cheek or tongue biting, irritation from a sharp filling or broken tooth, denture irritation, a traumatic event involving a sharp foreign object, or even toothbrush trauma from overzealous brushing with a hard-bristle toothbrush. "Cotton-roll" ulcers are produced when absorbent cotton rolls placed in the vestibular sulcus during dental treatment are removed. Traumatic stripping of the epithelium by the cotton roll results in fibrin-covered superficial erosions or ulcers.[115]

Chemical burns can be a consequence of deliberate or accidental ingestion of caustic agents, prolonged contact with aspirin or vitamin C tablets, use of undiluted oral antiseptics, contamination of prostheses with denture cleaners, or accidental contact with phosphoric, chromic, or trichloroacetic acid during dental treatment.[115] Chemical and thermal burns are rare, however, because the oral mucosa is quite resistant to heat and acid or alkaline compounds. Thermal burns usually affect the hard palate and are most commonly caused by ingestion of hot liquids or hot melted cheese (eg, pizza-cheese burn on the palate).

Electric burns are almost exclusively seen in children who chew electric wires. Another source of traumatic oral ulceration is therapeutic radiation for head and neck malignancies. As the offending cause or agent is usually quickly discontinued or removed, most traumatic injuries to the oral mucous membranes will be acute in nature.

## Cancer

Approximately 5% of all malignancies in patients in the United States are intraoral, and 90% of these are squamous cell carcinomas.[116,117] Annually in the United States, there are nearly 40,000 new cases and more than 9,000 deaths due to oral squamous cell carcinoma. There has been only a slight improvement in the overall 5-year survival rate, from about 45% to 50%, in the past several decades.[107,116] While not usually thought of as painful in its presentation, the accompanying mucosal discomfort usually prompts patients to seek medical care.[118]

Pain from cancer may result from disease progression, treatment, or from recurrent or uncontrolled disease following treatment.

Causes of cancer-related pain include ulceration and infection, stimulation of mucosal and submucosal nerve endings, or tumor infiltration of a peripheral nerve. When intraoral neoplasms become large, patients will typically complain of paresthesia or hypoesthesia, with accompanying symptoms of loose teeth, occlusal change, and/or restriction of tongue or jaw movement. Also, as with other orofacial pain conditions, the pain from cancer may be felt at the primary site, may be referred to another site, or both.

## Burning mouth syndrome

*Burning mouth syndrome* (BMS) is a common dysesthesia described as a burning sensation in the oral mucosa occurring in the absence of clinically apparent mucosal abnormalities or laboratory findings and often perceived as painful.[119] Although the tongue is most commonly affected, other mucosal surfaces may be symptomatic.

### Clinical characteristics

BMS has been divided into primary and secondary conditions. Secondary BMS is accompanied by potential precipitating or perpetuating factors, such as candidiasis, diabetes, anemia, vitamin deficiencies, oral parafunctional habits, use of angiotensin-converting enzyme inhibitors, dry mouth or use of medications that may cause dry mouth, and psychosocial stressors.[120] When all of these factors have been ruled out as playing a role in the maintenance of the symptoms or have been treated and the burning sensation persists, BMS is classified as primary. Women are more likely to have BMS than men, but the prevalence of BMS is unknown, owing to the wide variety of criteria used in prevalence studies. The occurrence is rare before the age of 30 years and is most frequent in those aged 50 years and older.[121-126]

Patients with BMS frequently complain of persistent or dysgeusic taste and altered taste perception.[119,127,129] The persistent taste alteration is usually identified as bitter, metallic, or a combination of both. Typically, the perception can be reduced by rinsing and eating.[127]

### Pathophysiology

The pathophysiology of BMS is largely unknown, but peripheral and central mechanisms have been proposed. Findings of altered salivary flow, altered salivary composition, dysgeusia, altered sensory thresholds, and degenerative changes in peripheral afferent fibers have prompted theories in favor of peripheral mechanisms.[129-131] Evidence implicating central mechanisms comes from neuroimaging studies showing decreased activity in the descending inhibitory control pathways.[132-134]

Diagnosis is based on a detailed history; clinical examination; laboratory studies that include complete blood cell count, vitamin, iron, and fasting blood glucose levels; fungal cultures; and exclusion of all other possible oral problems such as restorations and dental prostheses and the use of drugs that cause xerostomia.

### Management considerations

At this time, treatment of BMS remains anecdotal. There is no clear evidence to support pharmacologic treatment.[135] A recent systematic review of the literature revealed that there were no randomized controlled clinical trials of the systemic drugs frequently prescribed for BMS, such as tricyclic antidepressants (amitriptyline, desipramine), benzodiazepines (clonazepam), or gabapentin. Recent randomized controlled trials of α-lipoic acid, systemic capsaicin, and topical clonazepam have shown promising results for short-term relief of pain.[136–138] Caution should be taken in the interpretation of the results for α-lipoic acid, however, since all trials were performed by the same researchers. Clearly, more randomized controlled trials are needed to assess the efficacy of drugs currently used to treat BMS.

Cognitive behavioral therapy has been shown to be more effective for pain reduction in patients with BMS than placebo, with effects lasting more than 6 months.

## Geographic tongue

### Clinical characteristics

*Geographic tongue*, also known as *benign migratory glossitis* and *erythema migrans*, is usually an asymptomatic inflammatory disorder of the tongue mucosa characterized by multiple, well-demarcated zones of erythema located on the dorsum and lateral border of the tongue. This erythema is due to atrophy of the filiform papillae, and these atrophic areas are typically surrounded at least partially by a slightly elevated, yellowish white, serpentine or scalloped border.[114,139] Geographic tongue is a benign disorder of unknown origin that almost always affects the tongue, although it has been described in the buccal mucosa and lip.[140] Ulcerations are not seen, but fissures are frequently observed. Over several days or weeks, the atrophic and keratotic areas migrate across the surface of the tongue, producing a slightly different pattern. Lesions may completely disappear and return weeks to months later.[107]

While often asymptomatic, geographic tongue may present with a burning sensation often related to the consumption of food and drink, particularly that which is spicy or high in citric acid.[141,142]

### Etiology

Attempts to link this disease to stress and infection have been futile. It has been suggested, but not confirmed, that it is a manifestation of psoriasis. The association may be coincidental because of the relative prevalence of geographic tongue and psoriasis.[107]

### Management considerations

Reassurance and education is generally the only treatment indicated. In case of persistent pain, topically applied steroids may be helpful.

## Mucogingival pain of mucocutaneous/dermatologic or systemic origin

Painful oral conditions may be drug induced, as in contact stomatitis and fixed-drug eruption, or may occur subsequent to the xerostomic effect of many medications, including such diverse groups as the tricyclic antidepressants, antipsychotics, muscle relaxants, antihistamines, anticonvulsants, diuretics, anxiolytics, and antihypertensive agents. The painful lesions in contact stomatitis or fixed-drug eruption may vary from areas of mild-to-severe erythema to ulceromembranous erosions. A variety of dermatologic disorders, including erythema multiforme, lichen planus, benign mucous membrane (cicatricial) pemphigoid, bullous pemphigoid, pemphigus vulgaris, and lupus erythematosus, may present within the oral cavity with or without other obvious clinical manifestations outside the orofacial region. Pain is an expected concomitant finding and may be the symptom that makes the patient initially seek care.

A number of systemic diseases are known to present with painful erythematous, erosive/ulcerative, or hemorrhagic lesions in the oral cavity. These include uncontrolled diabetes mellitus, uremia, Crohn disease, and blood dyscrasias, such as leukemia and cytopenia, agranulocytosis cyclic neutropenia, and sickle cell anemia.

## HIV infection

Orofacial pain is commonly reported by patients with HIV/AIDS.[143] Pain may be due directly to HIV infection or to comorbid conditions, such as necrotizing periodontal diseases, herpetic gingivostomatitis, recurrent herpes zoster infections, and Kaposi sarcoma, among others, or to adverse reactions to antiviral agents. The dentist must also be aware that HIV-associated peripheral neuropathy may present as orofacial pain. Painful oral ulcerative conditions may be caused by a variety of pathogens, including various fungi, viruses, and bacteria.[144,145] Nonulcerative lesions can occur with nonspecific mucositis, burning pain with xerostomia, and nutritional deficiencies. As with all patients, a proper diagnostic workup and identification of disease processes must precede treatment (other than palliation). Referral to a neurologist may be required in some cases. A more detailed discussion of this topic can be found in several recent publications.[52,146-157]

Pain palliation with an NSAID or acetaminophen to control mild-to-moderate pain is generally indicated. If the pain is not adequately controlled, an opioid may be prescribed. Various chemotherapeutic or analgesics, mouthrinses, or topical agents may also be useful.

## References

1. Okeson J. Bell's Orofacial Pain, ed 6. Chicago: Quintessence, 2005.
2. Berman LH, Hartwell GR. Diagnosis. In: Cohen S, Hargreaves K (eds). Pathways of the Pulp, ed 9. St Louis: Mosby, 2006:1–39.
3. Addy M. Etiology and clinical implications of dentine hypersensitivity. Dent Clin North Am 1990;34(3):503–514.
4. Torneck CD. A report of studies into changes in the fine structure of the dental pulp in human caries pulpitis. J Endod 1981;7(1):8–16.
5. Cvek M. A clinical report on partial pulpotomy and capping with calcium hydroxide in permanent incisors with complicated crown fracture. J Endod 1978;4(8):232–237.
6. Cvek M. Endodontic treatment of traumatized teeth. In: Andreasen JO. Traumatic Injuries of the Teeth, ed 2. Philadelphia: Saunders, 1981.
7. Ritchey B, Mendenhall R, Orban B. Pulpitis resulting from incomplete tooth fracture. Oral Surg Oral Med Oral Pathol 1957;10(6):665–670.
8. Ingle JI. Alveolar osteoporosis and pulpal death associated with compulsive bruxism. Oral Surg Oral Med Oral Pathol 1960;13:1371–1381.
9. Langeland K, Rodrigues H, Dowden W. Periodontal disease, bacteria, and pulpal histopathology. Oral Surg Oral Med Oral Pathol 1974;37(2):257–270.
10. Robinson H, Boling L. The anachoretic effect in pulpitis. 1. Studies. J Am Dent Assoc 1941;28:265.
11. Ingle JI, Langeland K. Etiology and prevention of pulp inflammation, necrosis, and dystrophy. In: Ingle JI, Taintor JF (eds). Endodontics, ed 3. Philadelphia: Lea & Febiger, 1985:355.
12. Kim S. Neurovascular interactions in the dental pulp in health and inflammation. J Endod 1990;16(2):48–53.
13. Holland GR. The odontoblast process: Form and function. J Dent Res 1985;64(spec No):499–514.
14. Rossman LE, Hasselgren G, Wolcott J. Diagnosis and management of orofacial dental pain emergencies. In: Cohen S, Hargreaves K (eds). Pathway of the Pulp, ed 9. St Louis: Mosby, 2006:40–59.
15. Trowbridge HO. Intradental sensory units: Physiological and clinical aspects. J Endod 1985;11(11):489–498.
16. Bränströmm M, Aström A. The hydrodynamics of the dentine: Its possible relationship to dentinal pain. Int Dent J 1972;22:219–227.
17. Bränströmm M, Lindén L, Aström A. The hydrodynamics of the dental tubule and of pulp fluid: A discussion of its significance in relation to dentinal sensitivity. Caries Res 1967;1:310–317.

18. Van Hassel HJ. Physiology of the human dental pulp. Oral Surg Oral Med Oral Pathol 1971;32(1):126–134.

19. Lin L, Langeland K. Light and electron microscopic study of teeth with carious pulp exposures. Oral Surg Oral Med Oral Pathol 1981;51(3):292–316.

20. Torneck CD. Changes in the fine structure of the dental pulp in human caries pulpitis. 1. Nerves and blood vessels. J Oral Pathol 1974;3(2):71–82.

21. Walton RE, Pashley DH, Dowden WE. Pulp pathosis. In: Ingle JI, Taintor JF (eds). Endodontics, ed 3. Philadelphia: Lea & Febiger, 1985:416.

22. Falace DA, Cailleteau JG. Diagnosis of dental and orofacial pain. In: Falace DA (ed). Emergency Dental Care: Diagnosis and Management of Urgent Dental Problems. Baltimore: Williams & Wilkins, 1995:10–12.

23. Garfunkel A, Sela J, Ulmansky M. Dental pulp pathosis. Clinicopathologic correlations based on 109 cases. Oral Surg Oral Med Oral Pathol 1973;35(1):110–117.

24. Seltzer S. Classification of pulpal pathosis. Oral Surg Oral Med Oral Pathol 1972;34(2):269–287.

25. Seltzer S, Bender IB, Ziontz M. The dynamics of pulp inflammation: Correlations between diagnostic data and actual histologic findings in the pulp. Oral Surg Oral Med Oral Pathol 1963;16:846–871.

26. Glick DH. Locating referred pulpal pains. Oral Surg Oral Med Oral Pathol 1962;15:613–623.

27. Falace DA, Muse TL. Clinical characteristics and patterns of referred odontogenic pain [abstract]. J Dent Res 1993; 71:1187.

28. Wright EF, Gullickson DC. Dental pulpalgia contributing to bilateral preauricular pain and tinnitus. J Orofac Pain 1996;10(2):166–168.

29. Cailleteau JG. Diagnosis and management of toothaches of dental origin. In: Falace DA (ed). Emergency Dental Care: Diagnosis and Management of Urgent Dental Problems. Baltimore: Williams & Wilkins, 1995:26–57.

30. Orchardson R, Gillam DG. The efficacy of potassium salts as agents for treating dentin hypersensitivity. J Orofac Pain 2000;14(1):9–19.

31. Trowbridge HO, Silver DR. A review of current approaches to in-office management of tooth hypersensitivity. Dent Clin North Am 1990;34(3):561–581.

32. Kanapka JA. Over-the-counter dentifrices in the treatment of tooth hypersensitivity. Review of clinical studies. Dent Clin North Am 1990;34(3):545–560.

33. van Steenberghe D. The structure and function of periodontal innervation. A review of the literature. J Periodontal Res 1979;14(3):185–203.

34. Armitage GC. Development of a classification system for periodontal diseases and conditions. Ann Periodontol 1999;4(1):1–6.

35. Meng HX. Periodontal abscess. Ann Periodontol 1999;4(1):79–83.

36. Parameter on acute periodontal diseases. American Academy of Periodontology. J Periodontol 2000;71(5 suppl):S863–S866.

37. Abrams H, Jasper SJ. Diagnosis and management of acute periodontal problems. In: Falace DA (ed). Emergency Dental Care: Diagnosis and Management of Urgent Dental Problems. Baltimore: Williams & Wilkins, 1995:137–142.

38. Sharav Y. Orofacial pain. In: Wall PD, Melzack R (eds). Textbook of Pain, ed 4. New York: Churchill Livingstone, 1999:711–737.

39. Newman MG, Sims TN. The predominant cultivable microbiota of the periodontal abscess. J Periodontol 1979;50(7):350–354.

40. Topoll HH, Lange DE, Muller RF. Multiple periodontal abscesses after systemic antibiotic therapy. J Clin Periodontol 1990;17(4):268–272.

41. Herrera D, Roldan S, Gonzalez I, Sanz M. The periodontal abscess. I. Clinical and microbiological findings. J Clin Periodontol 2000;27(6):387–394.

42. Killoy WJ. Treatment of periodontal abscesses. In: Genco RJ, Goldman HM, Cohen DW (eds). Contemporary Periodontics. St Louis: Mosby, 1990:475.

43. Moore WE, Moore LV. The bacteria of periodontal diseases. Periodontol 2000 1994;5:66–77.

44. Offenbacher S. Periodontal diseases: Pathogenesis. Ann Periodontol 1996;1(1):821–878.

45. Birkedal-Hansen H. Role of cytokines and inflammatory mediators in tissue destruction. J Periodontal Res 1993;28(6 pt 2):500–510.

46. Jacobs MH. Pericoronal and Vincent's infections: Bacteriology and treatment. J Am Dent Assoc 1943; 30:392.

47. Perkins AE. Acute infections around erupting mandibular third molar. Br Dent J 1944;76:199–204.

48. Peterson LJ. Principles of management of impacted teeth. In: Peterson LJ, Ellis E, Hupp JR, Tucker MR (eds). Contemporary Oral and Maxillofacial Surgery, ed 4. St Louis: Mosby, 2003:187–188.

49. Ammons WF, Harrington GW. The periodontic-endodontic continuum. In: Newman MG, Takei H, Klokkevold P, Carranza FH (eds). Carranza's Clinical Periodontology, ed 10. St Louis: Saunders, 2006:875.

50. Wang H-L, Glickman GN. Endodontic and periodontic interrelationships. In: Cohen, S, Burns RC (eds). Pathways of the Pulp, ed 8. St Louis: Mosby, 2002:651–654.

51. Bergenholtz G, Hasselgren G. Endodontics and periodontics In: Lindhe J, Lang NP, Karring T, (eds). Clinical Periodontology and Implant Dentistry, ed 4. Ames, IA: Blackwell Publishing, 2003:346.

52. Narani N, Epstein JB. Classifications of oral lesions in HIV infection. J Clin Periodontol 2001;28(2):137–145.

53. Parameter on periodontitis associated with systemic conditions. American Academy of Periodontology. J Periodontol 2000;71(5 suppl):876–879.

54. Diabetes and periodontal diseases. Committee on Research, Science and Therapy. American Academy of Periodontology. J Periodontol 2000;71(4):664–678.

55. Klokkevold PR, Mealey BL. Influence of systemic disorders and stress on the periodontium. In: Newman MG, Takey HH, Klokkevold PR, Carranza FA (eds). Clinical Periodontology, ed 10. St Louis: Elsevier Saunders, 2006:284–311.

56. Bader JD, Martin JA, Shugars DA. Preliminary estimates of the incidence and consequences of tooth fracture. J Am Dent Assoc 1995;126(12):1650–1654.

57. Turp JC, Gobetti JP. The cracked tooth syndrome: An elusive diagnosis. J Am Dent Assoc 1996;127(10):1502–1507.

58. Ehrmann EH, Tyas MJ. Cracked tooth syndrome: Diagnosis, treatment and correlation between symptoms and post-extraction findings. Aust Dent J 1990;35(2):105–112.

59. Hiatt WH. Incomplete crown-root fracture in pulpal-periodontal disease. J Periodontol 1973;44(6):369–379.

60. Rosen H. Cracked tooth syndrome. J Prosthet Dent 1982;47(1):36–43.

61. Geurtsen W. The cracked-tooth syndrome: Clinical features and case reports. Int J Periodontics Restorative Dent 1992;12(5):395–405.

62. Abou-Rass M. Crack lines: The precursors of tooth fractures—Their diagnosis and treatment. Quintessence Int Dent Dig 1983;14(4):437–447.

63. Christensen GJ. The confusing array of tooth-colored crowns. J Am Dent Assoc 2003;134(9):1253–1255.

64. Okeson JP, Falace DA. Nonodontogenic toothache. Dent Clin North Am 1997;41(2):367–383.

65. Gross SG. Diagnostic anesthesia. Guidelines for the practitioner. Dent Clin North Am 1991;35(1):141–153.

66. Graff-Radford SB. Headache problems that can present as toothache. Dent Clin North Am 1991;35(1):155–170.

67. Wright EF. Referred craniofacial pain patterns in patients with temporomandibular disorder. J Am Dent Assoc 2000;131(9):1307–1315.

68. Simons DG, Travell JG, Simons LS. Travell & Simons' Myofascial Pain and Dysfunction: Upper Half of Body. Philadelphia: Lippincott Williams & Wilkins, 1998.

69. Silberstein SD, Lipton RB, Dalessio DJ. Wolff's Headache and Other Head Pain. New York: Oxford Univ Press, 2001.

70. Lilly JP, Law AS. Atypical odontalgia misdiagnosed as odontogenic pain: A case report and discussion of treatment. J Endod 1997;23(5):337–339.

71. Vickers ER, Cousins MJ, Walker S, Chisholm K. Analysis of 50 patients with atypical odontalgia. A preliminary report on pharmacological procedures for diagnosis and treatment. Oral Surg Oral Med Oral Pathol Oral Radiol Endod 1998;85(1):24–32.

72. Czerninsky R, Benoliel R, Sharav Y. Odontalgia in vascular orofacial pain. J Orofac Pain 1999;13(3):196–200.

73. Mattscheck D, Law A. The nonodontogenic toothache. In: Cohen S, Hargreaves KM (eds). Pathways of the Pulp, ed 9. St Louis: Mosby, 2006:59–79.

74. Kreiner M, Okeson JP. Toothache of cardiac origin. J Orofac Pain 1999;13(3):201–207.

75. Lang NP, Soskolne WA, Greenstein G, et al. Consensus Report: Necrotizing Periodontal Diseases. Ann Periodontol 1999;4(1):78.

76. Laskaris G. Oral manifestations of infectious diseases. Dent Clin North Am 1996;40(2):395–423.

77. Neville BW, Damm DD, Allen CM, Bouquot JE (eds). Bacterial infections. In: Oral and Maxillofacial Pathology. Philadelphia: WB Saunders, 1995:155.

78. Kingsbury J, Shafer DM, Weyman BA. Pediatric maxillofacial infections. In: Topazian RG, Goldberg MH, Hupp JR (eds). Oral and Maxillofacial Infections. Philadelphia: Saunders, 2002:418–419.

79. Loesche WJ, Syed SA, Laughon BE, Stoll J. The bacteriology of acute necrotizing ulcerative gingivitis. J Periodontol 1982;53(4):223–230.

80. Kornman KS, Wilson TG. Making a clinical diagnosis and treatment plan. In: Wilson TG, Kornman KS (eds). Fundamentals of Periodontics, ed 2. Chicago: Quintessence, 2003:305–329.

81. Axell T, Henricsson V. Association between recurrent aphthous ulcers and tobacco habits. Scand J Dent Res 1985;93(3):239–242.

82. Natah SS, Konttinen YT, Enattah NS, Ashammakhi N, Sharkey KA, Hayrinen-Immonen R. Recurrent aphthous ulcers today: A review of the growing knowledge. Int J Oral Maxillofac Surg 2004;33(3):221–234.

83. Bagan JV, Sanchis JM, Milian MA, Penarrocha M, Silvestre FJ. Recurrent aphthous stomatitis. A study of the clinical characteristics of lesions in 93 cases. J Oral Pathol Med 1991;20(8):395–397.

84. Wray D, Vlagopoulos TP, Siraganian RP. Food allergens and basophil histamine release in recurrent aphthous stomatitis. Oral Surg Oral Med Oral Pathol 1982;54(4):388–395.

85. Jurge S, Kuffer R, Scully C, Porter SR. Mucosal disease series. Number VI. Recurrent aphthous stomatitis. Oral Dis 2006;12(1):1–21.

86. Lehner T. Pathology of recurrent oral ulceration and oral ulceration in Behcet's syndrome: Light, electron and fluorescence microscopy. J Pathol 1969;97(3):481–494.

87. Akintoye SO, Greenberg MS. Recurrent aphthous stomatitis. Dent Clin North Am 2005;49(1):31–47, vii–viii.

88. Woo SB, Sonis ST. Recurrent aphthous ulcers: A review of diagnosis and treatment. J Am Dent Assoc 1996;127(8):1202–1213.

89. Balciunas BA, Kelly M, Siegel MA. Clinical management of common oral lesions. Cutis 1991;47(1):31–36.

90. Ship JA. Recurrent aphthous stomatitis. An update. Oral Surg Oral Med Oral Pathol Oral Radiol Endod 1996;81(2):141–147.

91. Siegel MA, Balciunas BA. Medication can induce severe ulcerations. J Am Dent Assoc 1991;122(9):75–77.

92. Porter SR, Kingsmill V, Scully C. Audit of diagnosis and investigations in patients with recurrent aphthous stomatitis. Oral Surg Oral Med Oral Pathol 1993;76(4):449–452.

93. Savage NW, Mahanonda R, Seymour GJ, Bryson GJ, Collins RJ. The proportion of suppressor-inducer T-lymphocytes is reduced in recurrent aphthous stomatitis. J Oral Pathol 1988;17(6):293–297.

94. Landesberg R, Fallon M, Insel R. Alterations of T helper/inducer and T suppressor/inducer cells in patients with recurrent aphthous ulcers. Oral Surg Oral Med Oral Pathol 1990;69(2):205–208.

95. Pedersen A, Klausen B, Hougen HP, Ryder LP. Peripheral lymphocyte subpopulations in recurrent aphthous ulceration. Acta Odontol Scand 1991;49(4):203–206.

96. Pedersen A, Ryder LP. Gamma delta T-cell fraction of peripheral blood is increased in recurrent aphthous ulceration. Clin Immunol Immunopathol 1994;72(1):98–104.

97. Khandwala A, Van Inwegen RG, Alfano MC. 5% amlexanox oral paste, a new treatment for recurrent minor aphthous ulcers. I. Clinical demonstration of acceleration of healing and resolution of pain. Oral Surg Oral Med Oral Pathol Oral Radiol Endod 1997;83(2):222–230.

98. Khandwala A, Van Inwegen RG, Charney MR, Alfano MC. 5% amlexanox oral paste, a new treatment for recurrent minor aphthous ulcers. II. Pharmacokinetics and demonstration of clinical safety. Oral Surg Oral Med Oral Pathol Oral Radiol Endod 1997;83(2):231–238.

99. Porter S, Scully C. Aphthous ulcers (recurrent). Clin Evid 2004(11):1766–1773.

100. Siegel MA. Strategies for management of commonly encountered oral mucosal disorders. J Calif Dent Assoc 1999;27(3):210–212, 215, 218–219 passim.

101. Wright EF. Clinical effectiveness of lysine in treating recurrent aphthous ulcers and herpes labialis. Gen Dent 1994;42(1):40–42; quiz 51–52.

102. Birek C. Herpesvirus-induced diseases: Oral manifestations and current treatment options. J Calif Dent Assoc 2000;28(12):911–921.

103. Stoopler ET. Oral herpetic infections (HSV 1-8). Dent Clin North Am 2005;49(1):15–29, vii.

104. Scott DA, Coulter WA, Lamey PJ. Oral shedding of herpes simplex virus type 1: A review. J Oral Pathol Med 1997;26(10):441–447.

105. Corey L, Spear PG. Infections with herpes simplex viruses. 2. N Engl J Med 1986;314(12):749–757.

106. Scully C. Ulcerative stomatitis, gingivitis, and skin lesions. An unusual case of primary herpes simplex infection. Oral Surg Oral Med Oral Pathol 1985;59(3):261–263.

107. Regezi JA, Sciubba JJ, Pogrel MA (eds). Atlas of Oral and Maxillofacial Pathology. Philadelphia: Saunders, 2000:8–31.

108. Corey L. Herpes simplex viruses. In: Kasper DL, Braunwald E, Hauser S, Longo D, Jameson JL, Fauci AS (eds). Harrison's Principles of Internal Medicine. New York: McGraw-Hill, 2005.

109. Spruance SL, Rea TL, Thoming C, Tucker R, Saltzman R, Boon R. Penciclovir cream for the treatment of herpes simplex labialis. A randomized, multicenter, double-blind, placebo-controlled trial. Topical Penciclovir Collaborative Study Group. JAMA 1997;277(17):1374–1379.

110. Wynn RL. New drug approvals in 1996. Gen Dent 1997;45(3):224–227.

111. Appleton SS. Candidiasis: Pathogenesis, clinical characteristics, and treatment. J Calif Dent Assoc 2000;28(12):942–948.

112. Staab JF, Bradway SD, Fidel PL, Sundstrom P. Adhesive and mammalian transglutaminase substrate properties of Candida albicans Hwp1. Science 1999;283(5407):1535–1538.

113. Farah CS, Ashman RB, Challacombe SJ. Oral candidosis. Clin Dermatol 2000;18(5):553–562.

114. Neville BW, Damm DD, Allen CM, Bouquot J. Oral & Maxillofacial Pathology, ed 2. Philadelphia: Saunders, 2002.

115. Tosti A, Piraccini BM, Peluso AM. Contact and irritant stomatitis. Semin Cutan Med Surg 1997;16(4):314–319.

116. Vokes EE. Head and neck cancer. In: Kasper DL, Braunwald E, Fauci AS, Hauser SL, Longo DL, Jameson JL (eds). Harrison's Principles of Internal Medicine, vol 1, ed 16. New York: McGraw-Hill, 2005:503–505.

117. Barasch A, Safford M, Eisenberg E. Oral cancer and oral effects of anticancer therapy. Mt Sinai J Med 1998;65(5-6):370–377.

118. Epstein JB. Oral and maxillofacial cancer pain. Spec Care Dentist 1986;6(5):223–227.

119. Sardella A, Lodi G, Demarosi F, Uglietti D, Carrassi A. Causative or precipitating aspects of burning mouth syndrome: A case-control study. J Oral Pathol Med 2006;35(8):466–471.

120. Patton LL, Siegel MA, Benoliel R, De Laat A. Management of burning mouth syndrome: Systematic review and management recommendations [review]. Oral Surg Oral Med Oral Pathol Oral Radiol Endod 2007;103(suppl):S50.e1–S50.e23.

121. Lamey PJ, Lewis MA. Oral medicine in practice: Burning mouth syndrome. Br Dent J 1989;167(6):197–200.

122. Hakeberg M, Berggren U, Hagglin C, Ahlqwist M. Reported burning mouth symptoms among middle-aged and elderly women. Eur J Oral Sci 1997;105(6):539–543.

123. Lipton JA, Ship JA, Larach-Robinson D. Estimated prevalence and distribution of reported orofacial pain in the United States. J Am Dent Assoc 1993;124(10):115–121.

124. Grushka M, Sessle BJ. Burning mouth syndrome. Dent Clin North Am 1991;35(1):171–184.

125. Basker RM, Sturdee DW, Davenport JC. Patients with burning mouths. A clinical investigation of causative factors, including the climacteric and diabetes. Br Dent J 1978;145(1):9–16.

126. Wardrop RW, Hailes J, Burger H, Reade PC. Oral discomfort at menopause. Oral Surg Oral Med Oral Pathol 1989;67(5):535–540.

127. Grushka M. Clinical features of burning mouth syndrome. Oral Surg Oral Med Oral Pathol 1987;63(1):30–36.

128. Ziskin DE, Moulton R. Glossodynia: A study of idiopathic orolingual pain. J Am Dent Assoc 1946;33:1423.

129. Grushka M, Sessle BJ, Howley TP. Psychophysical assessment of tactile, pain and thermal sensory functions in burning mouth syndrome. Pain 1987;28(2):169–184.

130. Hershkovich O, Nagler RM. Biochemical analysis of saliva and taste acuity evaluation in patients with burning mouth syndrome, xerostomia and/or gustatory disturbances. Arch Oral Biol 2004;49(7):515–522.

131. Lauria G, Majorana A, Borgna M, et al. Trigeminal small-fiber sensory neuropathy causes burning mouth syndrome. Pain 2005;115(3):332–337.

132. Jaaskelainen SK, Forssell H, Tenovuo O. Abnormalities of the blink reflex in burning mouth syndrome. Pain 1997;73(3):455–460.

133. Jaaskelainen SK, Rinne JO, Forssell H, et al. Role of the dopaminergic system in chronic pain—A fluorodopa-PET study. Pain 2001;90(3):257–260.

134. Albuquerque RJ, de Leeuw R, Carlson CR, Okeson JP, Miller CS, Andersen AH. Cerebral activation during thermal stimulation of patients who have burning mouth disorder: An fMRI study. Pain 2006;122(3):223–234.

135. Zakrzewska JM, Forssell H, Glenny AM. Interventions for the treatment of burning mouth syndrome. Cochrane Database Syst Rev 2005;(1):CD002779.

136. Femiano F, Scully C. Burning mouth syndrome (BMS): Double blind controlled study of alpha-lipoic acid (thioctic acid) therapy. J Oral Pathol Med 2002;31(5):267–269.

137. Gremeau-Richard C, Woda A, Navez ML, et al. Topical clonazepam in stomatodynia: A randomised placebo-controlled study. Pain 2004;108(1–2):51–57.

138. Petruzzi M, Lauritano D, De Benedittis M, Baldoni M, Serpico R. Systemic capsaicin for burning mouth syndrome: Short-term results of a pilot study. J Oral Pathol Med 2004;33(2):111–114.

139. Assimakopoulos D, Patrikakos G, Fotika C, Elisaf M. Benign migratory glossitis or geographic tongue: An enigmatic oral lesion. Am J Med 2002;113(9):751–755.

140. Van Der Waal I. The Burning Mouth Syndrome. Copenhagen: Munksgaard, 1990.

141. Scully C, Felix DH. Oral medicine—Update for the dental practitioner: Red and pigmented lesions. Br Dent J 2005;199(10):639–645.

142. Pass B, Brown RS, Childers EL. Geographic tongue: Literature review and case reports. Dent Today 2005;24(8):54, 56–57; quiz 57.

143. Schofferman J. Care of the terminally ill person with AIDS. Int Ophthalmol Clin 1989;29(2):127–130.

144. Pensfold J, Clark AJM. Pain syndromes in HIV infection: Brief review. Can J Anaesth 1992;39:724–730.

145. Bruce AJ, Rogers RS III. Oral manifestations of sexually transmitted diseases. Clin Dermatol 2004;22(6):520–527.

146. Campisi G, Pizzo G, Mancuso S, Margiotta V. Gender differences in human immunodeficiency virus-related oral lesions: An Italian study. Oral Surg Oral Med Oral Pathol Oral Radiol Endod 2001;91(5):546–551.

147. Cannon M, Cesarman E. Kaposi's sarcoma-associated herpes virus and acquired immunodeficiency syndrome-related malignancy. Semin Oncol 2000;27(4):409–419.

148. Depaola LG. Human immunodeficiency virus disease: Natural history and management. Oral Surg Oral Med Oral Pathol Oral Radiol Endod 2000;90(3):266–270.

149. Detels R, Tarwater P, Phair JP, Margolick J, Riddler SA, Munoz A. Effectiveness of potent antiretroviral therapies on the incidence of opportunistic infections before and after AIDS diagnosis. AIDS 2001; 15(3):347–355.

150. Dios PD, Ocampo A, Miralles C, Limeres J, Tomas I. Changing prevalence of human immunodeficiency virus-associated oral lesions. Oral Surg Oral Med Oral Pathol Oral Radiol Endod 2000;90(4):403–404.

151. Johnson RA. HIV disease: Mucocutaneous fungal infections in HIV disease. Clin Dermatol 2000;18(4): 411–422.

152. Brown DM, Jabra-Rizk MA, Falkler WA Jr, Baqui AA, Meiller TF. Identification of *Candida dubliniensis* in a study of HIV-seropositive pediatric dental patients. Pediatr Dent 2000;22(3):234–238.

153. Murray A, Alpagot T, Kao RT. Diagnosis and management of human immunodeficiency virus-associated periodontal diseases in adults. In: Hall WB (ed). Decision Making in Periodontology, ed 3. St Louis: Mosby, 1998:64–65.

154. Lynch DP. Oral manifestations of HIV disease: An update. Semin Cutan Med Surg 1997;16(4):257–264.

155. Mirowski GW, Bettencourt JD, Hood AF. Oral infections in the immunocompromised host. Semin Cutan Med Surg 1997;16(4):249–256.

156. Muzyka BC, Glick M. Major aphthous ulcers in patients with HIV disease. Oral Surg Oral Med Oral Pathol 1994;77(2):116–120.

157. Epstein JB, Sherlock CH, Wolber RA. Oral manifestations of cytomegalovirus infection. Oral Surg Oral Med Oral Pathol 1993;75(4):443–451.

# Temporomandibular Disorders

## Anatomy of the Masticatory Structures

Craniomandibular articulation occurs in the temporomandibular joints (TMJs), two of the most complex joints in the body. Each TMJ provides for hinging movements in one plane, which is a criterion for a ginglymoid joint, and gliding movements in another plane, which is a criterion for an arthrodial joint. Thus, the TMJ is technically considered a ginglymoarthrodial joint.[1] The TMJ is formed by the mandibular condyle fitting into the mandibular fossa of the temporal bone (Fig 8-1).[1] Separating these two bones from direct contact is the interposed articular disc (sometimes inappropriately referred to as a *meniscus*). The articular portion of the healthy disc is composed of dense fibrous connective tissue, devoid of any nerves or vessels, while the posterior attachment of the disc is richly vascularized and innervated.[2–4] Collateral ligaments also attach the disc to the condyle both medially and laterally. These ligaments permit rotational movement of the disc on the condyle dur-

ing opening and closing of the mouth. This so-called condyle-disc complex translates out of the fossa during extended mouth opening (Fig 8-2).[1] Therefore, in the normal joint, rotational movement occurs between the condyle and the inferior surface of the disc during early opening (the inferior joint space), and translation takes place in the space between the superior surface of the disc and the fossa (the superior joint space) during later opening. Movement of the joint is lubricated by synovial fluid, which also acts as a medium for transporting nutrients to and waste products from the articular surfaces.

Unlike most synovial joints, the articulating surfaces of the TMJs are lined with dense fibrocartilage instead of hyaline cartilage.[5] Because fibrocartilage has a greater ability to repair itself than hyaline cartilage, the management of arthritic conditions of the TMJ is different from that of other synovial joints.[6]

Movement of the TMJs is achieved by the muscles of mastication, which are comparable with other skeletal muscles in physiology and ergonomics.[7] Although the muscles

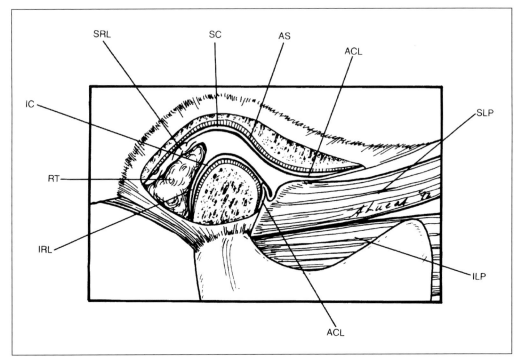

**Fig 8-1** Normal anatomy of the TMJ. RT = retrodiscal tissues; SRL = superior retrodiscal lamina (elastic); IRL = inferior retrodiscal lamina (collagenous); ACL = anterior capsular ligament (collagenous); SLP = superior lateral pterygoid muscle; ILP = inferior lateral pterygoid muscle; AS = articular surface; SC = superior joint cavity; IC = inferior joint cavity. (Reproduced with permission from Okeson.[1])

of mastication are the primary muscles involved in mandibular movement, other associated muscles of the head and neck furnish secondary support during mastication. The masticatory muscles include the masseter, medial pterygoid, and temporal muscles, which predominantly elevate the mandible (mouth closing); the digastric muscles, which assist in mandibular depression (mouth opening); the inferior lateral pterygoid muscles, which assist in protrud-ing the mandible; and the superior lateral pterygoid muscles, which provide stabilization for the condyle and disc during function.[8-11] The masticatory muscles are recruited for a variety of functional behaviors, such as talking, chewing, and swallowing.[12] A number of muscle behaviors are also apparently nonfunctional (parafunctional), defined under the broad term of *bruxism*, and include grinding, clenching, or rhythmic, empty-mouth chewing movements.[13,14]

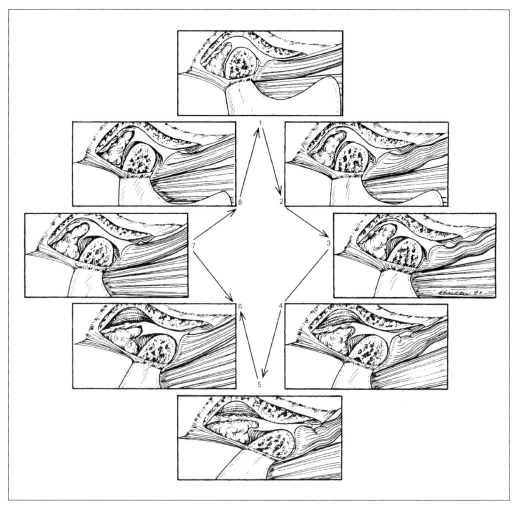

**Fig 8-2** Normal functional movement of the condyle and disc during the full range of opening and closing. Note that the disc is rotated posteriorly on the condyle as the condyle is translated out of the fossa. The closing movement is the exact opposite of opening. (Reproduced with permission from Okeson.[1])

# Defining Temporomandibular Disorders

*Temporomandibular disorders* (TMDs) is a collective term that embraces a number of clinical problems that involve the masticatory muscles, the TMJ, and the associated structures. The term is synonymous with *craniomandibular disorders*. TMDs have been identified as a major cause of nondental pain in the orofacial region and are considered to be a subclassification of musculoskeletal disorders.[15] TMDs represent clusters of related disorders in the masticatory system that have many common symptoms. The most

131

frequent presenting symptom is pain, usually localized in the muscles of mastication and/or the preauricular area and usually aggravated by chewing or other jaw activity. Patients with these disorders frequently have limited or asymmetric mandibular movements and TMJ sounds that are most frequently described as clicking, popping, grating, or crepitation.

Common patient complaints include jaw pain, earache, headache, and facial pain. Nonpainful masticatory muscle hypertrophy and abnormal occlusal wear associated with oral parafunction such as bruxism (jaw clenching and tooth grinding) may be related problems. Pain or dysfunction due to nonmusculoskeletal causes, such as otolaryngologic, neurologic, vascular, neoplastic, or infectious disease in the orofacial region, is not considered a primary TMD even though musculoskeletal pain may be present. However, TMDs often coexist with other craniofacial and orofacial pain disorders.

## Epidemiology of TMDs

Cross-sectional epidemiologic studies of selected nonpatient adult populations show that 40% to 75% of those populations have at least one sign of joint dysfunction (eg, movement abnormalities, joint noise, tenderness on palpation), and approximately 33% of selected nonpatient populations have at least one symptom of dysfunction (eg, face pain, joint pain).[16–19] Some signs appear to be relatively common in healthy populations: joint sounds or deviations on mouth opening occur in approximately 50% of nonpatient samples.[20] Other signs are relatively rare: mouth opening limitations occur in less than 5% of nonpatient populations.[18,21]

The results from cross-sectional epidemiologic studies vary considerably from study to study because of differences in descriptive terminology, data collection, analytic approaches (eg, single-factor versus multifactor analysis), and the individual factors selected for study. The interpretation of signs and symptoms is problematic because the correlation between signs and symptoms is poor.[18] Despite these limitations, several consistencies are apparent in the epidemiologic literature. Pain in the temporomandibular region is reported in approximately 10% of the population older than 18 years; it is primarily a condition of young and middle-aged adults, and approximately twice as common in women as in men.[22,23] TMDs are often remitting, self-limiting, or fluctuating over time.[24,25] While knowledge of the natural history or course of TMDs is limited, there is increasing evidence that progression to chronic and disabling intracapsular TMJ disease is uncommon.[25–27]

Signs and symptoms of TMDs are also observed in children and adolescents, although the prevalence tends to be lower than in adults.[22,28–30] (For a review, see Motegi et al.[31]) The incidence of joint sounds in these individuals can be as high as 17.5% over a 2-year period,[32] and clicking may come and go spontaneously with no predictable pattern.[33–35] While pain severity is the same across all age groups[36] and the frequency of morphologic irregularities has been correlated with age,[37,38] physical limitations and dysfunction steadily decrease in prevalence and severity in older age.[36,39–44] A more recent epidemiologic analysis showed significant variation of reported symptoms and clinically recorded signs in a group of young people followed from age 15 through age 35 in 5-year intervals. Progression to severe pain and dysfunction of the TMJs was rare.[45,46]

Prevalence of nonspecific measures of overall symptom levels (eg, Helkimo indices) in nonpatient surveys of adults is almost equal in men and women[39,47-53] In contrast, when individual symptoms were evaluated independently, women were found to have more headache, TMJ clicking, TMJ tenderness, and muscle tenderness than men.[18,41,54-61] These differences between men and women cannot explain clinical findings of a women-to-men ratio of 3:1 to 9:1 in persons seeking care for TMDs.[36,39,62,63] Women and men do not differ in pain-related sensitivity, in the meaning of their pain, or in pain-related illness behavior.[64] The predominance of women seeking treatment may be due to their greater health awareness.[64,65]

Despite the large percentages of the population having signs of TMJ dysfunction, the overall prevalence of TMD complaints in a general population is very small.[66,67] Only 3.6% to 7% of these individuals are estimated to be in need of treatment,[16,19,68-71] and the annual incidence rate is estimated to be 2%.[66,68,72] These estimates are supported by a study showing that only 7% of a patient population with benign TMJ clicking showed progression to bothersome clicking status over a 1- to 7.5-year period.[24] In another study, most patients with TMJ clicking remained stable or showed less or no clicking throughout the evaluation period even though most had only minimal conservative treatment interventions.[73] Furthermore, while TMJ clicking is fairly common, the progression to a potentially more serious nonreducing disc status is relatively uncommon.[20,27,74,75] Because joint sounds are common, often pain free, and not progressive, it is important to avoid overtreatment of benign chronic reducing and nonre-

ducing disc displacement in the absence of pain and impairment.[27]

The prevalence of a given TMD is difficult to determine due to the lack of a universally accepted classification scheme with diagnostic criteria. However, different investigators have used combinations of signs and symptoms to indirectly deduce the prevalence of differential diagnoses. Recent studies of patients seeking treatment for TMDs reported 26% to 31% with internal derangement and 30% to 33%[76] with a muscle disorder.[77] Schiffman and coworkers[69] used tested diagnostic criteria on a general population and found 33% with TMJ disorders and 41% with masticatory muscle disorders; only 7% of the sample had a disorder severe enough to be comparable with a clinic population. Thus, the indicated prevalence values may overstate the clinical significance of individual symptoms, because patients with mild transient signs and symptoms that do not require treatment are no doubt included. Similarly, it is estimated that 9% to 31% of asymptomatic joints appear to have asymptomatic disc displacements in magnetic resonance imaging (MRI) surveys.[78-80] A postmortem study revealed that 31 of 34 TMJs (of patients who had been previously clinically evaluated for signs and symptoms of TMDs) showed different types of changes, such as deviation in form, disc displacement, disc deformation, adhesions, and osteoarthritic changes, indicating that gross morphologic alterations can be present in the absence of TMDs.[81]

## Etiology of TMDs

The identification of an unambiguous universal cause of TMDs is lacking. For this reason, most of the factors discussed in this section, while thought to be direct causes of TMDs, await future research to document their etiologic significance.

Factors that increase the risk of TMDs are called *predisposing factors*, factors that cause the onset of TMDs are *initiating factors*, and factors that interfere with healing or enhance the progression of TMDs are *perpetuating factors*. Individual factors, under different circumstances, may serve any or all of these roles.[82–84] Long-term successful management usually depends on identifying the possible contributing factors and is often proportionate to the thoroughness and accuracy of the initial assessment. Thus, a comprehensive diagnostic approach requires clinicians to understand all potential contributing factors relevant to TMDs and chronic orofacial pain.

Many elements can affect the dynamic balance or equilibrium among the components of the masticatory system.[85] There are numerous factors driving the equilibrium either toward normal or adaptive physiologic health and function or toward dysfunction and pathology. Bone and TMJ soft tissue remodeling and muscle tone regulation are adaptive physiologic responses to insult or change. Loss of structural integrity, altered function, or biomechanical strains and stresses in the system can compromise adaptability and increase the likelihood of dysfunction or pathology.[86,87] Direct extrinsic trauma to any component of the masticatory system can spontaneously initiate loss of structural integrity and concomitant altered function, thereby reducing the adaptive capacity in the system. In addition, there are other contributing anatomic, systemic, and psychosocial factors that may sufficiently reduce the adaptive capacity of the masticatory system and result in TMDs.

## Trauma

*Trauma* is described as any force applied to the mastication structures that exceeds that of normal functional loading. Both intensity and duration need to be considered. Most trauma can be divided into three types: (*1*) *direct trauma* that results from a sudden and usually isolated blow to the structures, (*2*) *indirect trauma* that is associated with a sudden blow but without direct contact to the affected structures, and (*3*) *microtrauma* that results from prolonged, repeated force over time.

### Direct trauma

There is general agreement that direct trauma (*macrotrauma*) to the mandible or the TMJ produces injury and is accompanied in close temporal proximity with signs and symptoms of inflammation. If the forces lead to structural failure, loss of function may quickly follow. Mandibular stretching, twisting, or compressing forces during eating, yawning, yelling, or prolonged mouth opening have also been reported to trigger or aggravate TMDs.[85,88,89]

Patients with TMDs more often report physical trauma to the masticatory system than do nonpatients.[89–94] In one study, direct trauma to the mandible was associated with more localized symptoms with an onset between 24 and 72 hours after the event.[95] Cause is difficult or impossible to establish when symptom onset occurs long after the traumatic event, however.[91] Direct trauma was reported to be infrequently associated with the onset of disc displacement, according to one study.[96] A recent report indicated that third molar removal may be a risk factor for the development of TMDs.[97] Also, transient and permanent dysfunction of the TMJ following upper airway management procedures have been reported; however, controlled trials and longitudinal studies are not available in the English-language literature.[98,99]

### Indirect trauma

Flexion-extension injury (whiplash) with no direct blow to the face may cause symptoms consistent with TMDs.[90,100,101] There is some evidence that TMD signs and symptoms are more prevalent in those with a history of a flexion-extension injury.[90] Although symptoms in the mandible may be referred from injured cervical structures, a direct causal relationship between mandibular symptoms and indirect trauma has yet to be established.[102-104]

Computer simulation suggests that certain motor vehicle crashes do not cause flexion-extension injury to the TMJ.[105] In support of this finding, human volunteers in motor vehicle crash tests failed to demonstrate mandibular movement during a rear-end impact.[106] Thus, while evidence is lacking for mandibular strain without a direct blow to the mandible following a motor vehicle accident,[95,102] there are recognized pathways of heterotopic pain from the cervical area to the trigeminal area.[15,107,108] It is therefore not uncommon to observe symptoms of TMDs following flexion-extension injury to the neck without direct trauma to the face or mandible. The etiologic significance of nonimpact injuries is uncertain, and much misinformation is being provided to patients without scientific studies to support the claims.

### Microtrauma

Microtrauma has been hypothesized to originate from sustained and repetitive adverse loading of the masticatory system through postural imbalances or from parafunctional habits. It has been suggested that postural habits such as forward head position or phone-bracing may create muscle and joint strain and lead to musculoskeletal pain, including headache, in the TMD patient.[109]

Parafunctional habits have been most frequently assessed by indirect means such as self-report, questionnaires, reports by a bedroom partner, or tooth wear. These indirect measures of parafunctional habits have provided conflicting reports as to the relationship between TMD symptoms and the presence of parafunctional habits. The limitations of these measures have been noted.[110]

Parafunctional habits such as teeth clenching, teeth grinding, lip biting, and abnormal posturing of the mandible are common and usually do not result in TMD symptoms[76,111,112]; however, they have been suggested as initiating or perpetuating factors in certain subgroups of TMD patients.[14,112-122] Although the available research and clinical observations generally support this contention, the exact role of parafunctional habits in TMDs remains unclear because few studies have directly assessed these behaviors. Attrition severity secondary to bruxism cannot distinguish TMD patients from asymptomatic subjects,[123,124] and muscle hyperactivity has not been shown to be associated with arthrogenous TMDs.[125] Furthermore, clenching does not cause neuromuscular fatigue, because muscles compensate for sustained muscle activity by derecruitment of motor neurons or through slower firing rates.[126]

Despite the lack of evidence that non-experimentally induced parafunction or clenching can cause TMDs,[45,127] some studies have shown that experimentally induced parafunction can result in transient pain similar to that reported by patients with TMDs.[119,121,128] The impact of these studies is limited by their small sample size.

The intensity and frequency of oral parafunctional activity may be exacerbated by stress and anxiety, sleep disorders, and medications (eg, neuroleptics, alcohol),[14] although the relationship between nocturnal bruxism and psychologic factors has been questioned.[129,130] Some forms of masticatory muscle hyperactivity have been associated with emotional behavior and may be mediated via the cortex through the hypothalamus.[131] Intense and persistent parafunction can also occur in patients with neurologic disorders, such as cerebral palsy, and extrapyramidal disorders, such as orofacial dyskinesia and epilepsy.[132] Conversely, bruxism has not been related to facial type or head form.[133]

The most commonly believed indication of past nocturnal bruxism severity is dental attrition.[134] However, dental attrition can also be partly explained by overbite and overjet changes that correlate with age[135] and sex,[136,137] protrusive guidance schemes,[138,139] dentofacial morphology,[140] erosive diets,[141] bite force ability,[139,142] and environmental factors.[143,144] In addition, anthropologists argue that if bruxism, which is nearly universal in man, is pathologic, natural selection should have eliminated it by now.[145] Others have also suggested beneficial consequences of bruxism, by allowing better chewing efficiency from flattened occlusal surfaces.[146]

Another problem arises when attrition is used to suggest current bruxism levels.[115] Attrition appears to be episodic in nature and occurs in bursts due to as yet unspecified factors,[74,147] and thus may not necessarily represent ongoing habits. Continued research with more direct measurements of parafunction (eg, portable electromyography, sleep laboratory, and direct observation) will be necessary to clarify the specific role of current parafunction.[148-150]

## Anatomic factors

### Skeletal

Skeletal factors comprise adverse biomechanical relationships that can be genetic, developmental, or iatrogenic in origin. Severe skeletal malformations, interarch and intra-arch discrepancies, and past injuries to the teeth may play a role in TMDs. This role, however, may be less strong than previously believed. For example, while it is known that disc displacement is common in children with facial skeletal abnormalities such as retrognathia,[151] it cannot be said that these anatomic anomalies are etiologic. In addition, patients with internal derangement and other types of TMD in general do not have an increased prevalence of forward head posture.[76,152]

A steep articular eminence has also been proposed as an etiologic factor in internal derangement of the TMJ. In asymptomatic subjects, a steeper eminence was associated with an increased posterior rotation of the disc, posing a potential anatomic risk factor.[153] However, several studies have shown that, in TMJs with disc displacement without reduction and in TMJs with osseous changes, the eminence was less steep than in TMJs with disc displacement with reduction or TMJs without osseous changes, indicating adaptive remodeling.[152-156] In addition, unilateral joint sounds were associated with the side with the less steep condylar movement path.[34]

## Occlusal relationships

The dental profession historically has viewed occlusal variation as a primary etiologic factor for TMDs. Occlusal features such as working and nonworking posterior contacts and discrepancies between the retruded contact position (RCP) and intercuspal position (ICP) have been commonly identified as predisposing, initiating, and perpetuating factors. However, reviews of the literature and recent studies do not strongly support the etiologic role of occlusion in TMDs.[29,74,112,157–168]

The incidence of both osteoarthritic changes and tooth loss increases with age. While previous studies have correlated loss of molar support with arthritic changes in TMJs, these associations vanish when age is controlled.[37,169] Studies of living nonpatient populations do not provide evidence of an association between TMDs and lost molar support.[51,170–178] Further, a literature review did not reveal substantial evidence that moderate changes (approximately 4 to 6 mm) in occlusal vertical dimension cause masticatory muscle hyperactivity or TMD symptoms.[179] Although the results of animal studies need to be interpreted with caution, a recent animal study suggested that a rapid adaptive morphologic response to acute increases in the occlusal vertical dimension may be expected in the TMJs.[180] No recent studies with regard to the impact of vertical dimension on TMDs were found in the English-language literature.

Although occlusal guidance has been mentioned as influential for TMD signs and symptoms,[181,182] the majority of studies have not provided evidence for this association.[183–187]

Extensive overbite (vertical overlap of anterior teeth) has been associated with joint sounds[185] and broad masticatory muscle tenderness,[159,188] but most studies do not support these associations.[184–186] Reduced overbite, in particular, skeletal anterior open bite, however, has been associated with condylar changes[123,188,189] and with rheumatoid arthritis.[190,191]

Extensive overjet (horizontal overlap of anterior teeth) is mentioned as associated with TMD symptoms[192,193] and osteoarthritic changes,[123,194] but other studies fail to provide evidence of associations between overjet and TMDs.[184,186,189,192,194–198] Seligman and Pullinger[159] have shown that overjet greater than 5 mm is very uncommon in a healthy nonpatient population.

Crossbite per se has not been associated with TMDs.[159,185,188,195,199–202] Although anterior or posterior bilateral crossbites do not appear to be associated with TMDs, unilateral maxillary posterior lingual crossbite was found to be more common in TMD patients.[160]

It has been suggested that those occlusal factors that are more prevalent in TMD patients, such as large overjet, minimal overbite and anterior skeletal open bite, unilateral posterior crossbite, occlusal slides greater than 2 mm, and lack of firm posterior tooth contact, are possibly the result of condylar positional changes following intracapsular alterations associated with disease. Therefore, these occlusal factors may be the result of TMDs rather than the cause.[162,203] Previous studies have lacked reliable occlusal measurement techniques and data collection methods, which may explain the diversity of some findings. Nevertheless, whether considered individually or simultaneously, little evidence is available to strongly associate occlusal and other factors that are traditionally implicated in TMD etiology (eg, Angle malocclusions, deep overbite, minimal overjet, severe attrition, anterior and bilateral posterior crossbite, condyle position, discrepancy between RCP and ICP, and unilateral RCP contacts) with TMD symptoms. For example, contrary to traditional belief, class II division 2 occlusal relationships do not displace the mandible posteriorly.[204]

In summary, the contribution of occlusion to the etiology of TMDs appears small.[169] Some specific occlusal variants explain between 10% and 25% of specific diagnoses.[160] A small increased risk for osteoarthritic changes[160,194] and myofascial pain[160,205] is associated with RCP-ICP slides over 2 mm; internal derangements with unilateral maxillary lingual crossbite; osteoarthritic changes and myofascial pain with overjet over 6 mm; and internal derangement and osteoarthritic changes with more than six missing posterior teeth.[160] The greatest contribution was found for anterior open bite to define osteoarthritic changes and myofascial pain patients. However, most of the associations noted were judged to be secondary to joint alterations and not etiologic.[160]

## Pathophysiologic factors

### Systemic factors

Systemic pathophysiologic conditions may influence local TMDs and should generally be managed in cooperation with the patient's primary care physician or other medical specialist. These can include degenerative, endocrine, infectious, metabolic, neoplastic, neurologic, rheumatologic, and vascular disorders. Systemic factors can act simultaneously at a central and local level.[206,207] The interacting tissues may be nonadjacent and dissimilar; for example, degenerative muscle changes can result from intracapsular disease.[208]

Generalized joint laxity has been cited as a possible contributing factor to TMDs[209,210] and has been proven significantly more prevalent in patients with internal derangements than with other types of TMD or with normal controls.[18,74,211-213] Altered collagen metabolism may also play a role in joint laxity,[211] and the collagen composition in TMJs with painful disc displacement compared with asymptomatic joints has been found to differ.[214] Also, systemic joint laxity is significantly more prevalent in female than male adolescents,[211] although a more recent study of adults found no significant differences between the sexes.[215] Nevertheless, there is a weak correlation between the mobility of peripheral joints or the trunk and mandibular mobility,[216-218] and research has yet to demonstrate that joint laxity can predict the potential for developing TMDs.

### Local factors

Local pathophysiologic factors of TMDs, such as masticatory efficiency, appear to be multifactorial and involve such a large span of individual variation that it is difficult to establish norms.[219] While chewing efficiency is not affected by the extent of the occlusal contact area[146,220] or by the number and extensiveness of restorations,[219] it is enhanced by greater numbers of chewing units and fewer than five missing posterior teeth.[221] The threshold for impaired chewing is at fewer than three posterior chewing units.[172] In addition, chewing force is also influenced by sex,[222,223] age,[224] and pain levels.[225-229]

Masticatory muscle tenderness is not always related to variation in muscle activity[205,207] or the site or side of reported tenderness.[230,231] While the masseter muscle may react to proximal muscle pain, the anterior temporalis muscle does not, and any associations may be parallel developments rather than etiologic. Muscle tenderness does not appear to be the result of inflammation but is probably related to prolonged central hyperexcitability and altered central nervous system (CNS) processing following peripheral tissue injury.[231] Cervical muscle activity has been shown to influence masticatory muscle activity,[232,233] probably involving a primary afferent reflex response.[234] Thus, a primary cervical or TMJ disorder may precipitate a secondary masticatory muscle condition. Muscle hyperalgesia can also result from TMJ inflammation.[235]

Of great concern to the diagnostician is the distinction between pathologic and adaptive responses to disease in the TMJ. Histologic studies suggest that cartilage thickness and composition adapt to shearing stresses during functional loading.[236-239] Maintenance of an intact articular surface is to be expected, even in the face of osteoarthritic changes,[176,203,240] allowing for both stable morphologic relationships and histologic compatibility between the articulating components. Morphologic change, therefore, while mostly irreversible, usually achieves and maintains stability and should be considered adaptive.[241] The goal of treating osteoarthritic changes in this light should not be to restore earlier morphologic characteristics, but to encourage the body's adaptive response to pathophysiologic processes.

In early disc derangements, signs of osteoarthritis may not be apparent. Later internal derangements with osteoarthritic changes are possibly parallel but independent processes[242]; 50% of these derangements will show some active cellular osteoblast or osteoclast activity.[243] While disc displacement without reduction often leads to osteoarthritic changes over time,[27,74,242,244] almost half of patients with disc displacement with reduction will show a similar progression,[27,74] and the true incidence is likely to be much lower than 50%.[74] Disc displacement with reduction typically shows few histologic signs of early osteoarthritis because the other articular components are usually not greatly affected by the displacement.[242,245,246] TMJ clicking does not predict who will develop osteoarthritic changes over a 30-year period.[247]

It has been suggested that alterations in synovial fluid viscosity and inadequate lubrication may initiate clicking and derangement of the TMJ.[248,249] Synovial fluid analyses attempting to correlate biochemical signs of inflammation with pain reveal abnormal concentrations of plasma proteins[250-252] or neurotransmitters and inflammatory cytokines.[253-256] Other studies have evaluated the degradation of various enzymes and other metabolic byproducts, as well as the type of transmitters causing pain, inflammation, and degeneration in the TMJ.[257-269]

Frictional "sticking" of the disc has been proposed to cause TMJ internal derangement.[120] The forces depend on the type of clenching task, with greater impact at the ICP and during a unilateral molar clench.[270,271] According to experimental models and animal studies, the forces are also increased by reduced congruity between the opposing surfaces[272-275] and by flat unrounded surfaces,[271] and are affected by disc thickness and area[274] as well as by mandibular deformation during clenching.[276] Interestingly, nonworking tooth contacts have been hypothesized to reduce loads within the joint and act as a stress breaker for the clenching forces.[271]

Intracapsular pressure may also affect TMDs.[277,278] With joint movement, the alternating pressure acts as a pump for joint lubrication, nutrition, blood supply, drug delivery, waste removal, and even condylar growth. Thus, any interruption through immobilization or prolonged clenching may advance a TMD.

In contrast with disc displacement with reduction, disc displacement without reduction shows an ongoing synovitis,[279] and histologic evaluation shows moderate tissue involvement.[243] Nevertheless, signs and symptoms were not associated with disc position, and the arthrographic diagnosis could not predict the level of pain or dysfunction.[280] Thus, any pain and dysfunction, when present, may be unrelated to the disc displacement.

Female hormones have been mentioned as playing a role in TMJ disc disease; the presence of both estrogen and progesterone receptors within the articular disc has been both confirmed[281] and denied.[282] Randomized controlled trials (RCTs) indicate that estrogen does not play a role in the etiology of TMDs,[283,284] whereas cohort studies and case control studies show contrasting results.[285,286] Women do show higher intra-articular pressure than men, which may allow for more ischemia, disc friction, or prolongation of chronic inflammatory synovitis, partly explaining the prevalence of disc-related TMDs in women.[278]

The etiologic explanations for progression from disc displacement to osteoarthritis and osteoarthritic changes include failure of the reparative articular chondrocyte response due to metabolic dysfunction and relative or absolute overloading due to excessive mechanical forces, leading to articular cartilage biochemical failure.[287,288] Remodeling, in contrast, is a physiologic response to accommodate an altered disc position.[203] Thus, it is probable that a mechanical breakdown in the articular disc, such as a perforation, rather than an un-

usual disc position, leads to osteoarthritis and/or osteoarthritic changes following disc displacement.[289] It is not certain, however, that all gross abnormalities of the disc will lead to osteoarthritis, because the TMJ may be capable of healing disc perforations within a relatively short time according to one experimental animal study.[290]

Recent studies have proposed that mechanical stress leads to the accumulation of damaging free radicals in affected articular tissues of susceptible individuals. This condition is called *oxidative stress*.[291] Dijkgraaf and coworkers[292] proposed that free radicals may be responsible for adhesion formation in the TMJ through cross-linking of proteins.

## Genetic factors

Little research is available with regard to genetic susceptibility to TMDs. A recent study examined the relationship between catechol-O-methyl transferase (COMT) polymorphism, pain sensitivity, and the risk of TMD development. Three genetic variants (haplotypes) of the gene encoding COMT were identified and designated as *low pain sensitivity*, *average pain sensitivity*, and *high pain sensitivity*.[293] The haplotypes were associated with experimental pain sensitivity, and the presence of even a single haplotype for low pain sensitivity was shown to reduce the risk of developing myogenous TMD. Further studies are needed to identify how the presence of the different haplotypes relates to the risk of TMD development.

## *Psychosocial factors*

Psychosocial factors include individual, interpersonal, and situational variables that affect the patient's capacity to function adaptively. As a group, TMD and orofacial pain patients are significantly dissimilar both culturally and economically, so the relevant psychosocial factors present with tremendous diversity. However, individual TMD patients may have personality characteristics or emotional conditions that make managing or coping with life situations difficult.[61,158,294–297]

There is evidence that some patients with TMDs experience more anxiety than healthy control groups and that orofacial pain may be only one of several somatic manifestations of emotional distress.[298–302] Some muscle pain, for example, may be caused by excessive sympathetic nervous system activity as an overresponse to life stressors, and the attention focused on the pain can influence these pain levels.[303–306] Patients with such complaints often have a history of other stress-related disorders.[302,307] Depression and anxiety related to other major life events may alter the patient's perception of and tolerance to physical symptoms, causing them to seek more care.[308,309]

Patients with chronic TMDs have been found to have psychosocial and behavioral characteristics similar to patients with lower back pain and headache.[310,311] In general, TMD patients are not significantly different from other pain patients or healthy controls in personality type, response to illness, attitudes toward health care, or ways of coping with stress.[61,111,312–314] Any psychologic impairment may merely be associated with the presence of the pain.[225,309,315]

It is important to note that anxiety and depression may not only result from and predispose patients to TMDs, but that patients may present with mental disorders unrelated to TMDs.[316–319] *Mental disorders* are syndromes of psychologic or organic origin that impair adaptive functioning in areas of emotion, perception, cognition, behavior, or interpersonal adjustment. The clinical features of mental disorders have been outlined by the American Psychiatric Association in the *Diagnostic and Statistical Manual of Mental Disorders, Fourth Edition (DSM-IV)*.[320] Diagnostic criteria for psychotic syndromes, mood disturbances, anxiety disorders, organic mental disorders, and somatoform disorders are described. While the relationship of mental disorders to TMDs awaits research documentation, clinical reports suggest that the psychologic conflicts and emotional distress of preexisting psychiatric conditions may contribute to the cause of or exacerbate TMDs.[321–324]

Environmental contingencies can greatly complicate treatment by affecting an individual's perception of and response to pain and disease. Some patients may experience a lessening of distress to the extent that psychogenic symptoms decrease or resolve. This primary gain of symptom formation is to be distinguished from the secondary gain of social benefits experienced by patients once a disorder is established.[325–327] Secondary gain includes being exempt from ordinary daily responsibilities, being compensated monetarily from insurance or litigation, using the rationalization of "being ill" to avoid unpleasant tasks, and gaining attention from family, friends, or health care workers.[327,328]

The use of alcohol, minor tranquilizers, narcotics, barbiturates, and other pharmaceuticals contributes to the chronicity of many TMD patients. Every clinical assessment should pay careful attention to possible concurrent alcoholism or addiction in this patient group. The chemical dependency problems and pharmacologically induced depressions among TMD and chronic pain patients are frequently overlooked aspects that account for refractory responses to otherwise excellent treatment approaches.

Thus, psychosocial factors may predispose certain individuals to TMDs and may also perpetuate TMDs once symptoms have become established. A careful consideration of psychosocial factors is therefore important to the diagnostic evaluation and treatment of every TMD patient.

# Diagnostic Classification of TMDs

The classification of TMDs is hampered by limited knowledge of the cause and natural progression of these disorders, and yet advancement in our knowledge depends on an accepted taxonomy and corresponding diagnostic criteria.[329]

Diagnostic criteria allow comparisons of patient populations in different studies and provide a common language for developing a conceptual framework to use in the clinic.[330] Classification systems must be considered an evolving framework that will be modified by new findings and increased levels of understanding. Diagnostic criteria, which serve to operationalize the diagnostic classifications, are intended for use by the clinician in the daily practice of diagnosing and treating TMDs.

One set of diagnostic criteria will not satisfy all circumstances to which it might be applied.[331] For example, the requirements for diagnostic sensitivity and specificity in clinical research are different from those used in treating individual patients. The researcher needs inclusion criteria with high specificity at the expense of sensitivity, resulting in a homogeneous test population with a high probability of having the disease in question. In contrast, the clinician needs

to identify patients presenting with the entire spectrum of a particular disease, which requires higher sensitivity at the expense of reduced specificity. However, the clinician must be cautioned against unnecessary treatment of subclinical disease based on the presence of benign signs and symptoms that are very common in the general population.

The following diagnostic criteria can be modified to varied levels of sensitivity and specificity by adjusting the set points of the criteria. For example, the inclusion criteria for a clinical trial might require the presence of all four criteria for a specific disease, while a clinical diagnosis might require the presence of only two of four criteria. However, it is vital that the researcher or clinician carefully document and communicate the criteria that were used to establish the diagnosis.

The diagnostic criteria of the American Academy of Orofacial Pain are presented as an addendum to the International Classification of Headache Disorders.[332] It is hoped that this addendum will foster exchange between the dental and medical communities. TMDs are listed in the diagnostic classification of the International Headache Society (IHS) under the 11th major classification. (see Boxes 3-3, 3-4, and 3-5 for recommended subdivisions). TMDs are divided into TMJ disorders and masticatory muscle disorders. *The International Classification of Diseases, Ninth Revision (ICD-9)* codes, required by medical insurance, are given for each specific disorder.[333]

## *TMJ articular disorders*

### Congenital or developmental disorders (IHS 11.1.1.x)

Congenital or developmental disorders of the cranial bones and mandible include aplasia (agenesis), hypoplasia, hyperplasia, and neoplasms (see Box 3-3). Lesions and disorders of the jaws can be of either odontogenic or nonodontogenic origin and can be of systemic or metastatic nature. Most congenital or developmental disorders primarily cause problems with esthetics and/or function and are rarely accompanied by orofacial pain unless associated with neoplasia (eg, osteomyelitis, multiple myeloma, and Paget disease).

### Aplasia (IHS 11.1.1.1; *ICD-9* 754.0)

*Aplasia* is faulty or incomplete development of the cranial bones or mandible. Almost all aplasias of the mandible belong to the group of anomalies commonly known as *hemifacial microsomias* or *first* and *second branchial arch syndromes*.[334] The most common developmental defect is unilateral lack of growth of the condyle, usually resulting from incomplete development of the primordium of the condyle embryologically; in this case there is little or no articular fossa and a rudimentary or absent eminence.[335] The auditory apparatus is frequently affected. The most common signs and symptoms are facial asymmetry, malocclusion (open bite), dermal hypoplasia of the ear, torticollis, speech difficulties, feeding problems in infancy, and limited mandibular opening. The most common treatments are orthodontics, sagittal split osteotomy, distraction osteogenesis, and costochondral graft.[336]

### Hypoplasia (IHS 11.1.1.2; *ICD-9* 526.89)

*Hypoplasia* is a congenital or acquired condition in which there is incomplete development or underdevelopment of the cranial bones or the mandible. Growth is normal although proportionately reduced, but the deficiency is less severe in degree than it is in aplasia. Hypoplasia may be present at birth

or it can occur developmentally. Condylar hypoplasia may occur secondary to facial trauma. The most common signs and symptoms are sleep apnea, malocclusion, and micrognathia. The most common treatments are sagittal osteotomy, orthodontics, functional appliances that position the mandible forward to stimulate or accelerate growth, costochondral graft, distraction mesenchymogenesis, and distraction osteogenesis.[337,338]

### Hyperplasia (IHS 11.1.1.3; *ICD-9* 526.89)

*Hyperplasia* is the overdevelopment of the cranial bones or mandible as the result of a nonneoplastic increase in the number of normal cells and may be congenital or acquired. It can occur as a localized enlargement, such as condylar hyperplasia or coronoid hyperplasia, or as an overdevelopment of the entire mandible or side of the face.[339,340] Excessive size of the mandible is termed *mandibular prognathism* (*ICD-9* 524.10), which results in protrusion of the chin with no abnormality of condylar size, shape, or function.

### Dysplasia (IHS 11.1.1.4; *ICD-9* 526.89)

*Fibrous dysplasia* is a form of hyperplasia due to a benign slow-growing swelling of the mandible and/or maxilla characterized by the presence of fibrous connective tissue[341] with a whirled pattern and trabeculae of immature nonlamellar bone.[342] Radiographically the lesion may appear varied, from an opaque ground-glass to a lucent appearance, depending on the ratio of fibrous tissue to bone. There is usually no displacement of teeth, the cortical bone remains intact, and the occlusion of the dental arches remains undisturbed. The disease occurs particularly in children and young adults and usually becomes inactive when they reach skeletal maturity. The most common treatment is surgery.

## Neoplasia (IHS 11.1.2.1; ICD-9 213.1 [benign]; 170.1[malignant])

A *neoplasm* is new, often uncontrolled growth of abnormal tissue, in this case arising or involving the TMJ or supporting structures. Neoplasia in this area may be benign, malignant, or metastatic. Although neoplasm as an underlying cause of TMJ dysfunction is rare, it is well known in the literature.[343,344] Approximately 3% of malignant neoplasia metastasize to the mandible,[345-349] the most common of which are squamous cell carcinomas of the maxillofacial region and primary nasopharyngeal tumors[15,350-358] Neoplasia arising in the parotid gland, such as adenoid cystic carcinomas and mucoepidermoid carcinomas, also may produce TMJ pain and dysfunction.[359-361] The most common signs and symptoms are reduced opening, crepitation, occlusal changes, pain with function, and swelling.[362] If the condyle is involved, facial asymmetry will likely develop, with a midline shift similar to that seen in condylar hyperplasia.[363] The most common treatment is surgery.

## Disc derangement disorders (IHS 11.7.1.1.x; ICD-9 524.63)

*Articular disc displacement* is the most common form of TMJ arthropathy and is characterized by several stages of clinical dysfunction that involve the condyle-disc complex. It is characterized by an abnormal relationship or misalignment of the articular disc relative to the condyle. Although posterior[364,365] and mediolateral[366-369] displacements of the articular disc have been described, anterior or anteromedial displacements are more common.[370,371] Pain or mandibular movement

problems are not specific for disc derangement disorders,[372] and altered disc position is not necessarily related to any presenting symptoms.[373]

The causes of disc displacement are not agreed upon; however, it is postulated that in most cases, stretched or torn ligaments that bind the disc to the condyle allow for displacement.[374] An increased horizontal angle of the mandibular condyle is associated with more advanced TMJ internal derangement.[375,376] Lubrication impairment is also suggested to be a possible etiologic factor in disc displacement.[120,249]

For descriptive purposes, the severity of radiographic degenerative TMJ bone change is described according to the system proposed by Stegenga et al[377] despite its low sensitivity.[378] In this system, *moderate* is used when the condylar surface is locally flattened, irregular, or resorbed, with no clear trabecular pattern; when sclerosis is present but not extensive; or when there is no or only minor (< 4 mm) shortening of the condyle. *Extensive* is used when the condyle is small or shortened (> 4 mm) with extensive flattening and resorption, marginal hypertrophy (osteophytes), obvious sclerosis, or subcortical cystic translucencies.

Disc displacement is subdivided into disc displacement with reduction and disc displacement without reduction.

## Disc displacement with reduction (IHS 11.7.1.1.1; ICD-9 524.63)

A *disc displacement with reduction* is characterized by an abrupt alteration or interference of the disc with the condyle during mouth opening and closing. From a closed mouth position, the "temporarily" misaligned disc reduces or improves its structural relationship with the condyle when mandibular translation occurs during mouth opening, producing joint sounds described as clicking or popping (Fig 8-3). The clicking is termed *reciprocal* when the noise is heard during the opening movement as well as during the closing movement. The closing noise is usually of less magnitude and is produced by redisplacement of the disc.

The momentary jamming or misalignment of the disc may be due to articular surface irregularity, disc-articular surface adherence, synovial fluid degradation, disc-condyle incoordination as a result of abnormal muscle function, increased muscle activity across the joint, or disc deformation. Because disc displacement with reduction is so common, it may represent a physiologic accommodation without clinical significance.[3,4,20,288,374,379,390]

Clicking sounds in reducing disc displacement are not pathognomonic, because over one-third of an asymptomatic sample can have moderate to severe derangement,[80] and as many as a quarter of clicking joints show normal or only slightly displaced disc position.[373] Thus, asymptomatic clicking itself does not warrant treatment.[79,381,382]

Disc displacement with reduction may or may not be a painful condition. As the condition becomes more chronic or as the disc becomes progressively more displaced, it begins to interfere later in the translating (opening) movement. Previously used terms for this condition include *internal derangement*, *anterior disc displacement*, *reciprocal disc*, and *disc-condyle incoordination*.

*Diagnostic criteria for disc displacement with reduction.* All of the following must be present:
1. Reproducible joint noise that occurs usually at variable positions during opening and closing mandibular movements.
2. Soft tissue imaging reveals displaced disc that improves its position during mandibular opening, and hard tissue imaging

shows an absence of extensive degenerative bone changes. (Although in essence the diagnosis of disc displacement can only be confirmed with soft tissue imaging, the temperate nature of the disorder does not warrant routine soft tissue imaging.)

Any of the following may accompany the preceding items:
- Pain, when present, is precipitated by joint movement.
- Deviation during opening movement coincides with a click.
- No restriction in mandibular movement.
- Episodic and momentary catching during mouth opening (≤ 35 mm) that self-reduces with voluntary mandibular repositioning.

*Differential diagnosis:* anatomic variation, osteoarthritis

### Disc displacement without reduction (IHS 11.7.1.1.2; *ICD-9* 524.63)

*Disc displacement without reduction* is described as an altered or misaligned disc-condyle structural relationship that is maintained during mandibular translation. Thus, the disc is nonreducing or "permanently" displaced and does not improve its relationship with the condyle during translation (Fig 8-4). This condition is sometimes referred to as a *closed lock*. When acute, it is characterized by sudden and marked limited mouth opening because of a jamming or fixation of the disc secondary to disc adhesion, deformation, or dystrophy.[383] Pain is often present, especially on mouth opening. The acute stage is manifested clinically as a deflection to the affected side on opening, a marked limited laterotrusion to the contralateral side, and a lack of the prior click or pop in the affected joint. Disc displace-

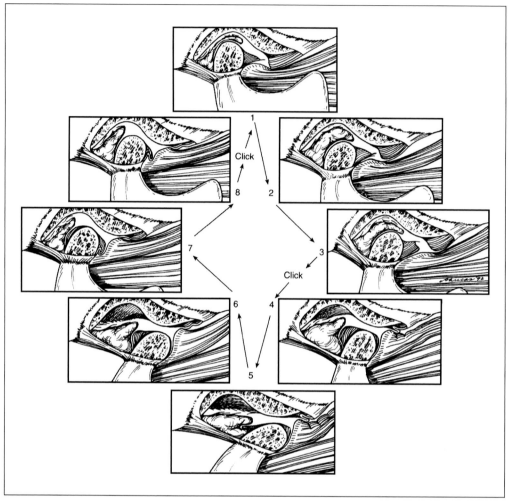

**Fig 8-3** Disc displacement with reduction. Note that during opening the condyle passes over the posterior border of the disc onto the intermediate area of the disc, thus reducing the displaced disc. (Reproduced with permission from Okeson.[1])

ment without reduction may be associated with overt trauma and, when acute, the accompanying pain is exacerbated by function. Although the arthroscopic appearance is generally reported to be consistent with synovitis, histologic evidence of synovitis is usually absent.[384,385]

As the acute condition becomes chronic, the pain is markedly reduced and, in many cases, relieved, and the opening range may approach normal dimensions over time.[385,389] If chronic, there usually is a history of joint noise and/or limitation of mandibular opening,[25,390] and the condition may progress to reveal osteoarthritic changes.[27,242,243,245]

*Diagnostic criteria for acute disc displacement without reduction.* All of the following must be present:

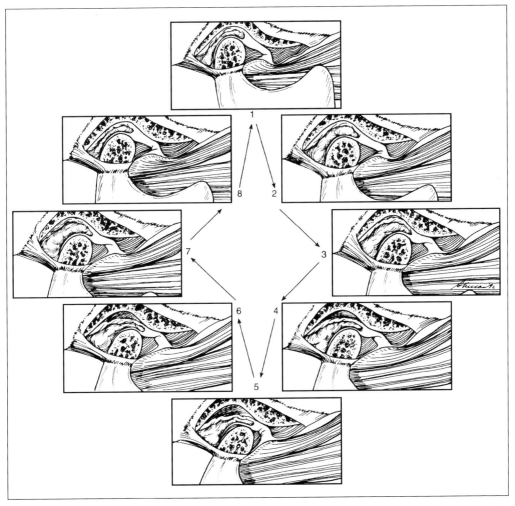

**Fig 8-4** Disc displacement without reduction. Note that the condyle never assumes a normal relationship on the disc, but instead causes the disc to move forward ahead of it. This condition limits the distance the condyle can translate forward. (Reproduced with permission from Okeson.[1])

1. Persistent markedly limited mouth opening (≤ 35 mm) with history of sudden onset.
2. Deflection to the affected side on mouth opening.
3. Markedly limited laterotrusion to the contralateral side (if unilateral disorder).
4. Soft tissue imaging reveals displaced disc without reduction. (Although in essence the diagnosis of disc displacement can only be confirmed with soft tissue imaging, the temperate nature of the disorder does not warrant routine soft tissue imaging.)

Any of the following may accompany the preceding items:
• Pain precipitated by forced mouth opening.
• History of clicking that ceases with locking.

- Pain with palpation of the affected joint.
- Ipsilateral hyperocclusion.
- No or mild osteoarthritic changes with hard tissue imaging.

*Differential diagnosis*: acute synovitis/capsulitis, acute myospasm

*Diagnostic criteria for chronic disc displacement without reduction.* All of the following must be present:
1. History of sudden onset of limited mouth opening.
2. Soft tissue imaging reveals displaced disc without reduction. (Although in essence the diagnosis of disc displacement can only be confirmed with soft tissue imaging, the temperate nature of the disorder does not warrant routine soft tissue imaging.)

Any of the following may accompany the preceding items:
- Pain, when present, is markedly reduced from the acute stage.
- History of clicking that resolved with sudden onset of the locking.
- Crepitation on mandibular movement.
- Gradual resolution of limited mouth opening.
- Mild to moderate osteoarthritic changes with imaging of hard tissues.

*Differential diagnosis*: osteoarthritis, polyarthritis, fibrotic ankylosis, neoplasm

## TMJ dislocation (IHS 11.7.1.2; *ICD-9* 830.0)

Also known as *open lock* or *subluxation, TMJ dislocation* is a condition in which the condyle is positioned anterior to the articular eminence and is unable to return to a closed position. It is manifested clinically as an inability to close the mouth. Dislocation may be the result of a physical jamming of the disc-condyle complex beyond the articular eminence that is maintained by muscle activity, or a true hyperextension of the disc-condyle complex beyond its normal maximum translation position. The duration of dislocation may be momentary or prolonged. When prolonged, the patient may need the clinician's assistance to reduce the dislocation and normalize mandibular function.[210] There is usually a clinical history of excessive range of motion that is not painful, but pain can occur at the time of dislocation, with residual pain following the episode.

*Diagnostic criteria for TMJ dislocation.* All of the following must be present:
1. Inability to close the mouth without a specific manipulative maneuver.
2. Radiographic evidence reveals condyle well beyond the eminence.

The following may accompany the preceding items:
- Pain at time of dislocation with mild residual pain after the episode.

*Differential diagnosis*: fracture

## Inflammatory disorders (IHS 11.7.1.3.x)

Primary inflammatory conditions of the TMJ include capsulitis, synovitis, and the polyarthritides. Polyarthritides are relatively uncommon and are associated primarily with rheumatologic disease. Synovitis and capsulitis frequently occur secondary to trauma, irritation, or infection, and often accompany other TMJ disorders.[391]

## Synovitis and capsulitis (IHS 11.7.1.3.1; ICD-9 524.62 or 726.90 or 716.98)

*Synovitis* is described as an inflammation of the synovial lining of the TMJ that can be due to infection, an immunologic condition secondary to cartilage degeneration, or trauma. The condition is characterized by localized pain that is exacerbated by function and superior or posterior joint loading. On occasion there will be a fluctuating swelling (due to effusion) that decreases the ability to occlude on the ipsilateral posterior teeth. Arthroscopically, synovial hyperplasia and the presence of lymph and blood capillaries define synovitis,[392,393] whereas histopathologically, proliferation of surface cells, an increase in vascularity, and a gradual fibrosis of the subsynovial tissue is observed.[394] Several proinflammatory cytokines have been detected in painful TMJs, which suggests that they may play a role in synovitis.[395] Other molecular markers of TMJs with synovitis include metalloproteinase 2,[264] metalloproteinase 3,[269,396,397] tenascin,[398] transforming growth factor β (TGF-β),[399] tumor necrosis factor α (TNF-α),[400] interleukin 1β (IL-1β)[401], interleukin-6 (IL-6)[402], serotonin,[401] and substance P.[403] The clinical and diagnostic value of such markers remains to be evaluated, since conflicting results exist,[402] and similar markers were found in TMJs with internal derangements and osteoarthritic changes.[396,397,401]

*Capsulitis*, an inflammation of the capsule related to sprain of capsular ligaments, is difficult if not impossible to clinically differentiate from synovitis and may also exhibit pain on joint distraction. Previously used terms include *arthritis, arthralgia, discitis,* and *retrodiscitis.*

*Diagnostic criteria for synovitis and capsulitis.* All of the following must be present:

1. Localized TMJ pain exacerbated by function, clinically reproduced with joint loading or palpation.
2. No extensive osteoarthritic changes with hard tissue imaging.

The following may accompany the preceding items:
- Localized TMJ pain at rest.
- Limited range of motion secondary to pain.
- Fluctuating swelling (due to effusion) that may decrease the ability to occlude on ipsilateral posterior teeth.
- A bright MRI (T2-weighted) signal when fluid is present.
- Ear pain.

*Differential diagnosis*: osteoarthritis, polyarthritis, ear infection, neoplasm

## Polyarthritides (IHS 11.7.1.3.2; ICD-9 714.9)

Joint inflammation and structural changes caused by a generalized systemic polyarthritic condition are referred to as *polyarthritides*. TMJ polyarthritides include rheumatoid arthritis, juvenile rheumatoid arthritis (Still disease), spondyloarthropathies (eg, ankylosing spondylitis, psoriatic arthritis, infectious arthritis, and Reiter syndrome), and crystal-induced disease (eg, gout and chondrocalcinosis). Other rheumatologically related diseases that may affect the TMJ include autoimmune disorders and other mixed connective tissue diseases (eg, scleroderma, Sjögren syndrome, and lupus erythematosus).[385] Polyarthritides are characterized by pain during acute and subacute stages, possible crepitation, limited range of motion secondary to pain and/or degeneration, and bilateral radiographic evidence of structural bony changes.[245] This group of arthritides comprises multiple diagnostic categories that are best diagnosed with the aid of serologic testing and managed by a rheumatologist. Bilateral resorption of condylar structures can result in an anterior open bite.

*Diagnostic criteria for polyarthritides.* All of the following must be present:
1. Pain with mandibular function.
2. Point tenderness on TMJ palpation.
3. Diagnosis of systemic disorder that may affect the TMJ.
4. Radiographic evidence of extensive TMJ changes.

The following may accompany the preceding items:
• Any of the characteristics of osteoarthritis (see IHS 11.7.1.4 below).
• Pain while the mandible is at rest.
• Bilateral TMJ and multiple other joint involvement.
• Limited range of motion secondary to pain.
• Crepitation on mandibular movement.

*Differential diagnosis*: osteoarthritis, neoplasm

## Noninflammatory disorders (IHS 11.7.1.4.x)

*Osteoarthritis* is a noninflammatory arthritic condition that is commonly found in a variety of synovial joints. Osteoarthritis is classified as either primary or secondary according to its origin.

### Primary osteoarthritis (IHS 11.7.1.4.1; ICD-9 715.18)

*Osteoarthritis*, ie, *osteoarthrosis* or *degenerative joint disease*, is defined as a degenerative condition of the joint characterized by deterioration and abrasion of articular tissue and concomitant remodeling of the underlying subchondral bone due to overload of the remodeling mechanism.[240,374,404-406] The progressive loss of articular cartilage in the osteoarthritic TMJ results from an imbalance between predominantly chondrocyte-controlled reparative and degradative processes.[86] The process accelerates as proteoglycan depletion, collagen fiber network disintegration, and fatty degeneration weaken the functional capacity of the articular cartilage. Different kinds of biochemical "markers" have been determined in the synovial fluid of TMJs with osteoarthritis. These include IL-6,[407] tissue inhibitor metalloproteinase 1,[261,407,408] matrix metalloproteinases,[266,409] heat shock protein,[410] TGF-β1,[411] bone morphogenetic protein 2,[412] chondroitin-4-sulfate and chondroitin-6-sulfate,[413] keratan sulfate,[414] and human leukocyte antigen-D related (HLA-DR).[415] The clinical and diagnostic value of these markers remains to be evaluated, since similar markers have also been present in other joint diseases. Radiographic evidence typically lags behind articular tissue changes.[416] The early changes in the synovial membrane, such as synovial intima hyperplasia and cell hypertrophy resulting in fibrous material in the intima matrix[394] and articular cartilage are only detectable with biopsy and arthroscopy.[287,417] For this reason, osteoarthrosis frequently escapes early clinical detection.[418]

Osteoarthritis is categorized as *primary* if there is no identifiable local or systemic etiologic factor.[419] Primary osteoarthritis is considered idiopathic. With improved understanding, some subsets of primary osteoarthritis will likely become secondary as new etiologic agents are identified.[331] Pain and dysfunction can vary greatly depending on the degree of associated inflammation and deformity. Minimal pain or dysfunction is commonly observed. Studies of clinical populations suggest that the ultimate course of the condition is fairly benign.[418-421] Therefore, treatment decisions should be based largely on the degree of pain and dysfunction present.

*Diagnostic criteria for primary osteoarthritis.* All of the following must be present:
1. No identifiable etiologic factor.
2. Pain with function.
3. Point tenderness on palpation.
4. Radiographic evidence of structural bony change (subchondral sclerosis, osteophytic formation, erosion) and joint space narrowing.

The following may accompany the preceding items:
• Limited range of motion and deviation to the affected side.
• Crepitation or multiple joint noises.

*Differential diagnosis*: inflammation, polyarthritides, neoplasm

### Secondary osteoarthritis (IHS 11.7.1.4.2; ICD-9 715.28)

*Secondary osteoarthritis* involves the same process of articular breakdown with osseous remodeling that occurs in the primary condition, although an associated prior event or disease responsible for overloading the remodeling mechanism can usually be identified. Potential etiologic factors include direct trauma to the TMJ (eg, traumatic arthritis), local TMJ infection, or history of active systemic arthritis (eg, rheumatoid arthritis). The identification of secondary osteoarthritis is useful clinically because

treatment of the causal condition may be indicated as the first step in treatment.

Osteoarthritis associated with TMJ disc derangement is also classified as secondary. Although there is some disagreement as to which is the precipitating condition, there is clearly a close relationship between the two disorders.[243,371,422-424]

One rare idiopathic degenerative condition, termed *condylysis*, occurs spontaneously, primarily in adolescent females,[425-427] and is suggested clinically by anterior bite opening and a rapid development of molar laterotrusive facets.[123] Normal condylar development proceeds until the sudden lytic event occurs, causing the condyle to become progressively smaller, and in some cases even disappear. Condylysis is not usually associated with ankylosis, erosive changes in the fossae, or a positive serologic test result.[428,429]

*Diagnostic criteria for secondary osteoarthritis.* All of the following must be present:
1. The presence of a clearly documented disease or event associated with osteoarthritis.
2. Pain with function.
3. Point tenderness on palpation.
4. Radiographic evidence of structural bony change (subchondral sclerosis, osteophytic formation, erosion) and joint space narrowing.

The following may accompany the preceding items:
• Limited range of motion and deviation to the affected side.
• Crepitation or multiple joint noises.

*Differential diagnosis*: synovitis and capsulitis, polyarthritis, neoplasm

## Ankylosis (IHS 11.7.1.5; *ICD-9 524.61*)

*Ankylosis* is defined as a restricted mandibular movement with deflection to the affected side on opening that is often a long-term sequela of trauma, including mandibular fracture.[430] It implies a firm, unyielding restriction due to intracapsular fibrous adhesions, fibrotic changes in the capsular ligaments (fibrous ankylosis), or, less frequently, the formation of a bony mass that results in fusion of the joint components (bony ankylosis). The condition usually is not associated with pain. The most frequent cause of TMJ ankylosis is macrotrauma[1]; less frequent causes are infection of the mastoid or middle ear, systemic disease, and inadequate surgical treatment of the condylar area.[431,432] Fibrous adhesions within the TMJ are thought to occur mainly in the superior compartment of the TMJ, where they cause decreased movement of the disc-condyle complex. Adhesions may occur secondary to joint inflammation resulting from direct trauma or systemic conditions such as a polyarthritic disease. Bony ankylosis results from the union of the bones of the TMJ by proliferation of bone cells, which may cause complete immobility of the joint. In fibrous ankylosis, no radiographic finding other than the absence of ipsilateral condylar translation on opening is found. Bony ankylosis is characterized by radiographic evidence of bone proliferation with marked deflection to the affected side and marked limited laterotrusion to the contralateral side.

*Diagnostic criteria for fibrous ankylosis.* All of the following must be present:
1. Limited range of motion on opening.
2. Marked deflection to the affected side.
3. Markedly limited laterotrusion to the contralateral side.

4. Radiographic findings that reveal absence of ipsilateral condylar translation on opening, but presence of a disc space.

*Diagnostic criteria for bony ankylosis.* All of the following must be present:
1. Extremely limited range of motion on opening when condition is bilateral.
2. Marked deflection to the affected side when condition is unilateral.
3. Markedly limited laterotrusion to the contralateral side when condition is unilateral.
4. Radiographic evidence of bone proliferation with obliteration of the disc space and absence of condylar translation.

*Differential diagnosis*: muscular contracture, disc dislocation without reduction

## Fracture (IHS 11.7.1.6; *ICD-9 802.2x closed; ICD-9 802.3x open*)

Direct traumatic force can injure all related bony components of the masticatory system (ie, temporal bone, maxilla, zygoma, sphenoid bone, and mandible). Trauma can be in the form of fracture, dislocation, contusion, and/or laceration of articular surfaces, ligaments, and disc, with or without intra-articular hemarthrosis. Sequelae may include adhesions, ankylosis, occlusal abnormalities, or joint degeneration.[277,433] Patients with nonsurgically treated dislocated fractures may be prone to symptoms of TMDs, functional disorders, and occlusal disorders.[433] Fractures of the condylar process may result in facial asymmetry, with greater skeletal changes when the fracture occurs earlier in life. Closed treatment methods have reportedly also resulted in facial asymmetry, even in adults.[434]

## Masticatory muscle disorders

Muscle disorders involving the masticatory muscles are analogous to skeletal muscle disorders throughout the body.[7] Some mechanisms behind muscle pain are overuse of a normally perfused muscle or ischemia of a normally working muscle,[435-438] sympathetic and fusimotor reflexes producing changes in the blood supply and muscle tone,[439,440] and psychologic or emotional states.[441,442] Neurons that mediate pain from skeletal muscles are subject to strong modulatory influences. Endogenous substances (bradykinin, serotonin, prostaglandins, neuropeptides, and substance P) can sensitize the nociceptive endings very easily. Painful muscle conditions not only result in increased sensitivity of peripheral nociceptors, but also produce hyperexcitability in the CNS and localized hyperalgesia.[19,435,443-445]

Most TMD patients are found to have tenderness of the elevator muscles during palpation, and many report pain on chewing.[21] Traditionally it has been hypothesized that these symptoms are associated with psychosocial factors[112] and increased postural electromyographic (EMG) activity.[446] Lund and coworkers,[447] however, questioned the common view that musculoskeletal pain is associated with tonic muscular hyperactivity, and showed that the activity of agonist muscles is often reduced by pain, with small increases in the level of antagonist muscle activity. As a result, maximum voluntary contraction, force production, endurance time, and the range and velocity of movement are often reduced.[447-450] In support of those findings, patients with bruxing and clenching habits were found to have very few tender muscles,[451] and only 30% of those with confirmed active bruxism had significant myalgia.[117]

Muscle disorders can be divided into those that affect a single muscle or group of muscles (regional) and those that affect all muscles (systemic). Systemic muscle disorders are not unique to the masticatory system and therefore not primarily managed by TMD therapies. The orofacial pain clinician needs to be aware of the common systemic conditions that cause muscle pain, and, when systemic disorders are identified, proper treatment or referral for treatment should be instituted.

Some systemic conditions that produce muscle pain are polymyalgia rheumatica, polymyositis, dermatomyositis, lupus erythematosus, and fibromyalgia. Fibromyalgia is of particular interest, since it may easily be confused with a regional masticatory muscle disorder.[452,453] *Fibromyalgia*, also termed *myofascitis*, *myofibrositis*, or *fibrositis*, is a generalized muscle pain condition that is characterized by continuous, aching pain associated with tenderness in many sites over the body. The severity of fibromyalgia may increase with age and be associated with sleep disturbances and depression.[454,454] It may also be associated with generalized fatigue, chronic headache, anxiety, subjective swelling, irritable bowel syndrome, and modulation of the symptoms by activity or the weather. Inclusionary criteria are pain in three of the four body quadrants for at least 3 months, tenderness in 11 of 18 specific sites, and normal EMG activity.[456-461] When fibromyalgia is suspected, referral to a rheumatologist is in order.

This section will focus on the local or regional muscle disorders that are responsible for producing orofacial pains (see Box 3-5). The multiple etiologic factors responsible for myalgia and the present lack of scientific data on the etiology and pathology of myalgia limits the ability to clearly distinguish

153

some groups of muscle pain disorders. Often the clinician must rely on clinical judgment to establish the diagnosis. It is hoped that new advancements in this field will lead to the establishment of refined, valid, and reliable diagnostic criteria.

## Local myalgia (IHS 11.7.2.1; ICD-9 729.1)

*Local myalgia* is characterized by sore masticatory muscles with pain in the cheeks and/or temples on chewing, opening wide, and often on waking. It is usually bilateral and described as a stiff, sore, achy pain, spasm, or cramp. The pain may be secondary to ischemia,[462] bruxism,[115] fatigue, metabolic alterations, autonomic effects, protective splinting (co-contraction), and delayed-onset muscle soreness.

   *Delayed-onset muscle soreness,*[15] also called *postexercise muscle soreness* or *muscle compartment syndrome*, is a painful condition caused by intense or unaccustomed use of a muscle.[463] This overuse appears to result in interstitial inflammation that produces a painful condition, with pain onset delayed between 8 and 24 hours. This condition may be considered a type of myositis; however, it does not present with typical signs of inflammation, such as swelling, increased EMG activity, trigger points, or referral of pain. Associated signs include loss of strength, reduced range of motion, and increase of pain on stretching and use. Whereas the symptoms may be attributed to myofibrillar damage and disruption of the cytoskeleton within muscle fibers,[464] recent studies suggested that the myofibrillar changes are a sign of active and adaptive remodeling of the myofibrils in response to exercise,[465,466] which might explain why repetitive training reduces or eliminates the

muscle soreness. Free radicals have also been suggested to play a key physiologic role in the adaptation and recovery process.[467]

*Diagnostic criteria for local myalgia.* All of the following must be present:
1. Regional dull, aching pain during function of the affected muscle(s).
2. No or minimal pain at rest.
3. Local muscle tenderness to palpation.
4. Absence of trigger points and pain referral patterns.

The following may accompany the preceding items:
• Sensation of muscle stiffness.
• Sensation of muscle weakness.
• Sensation of muscle fatigue.
• Mouth opening may be decreased, but passive stretching of the elevator muscles will increase mouth opening by more than 4 mm (soft end-feel).

*Differential diagnosis*: myositis, myofascial pain, neoplasm, fibromyalgia

## Myofascial pain (IHS 11.7.2.2; ICD-9 729.1)

*Myofascial pain* is characterized by a regional dull, aching muscle pain, and the presence of trigger points in muscles, tendons, or fascia.[468] When palpated, these trigger points may produce a characteristic pattern of regional referred pain and/or autonomic symptoms on provocation.[469-473] Previously used terms for myofascial pain include *myalgia, trigger-point pain*, and *myofascial pain dysfunction syndrome*. Since the referred pain is often felt as headache, this pain has also been associated with tension-type headache. The conditions show significant overlap in signs and symptoms, and may share similar pathophysiologic mechanisms, although different muscles are involved.[474]

Palpation of the active trigger points causes reproducible alteration of pain to a more extensive area that may or may not include the muscle containing the trigger points.[107,109,475] Inactivation of the trigger points with injection of local anesthetics, ice, or vapocoolant spray followed by stretch or transcutaneous electric nerve stimulation (TENS) relieves the larger area of pain. The pathogenesis of myofascial pain is not well understood, and the phenomenon of trigger points has been called questionable, because there is no to little evidence of histochemical differences between trigger points and adjacent muscle tissue. Recently, interest has focused on hyperalgesia due to changes in the CNS, including the sympathetic nervous system, as a mediator of myofascial pain.[468,476,477] Elevated levels of serotonin, norepinephrine, bradykinin, substance P, calcitonin-gene-related peptide, TNF-$\alpha$, and IL-1$\beta$ were demonstrated in human muscle tissue near active trigger points.[478] The presence of these well-known pain mediators could be indicators of peripheral and central sensitization as well as increased sympathetic activity.

*Diagnostic criteria for myofascial pain.* All of the following must be present:
1. Regional dull, aching pain at rest.
2. Pain is aggravated by function of the affected muscle(s).
3. Provocation of trigger points, which are frequently palpated within a taut band of muscle tissue or fascia, alters the pain complaint and often reveals a pattern of pain referral.
4. Greater than 50% reduction of pain with vapocoolant spray or local anesthetic injection into the trigger point, followed by stretch.

The following may accompany the preceding items:
• Sensation of muscle stiffness.
• Sensation of acute malocclusion not verified clinically.
• Ear symptoms, tinnitus, vertigo, toothache, tension-type headache.
• Mouth opening may be decreased, and passive stretching of the elevator muscles will increase mouth opening by more than 4 mm (soft end-feel).
• Hyperalgesia in the region of the referred pain.

*Differential diagnosis*: osteoarthritis, myositis, local myalgia, neoplasia, fibromyalgia

## Centrally mediated myalgia (IHS 11.7.2.3; *ICD-9* 729.1)

*Centrally mediated myalgia* is described as a chronic, continuous muscle pain disorder. The clinical presentation may resemble that of myositis, although there are no classic clinical signs of inflammation (reddening, swelling, etc). There are signs of neurogenic inflammation, however, which may result from prolonged nociceptive input to the CNS, which in turn may result in an antidromic effect on afferent peripheral neurons. These afferent neurons then carry the information from the CNS out to the peripheral tissues.[15] Antidromic stimulation of the peripheral nerves may result in the release of pain-modulating substances such as bradykinin and substance P, which cause pain.[479–482] Other central mechanisms may play a significant role in the cause or persistence of centrally mediated myalgia, such as chronic upregulation of the autonomic nervous system, chronic exposure to emotional stress, or other sources of deep pain input.

The continuity rather than the duration and intensity of the precipitating pain is more likely to produce chronic centrally mediated myalgia. Prolonged and constant muscle pain is more likely than intermittent muscle pain conditions to lead to the chronic condition.

Because the pain associated with centrally mediated myalgia is centrally generated, it will not respond to treatments directed at the painful muscle tissue itself; rather, therapies should be aimed at downregulation of the sensitized central mechanisms.[1]

*Diagnostic criteria for centrally mediated myalgia.* All of the following must be present:

1. History of prolonged and continuous muscle pain.
2. Regional dull, aching pain at rest.
3. Pain is aggravated by function of the affected muscle(s).
4. Pain is aggravated by palpation.

The following may accompany the preceding items:

- Trigger points and pain referral on palpation.
- Sensation of muscle stiffness, weakness, and/or fatigue.
- Sensation of acute malocclusion not verified clinically.
- Ear symptoms, tinnitus, vertigo, toothache, tension-type headache.
- Mouth opening may be decreased, and passive stretching of the elevator muscles may or may not increase mouth opening.
- Hyperalgesia.

*Differential diagnosis*: osteoarthritis, myositis, myofascial pain, local myalgia, neoplasm, fibromyalgia

## Myospasm (IHS 11.7.2.4; ICD-9 728.85)

*Myospasm* is an acute muscle disorder that involves a sudden, involuntary, tonic contraction of a muscle.[13] Previously used terms are *cramp* or *trismus*. Myospasm is characterized by a continuous muscle contraction (fasciculation) and can, therefore, be differentiated from most other muscle disorders by needle, fine wire, or surface EMG verification of sustained involuntary muscle contraction, even at rest.[483,484] A muscle in spasm is acutely shortened, grossly limited in range of motion, and painful.

Since myospasm involves the entire muscle (or a major portion of the muscle), the EMG recording is similar to, or greater than, the maximum voluntary contraction of the same muscle. A slight increase in resting EMG activity is not indicative of myospasm. Although myospasm was once considered to be a common source of masticatory muscle pain, present studies do not confirm this notion.[447,448,450] Instead, myospasm is likely to be a relatively rare finding in an orofacial pain population.

*Diagnostic criteria for myospasm.* All of the following must be present:

1. Acute onset of pain at rest as well as with function.
2. Markedly reduced range of motion due to continuous involuntary muscle contraction.
3. Pain is aggravated by function of the affected muscle(s).
4. Increased EMG activity grossly higher than at rest.
5. Sensation of muscle tightness or cramping or stiffness.

The following may accompany the preceding items:
• Acute malocclusion (dependent on the specific muscle involved).

*Differential diagnosis*: myositis, unclassified local myalgia, neoplasm

## Myositis (IHS 11.7.2.5; *ICD-9* 728.81)

*Myositis* is characterized by the clinical signs and symptoms associated with true tissue inflammation, such as swelling, tissue reddening, and increased temperature over the entire muscle.[15] This condition generally arises secondary to direct trauma to the muscle or a spreading infection and presents as a constant, acutely painful muscle(s). Since chemical substances produced in response to tissue damage and inflammation are presumably the principal causes of pain, elevated serum enzyme levels may be found as well as markers of inflammation. Clinically, the patient may exhibit a limited range of mandibular movement. Ossification of a muscle can occur secondary to inflammation, which results in myositis ossificans.[485,486] The inflammation may occur in the tendinous attachments of the muscle as well; this type of inflammation is termed either *tendinitis* or *tendomyositis*. Careful questioning of the patient usually reveals a history of trauma to the muscle or a source of adjacent infection (or both).

*Diagnostic criteria for myositis*. All of the following must be present:
1. Pain, usually continuous, in a localized muscle area following injury or infection.
2. Diffuse tenderness over the entire muscle.
3. Pain is aggravated by function of the affected muscle(s).

4. Moderately to severely limited range of motion due to pain and swelling.

## Myofibrotic contracture (IHS 11.7.2.6; *ICD-9* 728.9)

*Muscle contracture* refers to the painless shortening of a muscle. *Myofibrotic contracture* is the chronic resistance of a muscle to passive stretch as a result of fibrosis of the supporting tendons, ligaments, or muscle fibers themselves. Previously used terms are *chronic trismus*, *muscle fibrosis*, and *muscle scarring*. Myofibrotic contracture is not usually painful unless the muscle is extended beyond its functional length. This condition often follows a long period of limited range of motion as with intermaxillary fixation. History of infection or trauma to the muscle tissue is common.

*Diagnostic criteria for myofibrotic contracture*. All of the following must be present:
1. Limited range of mandibular motion.
2. Unyielding firmness on passive stretch (hard end-feel).
3. Little or no pain unless the involved muscle is forced to lengthen.

The following may accompany the preceding items:
• History of trauma, infection, or long period of disuse.

*Differential diagnosis*: TMJ ankylosis, coronoid hypertrophy

## Masticatory muscle neoplasia (IHS 11.7.2.7; *ICD-9*-CM 171.0)

Neoplasia of the masticatory muscles can be malignant or benign and may or may not be associated with pain. Tumors may be within the muscles themselves, within the masseter spaces, or most commonly, as extensions from adjacent structures or metastases from remote sites. Common presenting features are swelling, trismus, paresthesias, and pain that may refer to teeth. Masticatory muscles are uncommon end sites for tumor metastases, with only a handful of actual occurrences.[487-491] When suspected, confirmation through imaging and biopsy is mandatory.

# Management of TMDs

Management goals for patients with TMDs are similar to those for other orthopedic or rheumatologic disorders. They include decreased pain, decreased adverse loading, restoration of function, and resumption of normal daily activities. These management goals are best achieved by a well-defined program designed to treat the physical disorder(s) and to reduce or eliminate the effects of all contributing factors. The treatment options and sequences for TMDs outlined here are consistent with management of other musculoskeletal disorders.

As in many musculoskeletal conditions, the signs and symptoms of TMDs over time may be transient and self-limiting, resolving without serious long-term effects.[60,492-495] Little is known about which signs and symptoms will progress to more serious conditions in the natural course of TMDs. Therefore, special effort should be made to avoid early use of aggressive, irreversible treatments such as complex occlusal therapy or surgery. Conservative (reversible) treatment, such as self-management, behavioral modification, physical therapy, medications,

and orthopedic appliances are endorsed for the initial care of nearly all TMDs.[74,496-500]

## *Principles of management*

Most patients with TMDs achieve good symptom relief with conservative therapy.[24,63,501,502] Long-term follow-up of TMD patients shows that 50% to more than 90% of patients have few or no symptoms after conservative treatment. From a retrospective study of 154 patients, it was concluded that most TMD patients have minimal recurrent symptoms 7 years after treatment.[489] Furthermore, more than 85% to 90% of the patients in three longitudinal studies lasting 2 to 10 years had relief of symptoms after conservative treatment,[503-505] and stability was achieved in most cases between 6 and 12 months after the start of treatment.[505]

In many patients with TMJ disc displacement (reducing and nonreducing), painless mandibular function is possible with the displaced disc.[65,98,506] Patients with pain-free clicking TMJs generally do not need treatment except for reassurance and explanation of the condition, whereas patients with nonreducing discs typically respond well to conservative treatment.[96,506-508] The internal derangement of the TMJ often exhibits a natural progression of compensatory adaptation and remodeling.[391,420,509] Even with progression to osteoarthritic changes, the outcome is typically benign, with acceptable masticatory function.[423,510] Myogenous disorders more frequently require recurrent treatment than do TMJ articular disorders.[112,511]

Relevant precipitating and perpetuating contributing factors should be identified through the history and clinical examination. Factors such as bruxism and other parafunctional habits, trauma, adverse anatomic relationships, and pathophysiologic and psychosocial conditions may all have an impact on TMDs, but as most of these factors are highly prevalent in the general population, their presence in an individual case may be coincidental and not contribute to the TMD. Therefore, in addition to the physical diagnosis, the goal of each evaluation should be the development of a prioritized problem list of the relevant contributing factors, to guide the treatment plan and sequence.

Treatment prognosis can be affected by a number of considerations. Early treatment of acute musculoskeletal pain results in greater patient satisfaction, fewer work days lost, and reduced chance of developing a chronic pain condition.[512] In cases of chronic TMDs where the pain is less frequent and patients engage in greater daily activity, the prognosis improves.[513] The power of nonspecific effects in healing (eg, placebo effect) in the treatment of psychosocial and biologic conditions has been well documented.[514] These effects certainly play a role in the successful treatment of TMDs,[515] and the value of a good doctor-patient relationship is important as well.

Despite the documented success of the various forms of conservative care, some patients with TMDs do not improve. Reasons for treatment failure vary, but these patients typically fall into two groups: (1) those patients with incomplete or incorrect diagnosis,[63] and (2) those patients with unsuccessfully addressed or unrecognized contributing factors. When multiple contributing factors are present, and especially if the condition is chronic, a pain management program with a team of clinicians comprising appropriate specialists for each of the contributing factors may be needed. It is difficult for an in-dividual clinician to address the multiple factors that may be present in complex chronic pain patients.[516] Management goals are best achieved by using the optimal combination and sequence of treatment options indicated by the initial problem list. All management programs should be time limited and not left open-ended.

Treatment options include patient education and self-management, cognitive behavioral intervention, pharmacotherapy, physical therapy, orthopedic appliances, occlusal therapy, and surgery. In practice these treatment modalities should be used in combination depending on the needs of the patient. It is important to remember that Axis II (psychologic) factors need to be considered in the management of all TMDs. These factors will be reviewed in chapter 11.

## Patient education and self-management

The success of a self-management program depends on patient motivation, cooperation, and compliance, which in turn requires attentive listening on the part of the clinician, and sufficient time for the patient to present his or her concerns. The clinician must take the time to explain the clinical findings, diagnostic data, treatment options, and prognosis to the patient. The time spent on patient reassurance and education is a significant factor in developing a high level of rapport and treatment compliance. The clinician's explanation of the problem and treatment recommendations should use terminology the patient can understand.

A successful self-management program allows healing and prevents further injury to the musculoskeletal system, which may be enough to control the problem.[24,517,518] Self-management routine should include voluntary limitation of mandibular function, habit awareness and modification, and a home physiotherapy program. An explanation of the advantages of resting the affected muscular and articular structures, and functioning only within pain-free limits, much the same as an athlete resting an injured joint, is often helpful. Modification of functional behaviors (eg, avoidance of heavy mastication, gum chewing, wide yawning, and singing) and habit reversal of parafunctional behaviors (eg, clenching, bruxing, tongue thrusting, cheek biting, poor sleeping posture, object biting, and playing some musical instruments) should be emphasized.

Offending habits can be modified with habit awareness, motivation to change, knowledge of how to change, and commitment to self-management. A simple feedback mechanism, such as visual reminders adapted to the patient's daily activities, should be discussed and implemented (eg, small stickers strategically placed at home, in the automobile, and at work). Keeping a diary aimed at identifying circumstances and activities that foster the offending habits may also be helpful. Progress with this therapy should be discussed at each follow-up appointment.

A home physiotherapy program has also been proposed for the treatment of TMD pain and dysfunction, because it is simple, noninvasive, and cost-effective; allows an easy self-management approach; cultivates good doctor-patient communication; and can be managed by the general practitioner.[519,520] A program of heat and/or ice to the affected areas, massage of the affected muscles, and gentle range-of-motion exercises can decrease tenderness and pain and increase range of motion. A RCT compared heat transmission from superficial moist and dry heat application and found no significant difference.[521] Since compliance has been linked to convenience, the authors recommended instructing patients to use a dry heating pad unless a patient prefers moist heat. Heat applications transmit heat by conduction and are only useful for superficial heating (1 to 5 mm in depth). Heat stimulates muscle relaxation and vascular perfusion. Ice packs are used primarily for local analgesic and anti-inflammatory effects in muscle and joint tissues. Because the temperature differential is greater with cold application, a shorter duration may produce a greater response. Heat should not be used for acute injury (less than 72 hours), acute inflammation, or infection. Cold should not be used in patients with poor circulation (eg, due to diabetes, radiated tissues) or over open wounds.

## Cognitive behavioral intervention

Behavioral modification of maladaptive habits is an important part of the overall treatment program for TMD patients,[522] including those who have been refractive to conservative dental/physical medicine treatment approaches.[523] Although simple habits may be modified when the patient is made aware of them, changing persistent habits may require a structured program facilitated by a specialist in behavioral modification.[524,525] Significant modification of the patient's lifestyle is often necessary to alter the contributing factors. If a more structured approach is indicated, strategies such as a habit reversal program, lifestyle counseling, progressive relaxation, hypnosis, and biofeedback should be considered. Treatment should be individualized to best fit the patient's problems, preferences, and lifestyle. Several manuals and texts more fully describe this approach.[526-528]

*Biofeedback* is a structured therapy based on the theory that when an individual receives information about a desired change and is supported in making the change, the change is more likely to occur.[529,530] In general, biofeedback training requires equipment to measure biologic activity, for example, surface EMG to measure muscle activity. The equipment is designed with a "feedback" loop so that a patient can receive immediate feedback regarding performance. A number of controlled studies have demonstrated that relaxation training, with or without the use of surface EMG biofeedback, can decrease diurnal tonic muscle activity.[524,531,532] Most trials evaluating biofeedback for the treatment of TMDs have been undertaken with sample sizes of fewer than 20 subjects, and although there is cumulative evidence of effectiveness when biofeedback was compared with controls, there remains a need for large-sample, controlled-outcome trials.[533]

Biofeedback may be less effective in the treatment of nocturnal bruxism.[534] Nocturnal EMG biofeedback without a more comprehensive stress management program appears to decrease bruxism only temporarily[535,536]; therefore, its use may be limited to short-term management of acute conditions. Comprehensive stress management and counseling programs that involve a combination of EMG biofeedback, progressive relaxation, and self-directed changes in lifestyle appear to be more effective when used together than any single behavioral treatment. Use of behavioral therapies in conjunction with dental therapies also appears to enhance the overall therapeutic effects.[537,538]

## Pharmacologic therapy

Both clinical experience and controlled experimental studies suggest that pharmacologic agents may promote patient comfort and rehabilitation when used as part of a comprehensive program. Although there is a tendency for clinicians to rely on a single "favorite" agent, no one drug has proven efficacy for the entire spectrum of TMDs. It is important to become familiar with a variety of drugs, to realize maximal treatment effect, and to avoid unexpected complications and adverse drug interactions.

Drug misuse and abuse are of concern in the pharmacologic management of TMDs. Because opioid narcotics produce tolerance and dependence, they are most useful in short-term, acute pain conditions. Continued narcotic analgesic use in patients with chronic TMDs requires careful consideration.[539-541] Prescribing drugs on a pain-contingent basis, to be taken "as needed," is still common despite clear warnings in the literature that this approach is ineffective and may lead to abuse for some patients. Therefore, dependence-producing pharmaceuticals should only be used on a time-contingent basis.[542] All other avenues of treatment should be pursued rather than relying on narcotic medication.

The most widely used pharmacologic agents for the management of TMDs include analgesics, nonsteroidal anti-inflammatory drugs (NSAIDs), corticosteroids, benzodiazepines, muscle relaxants, and low-dose antidepressants.[543] The analgesics, corticosteroids, and benzodiazepines are indicated for acute TMD pain; NSAIDs and muscle relaxants may be used for both acute and chronic conditions; and tricyclic antidepressants are primarily indicated for long-term orofacial pain management.

## Analgesics

Analgesics, either opiate or nonopiate preparations, are used to reduce pain associated with TMDs. The nonopiate analgesics are a heterogeneous group of compounds that share certain therapeutic actions and side effects. They may be used for mild to moderate pain associated with TMDs. Aspirin, which inhibits prostaglandin synthesis, is the prototype for these compounds. All salicylate drugs are antipyretic, analgesic, and anti-inflammatory, but there are important differences in their effects. For patients who are sensitive to aspirin, a nonacetylated aspirin, choline magnesium trisalicylate, or salsalate may be effective.[544] Opioid narcotics act on specific opiate receptor sites in the central and peripheral nervous systems. Opioids have CNS depression qualities and addiction liabilities. They may be considered for short-term use for moderate to severe acute pain.[540]

## Nonsteroidal anti-inflammatory drugs

NSAIDs have been reported as effective for mild to moderate inflammatory conditions and acute postoperative pain.[540] A recent systematic review identified only one RCT of NSAID treatment for patients with chronic TMDs,[545] reporting no benefit of ibuprofen over placebo in myogenous TMDs.[546] NSAIDs may be effective for the treatment of arthrogenous TMD pain.[547]

There are several chemically dissimilar groups of NSAIDs, which differ in their antipyretic, analgesic, and anti-inflammatory efficacy.[548] Therefore, if one NSAID fails, another one may succeed. Because of the possible adverse affects of NSAIDs,[549] patients should be carefully monitored. Gastrointestinal complications pose the greatest risk associated with NSAID use. If gastroprotection is needed, a proton-pump inhibitor should be used in conjunction with NSAID therapy. Patients who do not have cardiovascular risk factors and are not taking aspirin also may use a cyclooxygenase-2 inhibitor if indicated, in conjunction with a proton-pump inhibitor.[550]

## Corticosteroids

Corticosteroids are potent anti-inflammatory drugs that are not commonly prescribed for systemic use in the treatment of TMDs because of their side effects. The exception is for acute severely painful joint inflammation or joint inflammation associated with the polyarthritides. Intracapsular TMJ injection of corticosteroids such as methylprednisolone has been recommended on a limited basis in cases of acute flare-up of severe joint pain where conservative treatment has been unsuccessful. Although there have been some concerns regarding long-term effects (eg, progression of joint destruction), the long-term prognosis appears good for alleviating TMJ pain and dysfunction with no or minimal increase in radiographically visible degenerative changes.[551–553] Injection of corticosteroids has also been reported to improve acute TMJ symptoms due to rheumatoid arthritis, with no long-term adverse sequelae.[552–554]

## Benzodiazepines

Benzodiazepines are antianxiety agents that are frequently administered to patients with chronic pain. These drugs are potentially habit forming, and there is a concern that they may worsen depression in patients with chronic pain.[543] However, several studies have demonstrated their therapeutic effects for musculoskeletal pain.[546,555,556] In addition, diazepam has been shown to reduce nocturnal bruxism as measured by EMG activity, and a 5-mg dose at bedtime has been recommended for the short-term management (1 to 2 weeks) of acute pain due to nocturnal bruxism.[14,557]

Benzodiazepine therapy should not be extended beyond a few weeks. Patients for whom a therapeutic course of a benzodiazepine in adjunction to conservative therapy fails to produce a therapeutic response should be reevaluated.

## Muscle relaxants

Muscle relaxants help prevent the increased muscle activity associated with TMDs.[558] Experimentally, muscle relaxants depress spinal polysynaptic reflexes preferentially over monosynaptic reflexes. Muscle relaxants affect neuronal activity associated with muscle stretch reflexes, primarily in the lateral reticular area of the brainstem. The oral doses of these drugs are well below the levels required to elicit experimental muscle-relaxant activity. Therefore, some investigators conclude that their activity is related only to their sedative effect.[543] Some central skeletal muscle relaxants are available in combination with analgesics.

Tizanidine proved to be an effective adjunct for the treatment of chronic daily headaches[559] but not for tension-type headaches.[560] Cyclobenzaprine proved to be effective for the treatment of acute lumbar and cervical spasms[561] but not for acute myofascial strain.[562] A recent meta-analysis[563] of the fibromyalgia literature identified five randomized, placebo-controlled trials that found that patients treated with cyclobenzaprine were three times as likely to report overall improvement in pain reduction, and moderate improvement in sleep, but no improvement in fatigue or tender points. A systematic review revealed strong evidence of the efficacy of muscle relaxants for nonspecified chronic low back pain.[564] No eligible trials were found comparing muscle relaxants with analgesics; hence, it is not known whether muscle relaxants yield better pain relief than analgesics. With regard to studies including TMD patients, cyclobenzaprine was found to be statistically superior to either placebo or clonazepam in reducing mandibular pain on awakening, but neither drug had any effect on sleep improvement.[565] Another study reported no difference in efficacy between short-term treatment of TMD patients with a splint or with orphenadrine.[566]

Because there is limited evidence of the efficacy of muscle relaxants in the treatment of TMDs, their use should probably be limited to a brief trial in conjunction with conservative management.

## Antidepressants

The tricyclic antidepressants, particularly amitriptyline, have analgesic properties independent of their anti-depressant effect and are prescribed for patients with chronic pain in addition to depression and sleep disturbance.[567-571] The therapeutic effect of these drugs is thought to relate to their ability to increase the availability of the biogenic amines serotonin and norepinephrine at the synaptic junction in the CNS. Doses as low as 10 mg are beneficial in the treatment of muscle contraction headaches and musculoskeletal pain.[572] Benefits include decrease in the number of awakenings, increase in stage 4 (delta) sleep, and notable decrease in rapid eye movement sleep. For these reasons, it was thought that tricyclic antidepressants might have potential in the treatment of certain types of nocturnal bruxism; however, three recent double-blind crossover studies[573-575] reported that amitriptyline did not significantly decrease EMG activity or pain levels but did decrease stress levels associated with nocturnal bruxism. Another placebo-controlled study found that amitriptyline significantly reduced the pain associated with both chronic muscular and TMJ dysfunction. More research needs to be done to determine the effectiveness of tricyclics in the treatment of bruxism and chronic myofascial pain. The therapeutic dose required to achieve an antidepressant action is significantly larger, and these drugs should only be prescribed by clinicians who are trained in the diagnosis and treatment of depression.

## Sodium hyaluronate

*Hyaluronic acid* is a naturally occurring polysaccharide belonging to the glycosaminoglycan family, and *sodium hyaluronate* is the salt of purified natural sodium hyaluronic acid. In healthy synovial joints, hyaluronic acid maintains the viscosity of synovial fluid and supports the lubricating and shock-absorbing properties of the articular cartilage. Sodium hyaluronate has been identified and tested in animals, with encouraging results.[576-578] The use of sodium hyaluronate for the treatment of disc displacements and disc dislocations without reduction seems promising,[579-585] as does its use for the treatment of pain and inflammation.[551,586-589] A systematic review of five meta-analyses on the management of arthritis with hyaluronic acid injections showed modest improvement of symptoms.[590] However, a review of the use of hyaluronate for TMDs showed equivocal results.[591] RCTs are needed to provide evidence of the efficacy of sodium hyaluronate over standard treatments for TMDs.

## *Physical therapy*

Physical therapy helps to relieve musculoskeletal pain and to restore normal function by altering sensory input; reducing inflammation; decreasing, coordinating, and strengthening muscle activity; and promoting the repair and regeneration of tissues. In most cases, physical therapy is used as an adjunct to other treatments. Coordination of physical therapy through a licensed professional therapist is recommended. Although well-controlled clinical trials have not been completed, physical therapy is well recognized as an effective, conservative method of treatment for TMDs.[108,471,519,592-598]

In chronic TMDs, a predetermined course of treatment should be implemented, with the ultimate goal of making the patient independent with a home program.[599] The home program includes self-management and an exercise regimen.

## Posture training

The goal of posture training is to prevent untoward activity of the head, neck, and shoulder muscles, as well as the masticatory and tongue muscles. Maintaining orthostatic posture prevents increased cervical and shoulder muscle activity and possible protrusion of the mandible. The more anterior the head is relative to the spinal column, the greater is its effective weight. Except during functional activity (eg, chewing, swallowing, and speaking), the mandible should be in a relaxed position with the teeth separated and the tongue resting in the floor of the mouth.

A RCT showed the effectiveness of posture training in myogenous TMD patients for both TMD and neck complaints.[600] Although posture training is a common physical therapeutic approach, its relationship to TMDs is not well understood and needs further study.[601]

## Exercise

Clinical experience suggests that an active exercise program is important to the development and maintenance of normal muscle and joint comfort, function, and stability. One of the objectives of an exercise program is to teach the patient how to avoid activities that are injurious to the involved synovial joints. In addition, exercise may be recommended to stretch and relax muscles,[108,602] mobilize and stabilize TMJs,[593] increase muscle strength,[603] and develop normal coordination arthrokinematics to reduce joint clicking.[604] Three types of exercise are generally recommended: (1) *repetitive exercises* to establish coordinated, rhythmic muscle function; (2) *isotonic exercises* to increase range of motion; and (3) *isometric exercises* to increase muscular strength. These exercises are prescribed to achieve specific goals and are modified as the patient progresses. Most patients will not exercise if it increases pain. Therefore, the therapist must initially help the patient achieve some symptom relief with physical agents or modalities. A maintenance level of exercise is recommended to ensure long-term resolution once the patient has reached the goals of treatment.

## Mobilization

Mobilization techniques are indicated for decreased range of motion and pain due to muscle contracture, disc displacement without reduction, and fibrous adhesions in the joint. In some cases, repeated manipulation by a physical therapist can restore a more physiologic resting muscle length or improve joint function to allow a normal range of mandibular motion.[371] Muscle relaxation and pain reduction are often required to enhance the effect of mobilization. Thus, a combination of heat, cold, ultrasound, and TENS is often administered before or in conjunction with mobilization. Acute disc displacement without reduction at times can be effectively reduced by manipulation of the mandible.[605] In addition to the use of adjunct modalities, local anesthetic injections may improve the outcome.[606]

Mobilization is accomplished through gripping the mandible firmly with the thumbs on the occlusal surfaces of the posterior teeth. The unaffected side is securely braced, and firm and controlled force is applied to the mandible in a downward, forward, and inward direction.[1,108] Another technique incorporates the patient's voluntary maximal lateral excursive mandibular movement to the unaffected side, followed by opening through the lateral border path.[108,607] Arthrographic studies indicate that manipulation does not produce complete anatomic reduction of the disc but does increase disc mobilization.[387,608] Following mobilization, therapy to maintain joint mobility should be considered, such as orthopedic appliance therapy, relaxation therapy, and exercises.

## Physical agents or modalities

### Electrotherapy
Electrotherapy devices can produce thermal, histochemical, and physiologic changes in the muscles and joints. These devices include electrogalvanic stimulation (EGS) and TENS. *EGS* uses a high-voltage, low-amperage,

monophasic current of varied frequency. This modality has been applied clinically to reduce or eliminate muscle spasm and soft tissue edema, as well as for muscle reeducation, trigger-point therapy, and increasing blood flow to tissues with decreased circulation.[609–612] *TENS* uses a low-voltage, low-amperage, biphasic current of varied frequency and is designed primarily for sensory counterstimulation in painful disorders.[613] Like EGS, this modality decreases muscle pain and hyperactivity and can aid in muscle reeducation. If significant motor stimulation occurs concurrently, it may impair the analgesic effect and exacerbate acute muscle pain.[614] Although TENS has traditionally been used outside of the temporomandibular area, application techniques for temporomandibular and cervical pain have been described. At present, primarily anecdotal clinical evidence supports the use of electrotherapy in the treatment of TMDs, and further research is needed.

## Ultrasound

Ultrasound is a frequently used physical treatment modality for musculoskeletal problems. When transmitted through the tissue, the high-frequency oscillations of the transducer head are converted to heat, which can reach a depth of 5 cm.[615] It has been proposed that ultrasound may be used to produce deep heat in the joints; treat joint contracture by increasing the stretch of the extracapsular soft tissue; decrease chronic pain, muscle contraction, and tendonitis; and facilitate resorption of the calcium deposits of bursitis.[615–617] Ultrasound is also commonly used to carry medication into the tissue through phonophoresis, although the mechanism and efficacy of drug delivery are unknown.[618] A systematic review on the efficacy of ultrasound for musculoskeletal

disorders revealed that only 2 of 18 placebo-controlled trials showed statistically and clinically significant benefits of ultrasound. The 4 trials related to TMDs did not reach the quality standard used in the review, however, and no significant benefit of ultrasound was achieved.[619]

## Iontophoresis

*Iontophoresis* is a technique to enhance the transport of drug ions across a tissue barrier. A weak current carries the drug ions, usually corticosteroids, through the skin into the deeper tissues, where the drug exerts its effect.[620] However, recent studies question the efficacy of this modality to provide pain relief.[621, 622]

## Vapocoolant spray

Application of vapocoolant spray followed by muscle stretching decreases muscle soreness and tightness and is thought to inactivate myofascial trigger points.[111,623] To date, there are no RCTs showing efficacy of such therapy.

## Anesthetic block/trigger-point injections

Local anesthetic injection into myofascial trigger points, alone or in conjunction with muscle stretching or mobilization, has been shown to be useful for the management of myofascial pain. Although the anesthetic is useful in pain reduction,[624] it appears that the mechanical disruption of the trigger point by the needle provides the therapeutic effect.[625,626]

Trigger-point injections should be used adjunctively with other modalities, such as pharmacotherapy, physical therapy, and, in many cases, behavioral modification.[627] The injections are usually given in a series of three to five treatments to a muscle group(s), initially at weekly intervals. Depending on their degree of effectiveness, they are either discontinued or administered at longer intervals. Procaine (1% to 2% without epinephrine, diluted to 0.5% with sterile saline) is recommended for trigger-point injections because of its low myotoxicty.[628] However, because this medication is no longer packaged for use in dental syringes, 2% lidocaine without epinephrine is appropriate if a dental syringe is used. A longstanding anesthetic such as bupivacaine should not be used for muscle injections because of increased risk for myotoxicity.

### Acupuncture

Although the precise mechanism of action is unknown, acupuncture has been used for the treatment of chronic musculoskeletal pain and studies of its application for TMDs suggest that it is beneficial.[513,629–633] The early benefits seem comparable with the more conventional TMD treatments, with reduction in pain and an increase in joint function.[513] Rigorous clinical trials evaluating acupuncture as an adjunctive therapy are needed before definitive recommendations regarding its application can be made.

### Laser treatment

Low-level laser therapy recently has been advanced for the treatment of TMDs. It is suggested to have biostimulating and analgesic effects through direct irradiation, without causing a thermal response.[635] Laser treatment has been studied in several musculoskeletal pain syndromes, and contradictory results were reported in two major meta-analyses.[636,637] Several studies have investigated the efficacy of laser therapy in TMDs.[638–644] The studies used different types, frequencies, and durations of laser radiation in the various patient groups, however, and treatment parameters could not be

standardized, nor could effectiveness be evaluated because of the poor methodological designs. More recent placebo-controlled studies involving small samples of TMD patients reported significant reduction in pain and dysfunction with the use of low-level laser therapy.[645,646] Because of the small sample size of these studies, further research is needed to support the use of low-level laser therapy in TMD treatment.

### Orthopedic appliance therapy

Interocclusal splints, orthotics, orthoses, biteguards, bite planes, nightguards, and bruxism appliances are routinely used in the treatment of TMDs. Removable acrylic resin appliances that cover the teeth have traditionally been used to alter occlusal relationships and redistribute occlusal forces,[647,648] to prevent wear and mobility of the teeth,[649] to reduce bruxism and parafunction,[650] to treat masticatory muscle pain and dysfunction,[492,537,651–655] to treat painful TMJs,[655–659] and to alter structural relationships in the TMJ.[660–663] Researchers do not agree, however, on how the appliances work or what the most effective occlusal design is.[656,663,664]

Generally, studies of appliance therapy have reported a reduction in orofacial pain and other symptoms associated with TMDs.[537,655,656,665,666] However, most studies have been limited by small sample size, short-term outcome, inadequate control groups, and failure to compare appliance therapy with other forms of treatment. Furthermore, several recent review articles[667–673] concluded that when these appliances were compared with an inactive placebo, they were mildly favorable, performing no better than nonoccluding appliances or other types of TMD therapies, such as behavioral modification or self-management strategies.

The complications that can occur with the excessive or incorrect use of any appliance include caries, gingival inflammation, mouth odors, speech difficulties, occlusal changes, and psychologic dependence on the appliance. Serious complications can include major, irreversible changes in functional and morphologic occlusal features as a result of long-term, full-time use of these appliances,[674,675] particularly with partial-arch coverage appliances.

**Stabilization appliances**

Also termed *flat plane*, *gnathologic*, or *muscle-relaxation appliances*, stabilization appliances cover all of the maxillary or mandibular teeth. Stabilization appliances are used as an adjunct for managing symptoms associated with myogenous[492,537,651-654] as well as arthrogenous TMDs.[676-678] Preferably, they are used at night only. Because acrylic is softer than enamel, these appliances have been used to reduce the chance of further tooth attrition in patients with nocturnal bruxism. Stabilization appliances can also be used for the management of an unstable occlusion, for example, missing multiple bilateral posterior tooth contacts. Occasionally, they are used to reduce clenching-induced earache, tooth pain, as well as some forms of temporal headache.[679-685]

Nocturnal EMG monitoring of the masseter muscle has shown a short-term decrease in the level of bruxism activity when an appliance is worn.[650,686,687] However, recent studies demonstrate that the response is variable and that bruxism is not eliminated with stabilization appliances.[134,651,688] These studies emphasize the variability of the clinical response to the appliances and the need for careful follow-up. The occlusal surface of the appliance should be adjusted to provide a stable physiologic mandibular posture by creating bilateral, even, posterior occlusal contacts for the opposing teeth on closure.[134] Appliances adjusted to a "neuromuscularly determined" mandibular position seem to show no advantage over conventional stabilization appliances.[303] Anterior guidance is usually provided by acrylic guide ramps in the canine or anterior areas of the appliance to separate the opposing posterior teeth from the appliance in all excursive movements of the mandible. Clinical experience suggests that the occlusal surface of the appliance should be adjusted initially and periodically to compensate for changes in the maxillomandibular relationship such as pain, muscle activity, inflammation, edema, or structural change in soft tissues.

In acute cases, the appliance may be worn full time for a specified period, and then only at night as symptom reduction occurs. In the case of ongoing nocturnal bruxism with morning pain, nighttime use is preferred. Patients who do not show a positive response within 3 to 4 weeks should be reevaluated. Failure to show an initial positive response does not necessarily indicate a need for more aggressive or prolonged therapy. Other factors should be considered, such as chronic pain behavior, noncompliance, misdiagnosis, or degree of pathologic changes in the TMJ.

Research on the use of stabilization appliances made with a soft, resilient material has provided mixed results regarding the effect of these appliances in reducing nocturnal bruxism and the signs and symptoms of TMDs.[686,689-692] Concern has been raised regarding the effect of using unadjusted appliances on occlusal contacts.[693] One study suggests that efficacy may be related to the stability of the appliance.[518] Recent studies compared soft appliances with hard acrylic appliances and found both to be equally effective in reducing painful symptoms[691,692]; however, they were no more effective than self-management techniques without appliance therapy.[692] At the present time, these appliances seem best suited for short-term treatment and for treatment of children with mixed dentition, as the soft appliance seems to have minimal effect on dental development.[689]

### Partial-coverage appliances

A recently popular partial-coverage appliance covers only the maxillary central incisors and contacts with only one or two opposing mandibular anterior teeth.[694,695] The working hypothesis was that occlusal forces applied to a few anterior teeth would be lighter than forces applied to a full occlusion. In a 3-month follow-up study, no differences in improvement were observed between TMD patients wearing this appliance and patients wearing a stabilization appliance,[696] but a 6-month follow-up study reported that more patients in the stabilization appliance group improved.[697]

Another example of a partial-coverage oral appliance covers only the posterior teeth. The posterior bite plane is usually fabricated for the mandibular teeth and consists of areas of hard acrylic positioned over the posterior teeth connected by a cast metal lingual bar. It has been advocated in cases of loss of vertical dimension or when there is a need to make major changes in anterior positioning of the mandible.[698] The efficacy of this type of appliance has been studied in only one small controlled trial.[699]

Studies supporting the efficacy of partial-coverage appliances in reducing TMD symptoms are limited by number and sample size. These appliances have the potential to produce a malocclusion[697] and possible internal TMJ changes. There is no evidence to state that they more effectively reduce TMD symptoms than full-arch appliances.

### Anterior positioning appliances

Anterior positioning appliances, also called *anterior repositioning appliances* or *mandibular orthopedic repositioning appliances*, can be fabricated for either dental arch, although the maxillary appliance is usually more effective at guiding the mandible into the protrusive position. All teeth in the arch are covered, and the opposing teeth are provided with minimal posterior occlusal indentations and a reverse guidance incline in the anterior segment of the appliance.[699,700] This design is aimed at encouraging a more comfortable therapeutic condyle-disc-fossa relationship. Anterior positioning appliances are used to decrease joint pain, joint noise (clicking), and associated secondary muscle symptoms in TMDs.[661-663,699,701,702] The primary indication for anterior positioning appliance therapy is acute joint pain associated with disc displacement with reduction.[537,701,703-705] Originally, full-time use of the appliance was suggested, with the intent to establish a new mandibular position with the disc "recaptured."[706,707] Although short-term success with full-time wear of anterior positioning appliances was good,[663,699] long-term success at establishing a new occlusal position with the disc recaptured has not been realized.[75,702,704,707-710] Therefore, attempts to achieve a new therapeutic mandibular position aimed at restoring the disc-condyle relationship with anterior positioning appliances should be restricted to few selected cases of articular pain that can only be managed by maintained mandibular positioning. In these cases, the patient needs to understand in advance the time and expense involved. Whether the appliance will be used full time or part time, the potential occlusal consequences need to be discussed with the patient prior to treatment, since mandibular repositioning can result in irreversible changes in the occlusion, such as a posterior open bite.[711]

An anterior positioning appliance may be effective in reducing symptoms associated with disc displacement with reduction. Nocturnal use of the appliance is also often effective for preventing intermittent disc displacement without reduction on awakening and reducing joint pain. Because the appliance is used only at night, the potential for occlusal changes is greatly reduced.

Full-time, short-term wear of the anterior repositioning appliance should be limited to cases with acute disc displacement without reduction (acute closed lock) if the dentist is able to reduce the disc (unlock the mandible). In such cases, restoring the disc-condyle relationship full-time for 5 to 7 days may reduce or prevent additional locking episodes and encourage adaptation. Once joint pain and dysfunction are decreased, the appliance use may be gradually reduced to nighttime wear only, and, if needed, eventually replaced with a stabilization appliance. These measures should allow the mandible to approximate the pretreatment occlusal position. This approach is strongly recommended to avoid or minimize the need for unnecessary restorative or orthodontic treatment, and is not intended to correct the disc-condyle relationship but to facilitate control of symptoms.[506] Clicking is not usually eliminated but may be decreased in intensity. In some instances, returning the patient to the preexisting occlusal condition reinitiates the painful joint symptoms, likely due to the lack of adaptation of the retrodiscal tissues. In most instances, immediately returning the patient to anterior positioning appliance therapy

will once again reduce the symptoms, and, in such cases, more time should be allowed for tissue adaptation to minimize the need for any permanent occlusal therapy. Only after repeated unsuccessful attempts to return the joint to an orthopedically stable position in the fossa should permanent occlusal therapy be considered.

Use of a stabilization appliance with adjunctive therapy for pain relief and improved function are also viable treatment options for TMJ internal derangement.[712-714] Asymptomatic clicks by themselves do not warrant treatment, and recent studies using TMJ imaging throw doubt on the need for a "perfect" disc position.[80] If improvement is not realized with orthopedic appliance therapy and adjunctive measures, and significant pain and mechanical symptoms persist, arthroscopy or open-joint surgery may be necessary.

## Occlusal therapy

The topic of occlusion remains an enigma to those interested in studying the pathophysiology of TMDs and the therapeutic concepts related to occlusal discrepancies. It is difficult to establish any significant cause and effect relationships due to the many variables involved with these multifactorial problems.[715,716] There are valid reasons for occlusal treatment for many dental conditions, such as lack of interarch/intra-arch tooth stability; tooth mobility; fremitus; occlusally related fracture of a tooth or restoration; tooth sensitivity; altered or compromised masticatory function, swallowing, or speech; and compromised supporting tissues due to adverse loading. Although occlusally related dental treatment may be necessary for patients with TMDs, it is believed to be infrequently necessary for the purpose of treating TMDs.[721]

The use of anterior positioning appliances to correct the disc-condyle relationship in TMJ disc displacement has led to the concept of two-phased treatment. This treatment approach was especially popular in the late 1970s and during the 1980s. Phase I involved the use of the anterior positioning appliance and any adjunctive therapies, and phase II involved rearticulation of the teeth in the newly acquired therapeutic mandibular position through definitive, irreversible occlusal treatment, including occlusal adjustment, restorative dental treatment, and orthodontic or orthognathic treatment. It is strongly suggested that use of the terms *phase I* and *phase II* in the treatment of TMDs be discontinued, as they imply that phase II inevitably follows phase I. The scientific literature does not support the need for two-phase treatment because definitive occlusal therapy is not required for the effective treatment of most TMDs.[717] Despite the lack of scientific support, the two-stage philosophy continues to be promoted by many continuing education courses, and the concept of an occlusal etiology for TMDs is adhered to by many dental professionals.[718]

Primary occlusal therapy should be used with caution, because there is no clear evidence that natural occlusal morphologic variation is a common cause of TMDs.[159-161,717,719] Based on current evidence, the routine emphasis of treating chronic malocclusions to treat TMDs is unsupported. Because TMDs, especially involving TMJ pathology, may affect the dental occlusion, malocclusion may be a consequence of a TMD rather than a cause.[162,421] The clinician should not proceed with occlusal treatment to correct the resultant malocclusion until reasonably assured that the TMJ pathology is stable and no further changes are likely. Evidence of stability may be obtained through longitudinal monitoring of pain symptoms, occlusal relationships, TMJ imaging, and cephalometric analysis. The risk of recurrence or progression should be clearly communicated to the patient before initiating the definitive occlusal treatment.

The clinician is advised to proceed cautiously, using the least invasive procedures possible.[499] The pretreatment intercuspal relationship should be preserved whenever possible. There is no evidence that anterior guidance is superior to other forms of guidance for treating TMD symptoms related to nocturnal bruxism,[720,721] and anterior guidance may not provide optimal joint loading for all TMD articular conditions.[273,722] Thus, altering the occlusion to provide anterior guidance for patients with TMDs is questionable. In general, there is a lack of evidence that complex occlusal therapy to provide an idealized dental occlusion is necessary for routine TMD management.[155,713,719,723]

### Occlusal adjustment

Occlusal adjustment was at one time considered beneficial for TMDs, and occlusal interferences were implicated in the cause of TMDs. However, there is no agreement or evidence on which type of occlusal interference, if any, might impede mandibular function or play an etiologic role in the development of TMDs.[168] Review of studies revealed that artificial occlusal interferences failed to induce TMD symptoms[168,724] but did reduce masseter activity.[724] A Cochrane Database systematic review[725] and several other systematic reviews of RCTs[168,672,726] showed that there was not enough evidence to conclude that occlusal adjustments are useful to prevent or treat TMDs. For these reasons and because occlusal adjustment is an irreversible treatment modality, it should rarely be considered for primary treatment in TMDs. The reviews agree that occlusal adjustment may be considered as a treatment option to improve mandibular stability in cases where specific TMD disturbances have resulted in an unstable occlusal relationship, or when an occlusal interference related to a recent restoration precipitates symptoms.

**Restorative therapy**

Restorative dental care should never be a primary treatment option for TMDs.[717] Once stability and symptom resolution are achieved, restorative therapy has been suggested for patients who might benefit from reduction of adverse loading and redistribution of occlusal forces, as suggested by earlier studies.[727-729] However, as with other irreversible occlusal therapies like occlusal adjustment, their efficacy for TMDs is not predictable, and further research on the influence of dental occlusion on TMJ loading is needed. There are a few instances when the occlusal condition is associated with TMD symptoms by way of functional mandibular instability. In these instances, the occlusal condition must be addressed, but any extensive restorative therapy in TMD patients should be undertaken with caution. Sudden, radical changes in occlusion in these patients carry some risk, although the occlusal alterations are usually well tolerated according to human[175,730] and animal[180] studies.

**Orthodontic-orthognathic therapy**

Orthodontic treatment is often the treatment of choice when major occlusal alterations are considered to be advantageous. Fixed, removable, functional, and extraoral orthodontic appliances are all capable of improving occlusal and mandibular stability.[731] Orthodontics has been suggested as a follow-up treatment to anterior positioning appliance therapy to correct TMJ disc displacement. However, this treatment has not proven to be as successful on a longitudinal basis as anterior positioning appliance therapy alone.[708,732] Orthodontic therapy does present some risk of destabilizing the masticatory system during treatment[733] and, therefore, the orthodontic diagnosis and treatment plan must consider possible influences of resulting occlusal instability during treatment on preexisting TMDs.[734,735]

Many retrospective clinical studies have examined the relationship between orthodontic treatment and TMDs and have found no significant correlation on a population basis.[198,736-747] Additionally, several recent prospective long-term studies also confirm no correlation between orthodontic treatment in childhood and increased risk of developing TMDs later in life.[682,748-751] Orthodontic treatment with premolar extraction has been specifically implicated in the development of TMDs through incisor retraction and subsequent distalization of the mandible.[752] However, studies comparing orthodontic treatments with and without premolar extraction have found no difference in posttreatment condylar position,[753-756] overbite,[755] discrepancy between ICP and RCP,[757] mandibular position,[758] or symptoms of TMDs.[745,758-760]

A prospective study of posttreatment changes in the TMJ found no statistically significant correlation between changes in the condyle-fossa relationship based on age, sex, skeletal or dental variables, signs or symptoms of TMDs, headgear use, type of elastics, or nonextraction versus extraction treatment.[761] In addition, some longitudinal studies suggest that a history of orthodontic treatment tends to be associated with a lower prevalence of TMD signs and symptoms than no history of orthodontic treatment.[682,738,762] A recent review of the literature concluded that, based on the available evidence, orthodontic treatment "neither causes nor cures TMD."[763]

Although as a group there is little evidence that orthodontically treated patients have a greater prevalence of TMD symptoms, the individual patient response to the dental instabilities associated with orthodontic treatment may be quite different. Thus, the orthodontist must be alert for, and be prepared to deal with, the onset or exacerbation of TMD signs and symptoms that may occur during orthodontic tooth movement. The potential for problems clearly mandates a pretreatment TMD screening examination for all orthodontic patients.[764]

Orthognathic surgery may be considered in conjunction with orthodontic or restorative treatment for correction of skeletal malocclusions. However, when it is considered in TMD patients, orthognathic surgery should always be preceded by a careful evaluation to confirm reasonable symptom resolution and stability of the maxillomandibular relationship as well as to assess and manage any other contributing factors. Surgical treatment for skeletal asymmetries and growth anomalies with the intent of alleviating pain associated with TMDs is rarely indicated. However, in those TMD patients with severe skeletal malocclusion who desire greater occlusal stability or improved esthetics, orthognathic treatment is often the method of choice.[741,765–767] Two retrospective studies showed no increase in TMD signs and symptoms in patients with juvenile rheumatoid arthritis[768] or patients with anterior open bites[769] who underwent or-

thognathic surgery. One other study showed that in patients with rigid fixation, symptoms of clicking and muscle pain improved after orthognathic surgery, whereas these symptoms increased in patients with nonrigid fixation.[770] While prospective studies and systematic reviews are lacking, the available literature indicates that orthognathic surgery in patients with TMDs does not generally exacerbate or improve the condition and, hence, is a feasible option for those who desire it.

## Surgery

TMJ surgery is effective for specific articular disorders. However, the complexity of surgical techniques, potential complications, prevalence of behavioral and psychosocial contributing factors, and availability of nonsurgical approaches suggest that TMJ surgery should only be used in selected cases.

The decision to treat the patient surgically depends on the degree of pathology or anatomic derangement present within the joint, the potential for repair of the condition, the outcome of appropriate nonsurgical treatment, and the degree of impairment the problem creates for the patient. The appropriate duration and complexity of nonsurgical treatment prior to consideration of surgery is determined by a combination of factors including the expected prognosis in comparison with actual improvement, the degree of impairment, and patient compliance. Patients with complicating factors, such as pending litigation, depression, or uncontrolled nocturnal bruxism, may have a poor surgical prognosis. The clinician must have a full knowledge and appreciation of the potential for surgical failure and complications, including neuropathic pain disorders (eg, deafferentation pain). A realistic discussion of the prognosis, the patient's expectations, and the complicating factors can provide the patient with the information necessary to make an informed decision.

Preoperative and postoperative nonsurgical management must be integrated into the overall surgical treatment plan.[771] This therapy is directed at decreasing the functional load placed on the joint, eliminating or modifying contributing factors such as parafunctional oral habits, and providing appropriate psychologic and medical support. The clinical practice guidelines for TMJ surgery of the American Association of Oral and Maxillofacial Surgeons state that TMJ surgery is only indicated when nonsurgical therapy has been ineffective and is not indicated for asymptomatic or minimally symptomatic cases.[772] In addition, surgery should not be performed for preventive reasons. Indications for surgery include moderate to severe pain and/or dysfunction that is disabling.[772] Surgical management may include joint lavage (arthrocentesis), closed surgical procedures (arthroscopy), and open surgical procedures (arthrotomy/arthroplasty).

### Arthrocentesis

*Arthrocentesis* involves simple intra-articular irrigation or lavage of the TMJ with or without deposition of corticosteroids. It has been suggested that this method may be as effective as arthroscopy when used with joint mobilization in the treatment of intra-articular joint restrictions of mandibular movement such as internal derangement without reduction.[773,774] However, it also can be used as a palliative procedure for patients with acute episodes of degenerative[775] or rheumatoid[776] arthritis and to relieve the pain in patients who have painful clicking in the TMJ that does not respond to medical management. A recent review identified 19 studies that evaluated the outcomes of arthrocentesis in patients with different types of internal derangement.[777] The review revealed successful treatment outcomes in 83% of the cases but noted that most studies had methodological flaws. Many were uncontrolled case series, and only one of the studies was an RCT. Before the efficacy of this procedure can be confirmed, more RCTs are needed.

### Arthroscopy

Arthroscopy allows direct observation and sampling of the joint tissues[778,779] and holds promise as a modality for treating painful joints and joints with hypomobility secondary to a persistent nonreducing displaced disc. Arthroscopic revision of previous open surgery has been found to be helpful in alleviating postoperative pain and intracapsular fibrosis.[780] At this time, arthroscopy is primarily performed in the upper joint space and is used for minor debridement and lavage, cutting of minor adhesions, and biopsies. Reduction of symptoms following arthroscopic surgery is not due to improved disc position.[781,782] Postsurgical MRIs reveal that most patients have persistent anterior disc displacement but increased disc mobility.[783-788] The prognosis of arthroscopy appears comparable with that of discectomy and discoplasty.[789-794] Because it is less invasive than open joint surgeries, arthroscopic surgery should have preference whenever possible. A recent meta-analysis reported the efficacy of arthrocentesis and arthroscopy as treatment for disc displacement without reduction that was refractory to nonsurgical modalities.[795]

## Arthrotomy

Open surgical intervention of the TMJ (arthrotomy) is usually required for bony or fibrous ankylosis, neoplasia, severe chronic dislocations, persistent painful disc derangement, and severe osteoarthritis refractory to conservative modalities of treatment.[779] Surgery is less often indicated for displaced condylar fractures, agenesis of the condyle, and severe, painful chronic arthritides. Surgery is seldom, if ever, indicated for inflammatory joint disorders (synovitis or capsulitis), condylysis, and nonpainful degenerative arthritis. Arthrotomy is generally indicated for the patient with advanced TMJ disease who meets the surgical criteria and has disease refractory to or not amenable to arthroscopic surgical techniques.

Open-joint surgical procedures include discoplasty, disc repositioning, discectomy with or without replacement, arthroplasty including high condylectomy, and total joint reconstruction/replacements. Discoplasty and disc repositioning with plication have been reported to have an 80% to 90% success rate in reducing joint pain and noise and increasing mouth opening, although short of normal ranges.[789,796-799]

Discectomy without replacement has the longest history and the most reports of long-term success (up to 30 years).[800-803] Use of a dermal graft in discectomy does not appear to prevent remodeling but may be beneficial in eliminating or preventing joint noises.[804]

The success obtained with less invasive procedures has greatly reduced the need for arthroplasty. Condylectomy (subcondylar osteotomy) and condylotomy are performed infrequently. These procedures have been indicated for more complex disease or traumatic conditions,[805,806] and the risk of postsurgical complications, including marked occlusal changes, is higher with these procedures. Modified condylotomy (using an intraoral vertical ramus osteotomy) in the treatment of TMJ internal derangement can reduce related pain and predictably correct disc position.[807-809] Further controlled investigations are needed to test these applications.

# Clinical Research

Decisions regarding the clinical management of disease are commonly based on empirical observation and experience. This process is appropriate within limits but is compromised by personal biases and preferences. Clinical research on various treatment strategies is required to overcome these personal prejudices and aid in setting general standards of care. The most powerful clinical test for alternative treatment methods is the RCT.[810,811] Such a prospective clinical trial requires well-defined criteria for the study population, randomized assignment to competing treatments, an untreated control group, blinded pre- and posttreatment examination using reliable and valid outcome measurements, and inferential statistical analysis. Technical barriers, expense, and moral restraints at times limit the application of this method, but the design serves as a model for all clinical investigations of treatment, including retrospective patient surveys.[811] Feinstein[812,813] has described methods to adapt this rigid experimental design to the clinical setting.

At this time, the term *evidence-based* is very popular in research. Many systematic reviews have been conducted to evaluate whether the different treatment modalities offered to patients actually have scientific proof of efficacy. While this is a good start, there is no consensus with regard to the best methods of accomplishing such a systematic review. Hence, different systematic reviews may use dissimilar inclusion and evaluation criteria and statistical methods, which may lead to opposing views on the conclusions reached. Caution should be taken when interpreting the conclusions of these studies. Just because several systematic reviews conclude that there is a lack of evidence that a certain treatment is effective does not necessarily mean that the treatment modality is ineffective; rather, it may mean that there have not been any or enough well-done clinical RCTs.

Despite increasing evidence that TMDs are best managed with conservative reversible treatments, some clinicians continue to choose treatments based on personal biases rather than controlled scientific investigation.[718,733] There continues to be a need for RCTs for nonsurgical and surgical treatments for TMDs. In addition, studies designed to elucidate the cause of TMDs are much needed. Practicing clinicians, who are involved in the treatment of TMDs on a daily basis, should be knowledgeable in clinical trial methodology and be able to critically appraise the literature on which they base their treatment decisions. As readers and clinicians become more discriminating, TMD patients will benefit.

# References

1. Okeson JP. Management of Temporomandibular Disorders and Occlusion, ed 5. St Louis: Mosby, 2003.
2. Fred L. Anatomy of the Head, Neck, Face and Jaws. Philadelphia: Lea & Febiger, 1980.
3. Scapino RP. The posterior attachment: Its structure, function, and appearance in TMJ imaging studies. Part I. J Craniomandib Disord Facial Oral Pain 1991;5:83–95.
4. Scapino RP. The posterior attachment: Its structure, function, and appearance in TMJ imaging studies. Part 2. J Craniomandib Disord Facial Oral Pain 1991;5:155–166.
5. Dubrul E. The craniomandibular articulation. In: Sicher's Oral Anatomy, ed 7. St Louis: Mosby, 1980: 147–209.
6. Meikle MC. Remodeling. In: Sarnat BG, Laskin DM, (eds). The Temporomandibular Joint. A Biological Basis for Clinical Practice, ed 4. Philadelphia: Saunders, 1992:93–107.
7. Waltimo A, Kemppainen P, Kononen M. Maximal contraction force and endurance of human jaw-closing muscles in isometric clenching. Scand J Dent Res 1993;101:416–421.
8. McNamara JA Jr. The independent functions of the two heads of the lateral pterygoid muscles. Am J Anat 1973;13:197–206.
9. Meyenberg K, Kubik S, Palla S. Relationships of the muscles of mastication to the articular disc of the temporomandibular joint. Helv Odontol Acta 1986; 30:1–20.
10. Wilkinson TM. The relationship between the disc and the lateral pterygoid muscle in the human temporomandibular joint. J Prosthet Dent 1988;60:715–724.
11. Heylings DJ, Nielsen IL, McNeill C. Lateral pterygoid muscle and the temporomandibular disc. J Orofac Pain 1995;9:9–16.
12. Hylander WL. Functional anatomy. In: Sarnat BG, Laskin DM (eds). The Temporomandibular Joint: A Biological Basis for Clinical Practice, ed 4. Philadelphia: Saunders, 1992:60–92.
13. Glaros AG, Rao SM. Effects of bruxism: A review of the literature. J Prosthet Dent 1977;38:149–157.
14. Rugh JD, Harlan J. Nocturnal bruxism and temporomandibular disorders. Adv Neurol 1988;49:329–341.
15. Okeson JP. Bell's Orofacial Pain, ed 5. Chicago: Quintessence, 2005.
16. Rugh JD, Solberg WK. Oral health status in the United States. Temporomandibular disorders. J Dent Educ 1985;49:398–404.
17. Schiffman E, Fricton JR. Epidemiology of the TMJ and craniofacial pain. In: Fricton JR, Kroening RJ, Hathaway KM (eds). TMJ and Craniofacial Pain: Diagnosis and Management. St Louis: IEA, 1988:1–10.
18. De Kanter RJAM, Truin GJ, Burgersdijk RCW, et al. Prevalence in the Dutch adult population and a meta-analysis of signs and symptoms of temporomandibular disorders. J Dent Res 1993;72:1509–1518.
19. Dworkin SF, Huggins KH, LeResche L, et al. Epidemiology of signs and symptoms in temporomandibular disorders: Clinical signs in cases and controls. J Am Dent Assoc 1990;120:273–281.
20. Wabeke KB, Spruijt RJ. On Temporomandibular Joint Sounds: Dental and Psychological Studies [thesis]. Amsterdam: Univ of Amsterdam, 1994.

21. Huber NU, Hall EH. A comparison of the signs of temporomandibular joint dysfunction and occlusal discrepancies in a symptom-free population of men and women. Oral Surg Oral Med Oral Pathol 1990; 70:180-183.

22. LeResche L. Epidemiology of temporomandibular disorders: Implications for the investigation of etiologic factors. Crit Rev Oral Biol Med 1997;8:291-305.

23. Anastassaki A, Magnusson T. Patients referred to a specialist clinic because of suspected temporomandibular disorders: A survey of 3194 patients in respect of diagnoses, treatments, and treatment outcome. Acta Odontol Scand 2004;62:183-192.

24. Randolph CS, Greene CS, Moretti R, Forbes D, Perry HT. Conservative management of temporomandibular disorders: A posttreatment comparison between patients from a university clinic and from private practice. Am J Orthod Dentofac Orthop 1990;98:77-82.

25. Nickerson JW, Boering G. Natural course of osteoarthrosis as it relates to internal derangement of the temporomandibular joint. Oral Maxillofac Surg Clin North Am 1989;1:1-19.

26. Egermark I, Carlsson GE, Magnusson T. A 20-year longitudinal study of subjective symptoms of temporomandibular disorders from childhood to adulthood. Acta Odontol Scand 2001;59(1):40-48.

27. De Leeuw R, Boering G, Stegenga B, de Bont LGM. Temporomandibular joint osteoarthrosis: Clinical and radiographic characteristics 30 years after nonsurgical treatment. A preliminary report. Cranio 1993;11:15-24.

28. Keeling SD, McGorray S, Wheeler TT, King GJ. Risk factors associated with temporomandibular joint sounds in children 6 to 12 years of age. Am J Orthod Dentofac Orthop 1994;105:279-287.

29. Verdonck A, Takada K, Kitai N, et al. The prevalence of cardinal TMJ dysfunction symptoms and its relationship to occlusal factors in Japanese female adolescents. J Oral Rehabil 1994;21:687-697.

30. Suvinen TI, Nystrom M, Evalahti M, Kleemola-Kujala E, Waltimo A, Kononen M. An 8 year follow-up study of temporomandibular disorder and psychosomatic symptoms from adolescence to young adulthood. J Orofac Pain 2004;18:126-130.

31. Motegi E, Miyasaki H, Oguka I. An orthodontic study of temporomandibular joint disorders. Part I. Epidemiological research in Japanese 6-18 year olds. Angle Orthod 1992;62:249-256.

32. Wanman A, Agerberg G. Temporomandibular joint sounds in adolescents: A longitudinal study. Oral Surg Oral Med Oral Pathol 1990;69:2-9.

33. Magnusson T, Egermark I, Carlsson GE. Five year longitudinal study of signs and symptoms of mandibular dysfunction in adolescents. Cranio 1986;4:338-344.

34. Wabeke KB, Spruijt RJ, Habets LL. Spatial and morphologic aspects of temporomandibular joints with sounds. J Oral Rehabil 1995;22(1):21-27.

35. Nilner M, Kopp S. Distribution by age and sex of functional disturbances and diseases of the stomatognathic system in 7-18 year olds. Swed Dent J 1983;7: 191-198.

36. Levitt SR, McKinney MW. Validating the TMJ scale in a national sample of 10,000 patients: Demographic and epidemiologic characteristics. J Orofac Pain 1994; 8:25-35.

37. Widmalm SE, Westesson PL, Kim IK, Pereira FJ Jr, Lundh H, Tasaki MM. Temporomandibular joint pathosis related to age, sex, and dentition in autopsy material. Oral Surg Oral Med Oral Pathol 1994;78:416-425.

38. Pereira FJ Jr, Lundh H, Westesson PL. Morphologic changes in the temporomandibular joint in different age groups. An autopsy investigation. Oral Surg Oral Med Oral Pathol 1994;78:279-287.

39. Howard JA. Temporomandibular joint disorders, facial pain and dental problems of performing artists. In: Sataloff R, Brandfonbrener A, Lederman R (eds). Textbook of Performing Arts Medicine. New York: Raven Press, 1991:111-169.

40. Koidis PT, Zarifi A, Grigoriadou E, Garefis P. Effect of age and sex on craniomandibular disorders. J Prosthet Dent 1993;69:93-101.

41. Lipton JA, Ship JA, Larach-Robinson D. Estimated prevalence and distribution of reported orofacial pain in the United States. J Am Dent Assoc 1993;125:125-135.

42. Osterberg T, Carlsson GE, Wedel A, Johansson V. A cross-sectional and longitudinal study of craniomandibular dysfunction in an elderly population. J Craniomandib Disord Facial Oral Pain 1992;6:237-246.

43. Greene CS. Temporomandibular disorders in the geriatric population. J Prosthet Dent 1994;72:507-509.

44. Kaunisaho K, Hiitunen K, Ainamo A. Prevalence of symptoms of craniomandibular disorders in a population of elderly inhabitants in Helsinki, Finland. Acta Odontol Scand 1994;52:135-139.

45. Magnusson T, Egermark I, Carlsson GE. A longitudinal epidemiologic study of signs and symptoms of temporomandibular disorders from 15-35 years of age. J Orofac Pain 2000;14:310-319.

46. Magnusson T, Egermark I, Carlsson GE. A prospective investigation over two decades on signs and symptoms of temporomandibular disorders and associated variables. A final summary. Acta Odontol Scand 2005; 63:99-109.

47. Agerberg G, Carlsson GE. Functional disorders of the masticatory system. I. Distribution of symptoms according to age and sex as judged from investigation by questionnaire. Acta Odontol Scand 1972;30:597-613.

48. Helkimo M. Studies on function and dysfunction of the masticatory system. I. An epidemiological investigation of symptoms of dysfunction in Lapps in the North of Finland. Proc Finn Dent Soc 1974;70:37–49.

49. Helkimo M. Studies on function and dysfunction of the masticatory system. II. Index for anamnestic and clinical dysfunction and occlusal state. Swed Dent J 1974;67:101–121.

50. Hansson T, Nilner M. A study of the occurrence of symptoms of diseases of the temporomandibular joint, masticatory musculature, and related structures. J Oral Rehabil 1975;2:313–324.

51. Swanljung O, Rantanen T. Functional disorders of the masticatory system in southwest Finland. Community Dent Oral Epidemiol 1979;7:177–182.

52. Heft MW. Prevalence of TMJ signs and symptoms in the elderly. Gerontology 1984;3:125–130.

53. Glass EG, McGlynn FD, Glaros AG, Melton K, Romans K. Prevalence of temporomandibular disorder symptoms in a major metropolitan area. Cranio 1993;11:217–220.

54. Agerberg G, Bergenholz A. Craniomandibular disorders in adult populations of West Bothnia, Sweden. Acta Odontol Scand 1989;47:129–140.

55. Salonen L, Hellden L. Prevalence of signs and symptoms of dysfunction in the masticatory system: An epidemiologic study in an adult Swedish population. J Craniomandib Disord Facial Oral Pain 1990;4:241–250.

56. Sigueria JTT, Ching LH. Orofacial pain in totally edentulous patients with temporomandibular disorders: A retrospective longitudinal study. Rev Paul Odontol 1999;21(3):32–37.

57. Solberg WK, Woo MW, Houston JB. Prevalence of mandibular dysfunction in young adults. J Am Dent Assoc 1979;98:25–34.

58. Pullinger A, Seligman DA, Solberg W. Temporomandibular disorders. Part I. Functional status, dentomorphologic features, and sex differences in a nonpatient population. J Prosthet Dent 1988;59:228–235.

59. Agerberg G, Inkapool I. Craniomandibular disorders in an urban Swedish population. J Craniomandib Disord Facial Oral Pain 1990;4:154–164.

60. Magnusson T, Carlsson GE, Egermark I. Changes in subjective symptoms of craniomandibular disorders in children and adolescents during a 10-year period. J Orofac Pain 1993;7:76–82.

61. De Leeuw JR Jr, Steenks MH, Ros WJG, Bosman F, Winnubst JA, Scholte AM. Psychosocial aspects of craniomandibular dysfunction. An assessment of clinical and community findings. J Oral Rehabil 1994;21: 127–143.

62. Centore L, Bianchi P, McNeill C. The relationships between non-organic multiple physical complaints and narcissism [abstract 1084]. J Dent Res 1989;68(special issue):317.

63. Skeppar J, Nilner M. Treatment of craniomandibular disorders in children and young adults. J Orofac Pain 1993;7:362–369.

64. Bush FM, Harkins SW, Harrington WG, Price DD. Analysis of gender effects on pain perception and symptom presentation of temporomandibular pain. Pain 1993;53:73–80.

65. Phillips JM, Gatchel RJ, Wesley AL, Ellis E. Clinical implications of sex in acute temporomandibular disorders. J Am Dent Assoc 2001;132:49–57.

66. Luz JGC, Oliviera NG. Incidence of temporomandibular joint disorders in patients seen at a hospital emergency room. J Oral Rehabil 1994;21:349–351.

67. Turp JC, Schindler HJ. Chronic temporomandibular disorders. Schmerz 2004;18:109–117.

68. Dworkin SF, Le Resche L. Temporomandibular disorder pain: Epidemiologic data. APS Bulletin 1993;3 (April/May):12–13.

69. Schiffman E, Fricton JR, Haley D, Shapiro BL. The prevalence and treatment needs of subjects with temporomandibular disorders. J Am Dent Assoc 1989; 120:295–304.

70. Greene CS, Marbach JJ. Epidemiologic studies of mandibular dysfunction: A critical review. J Prosthet Dent 1982;48(2):184–190.

71. De Kanter RJ, Kayser AF, Battistuzzi PG, Truin GJ, Van'T Hof MA. Demand and need for treatment of craniomandibular dysfunction in the Dutch adult population. J Dent Res 1992;71:1607–1612.

72. Von Korff M, LeResche L, Dworkin SF. First onset of common pain symptoms: A prospective study of depression as a risk factor. Pain 1993;55:251–258.

73. Magnusson T, Egermark I, Carlsson GE. Treatment received, treatment demand, and treatment need for temporomandibular disorders in 35-year old subjects. Cranio 2002;20:11–17.

74. Magnusson T, Carlsson GE, Egermark I. Changes in clinical signs of craniomandibular disorders from the age of 15-25 years. J Orofac Pain 1994;8:207–215.

75. Lundh H, Westesson PL, Kopp S. A three-year follow-up of patients with reciprocal temporomandibular joint clicking. Oral Surg Oral Med Oral Pathol 1987; 63:530–533.

76. Lobbezoo-Scholte AM, de Leeuw JR, Steenks MH, et al. Diagnostic subgroups of craniomandibular disorders. Part I. Self-report data and clinical findings. J Orofac Pain 1995;9:24–36.

77. Pullinger A, Seligman DA. Overbite and overjet characteristics of refined diagnostic groups of temporomandibular disorders. Am J Orthod Dentofac Orthop 1991;100:401–415.

78. Alexander SR, Moore RN, DuBois LM. Mandibular condyle position. Comparison of articular mountings and magnetic resonance imaging. Am J Orthod Dentofac Orthop 1993;104:230–239.

79. Romanelli GG, Harper R, Mock D, Pharoah MJ, Tenenbaum HC. Evaluation of temporomandibular joint internal derangement. J Orofac Pain 1993;7:254–262.

80. Kircos LT, Ortendahl DA, Mark AS, Arakana M. Magnetic resonance imaging of the TMJ disc in asymptomatic volunteers. J Oral Maxillofac Surg 1987;45:852.

81. Pereira FJ Jr, Lundh H, Westesson PL, Carlsson LE. Clinical findings related to morphologic changes in TMJ autopsy specimens. Oral Surg Oral Med Oral Pathol 1994;78:288–295.

82. McNeill C. Craniomandibular (TMJ) disorders—The state of the art. Part II. Accepted diagnosis and treatment modalities. J Prosthet Dent 1983;49:393–397.

83. McNeill C, Danzig WM, Farrar WB, et al. Craniomandibular (TMJ) disorders—The state of the art. Position Paper of the American Academy of Craniomandibular Disorders. J Prosthet Dent 1980;44:434–437.

84. Fricton JR, Kroening RJ, Hathaway KM (eds). TM Disorders and Craniofacial Pain: Diagnosis and Management. St Louis: Ishiaku Euro America, 1988.

85. Parker MW. A dynamic model of etiology in temporomandibular disorders. J Am Dent Assoc 1990;120: 283–289.

86. Dijkgraaf LC, De Bont LG, Boering G, Liem RS. The structure, biochemistry, and metabolism of osteoarthritic cartilage: A review of the literature. J Oral Maxillofac Surg 1995;53:1182–1192.

87. Dijkgraaf LC, De Bont LGM, Boering G, Liem RS. Normal cartilage structure, biochemistry, and metabolism: A review of the literature. J Oral Maxillofac Surg 1995;53:924–929.

88. Harkins SJ. Extrinsic trauma and temporomandibular dysfunction. Cranio 1986;4:1–2.

89. Harkins SJ, Marteney JL. Extrinsic trauma: A significant precipitating factor in temporomandibular dysfunction. J Prosthet Dent 1985;54:271–272.

90. Braun BL, Di Giovanna A, Schiffman E, Bonnema J, Fricton JR. A cross-sectional study of temporomandibular joint dysfunction in post-cervical trauma patients. J Craniomandib Disord Facial Oral Pain 1992;6:24–31.

91. Katzberg RW, Tallents RH, Hayakawa K, Miller TL, Goske MJ, Wood BP. Internal derangements of the temporomandibular joint: Findings in the pediatric age group. Radiology 1985;154:125–127.

92. Pullinger A, Seligman DA. TMJ osteoarthrosis: A differentiation of diagnostic subgroups by symptom history and demographics. J Craniomandib Disord Facial Oral Pain 1987;1:251–256.

93. Pullinger A, Seligman DA. Trauma history in diagnostic groups of temporomandibular disorders. Oral Surg Oral Med Oral Pathol 1991;71:529–534.

94. De Boever JA, Keersmaekers K. Trauma in patients with temporomandibular disorders: Frequency and treatment outcome. J Oral Rehabil 1996;23:91–96.

95. Burgess J. Symptom characteristics in TMD patients reporting blunt trauma and/or whiplash injury. J Craniomandib Disord Facial Oral Pain 1991;5:251–257.

96. Vichaichalermvong S, Nilner M, Panmekiate S, Petersson A. Clinical follow-up with different disc positions. J Orofac Pain 1993;7:61–67.

97. Huang GJ, Rue TC. Third-molar extraction as a risk factor for temporomandibular disorder. J Am Dent Assoc 2006;137:1547–1554.

98. Gould DB, Banes CH. Iatrogenic disruptions of right temporomandibular joints during orotracheal intubation causing permanent closed lock of the jaw. Anesth Analg 1995;81(1):191–194.

99. Domino KB, Posner KL, Caplan RA, Cheney FW. Airway injury during anesthesia: A closed claims analysis. Anesthesiology 1999;91:1703–1711.

100. Weinberg S, Lapointe H. Cervical extension-flexion injury (whiplash) and internal derangement of the temporomandibular joint. J Oral Maxillofac Surg 1987;45:653–666.

101. Kronn E. The incidence of TMJ dysfunction in patients who have suffered a cervical whiplash injury following a traffic accident. J Orofac Pain 1993;7:209–213.

102. Goldberg HL. Trauma and the improbable anterior displacement. J Craniomandib Disord Facial Oral Pain 1990;4:131–134.

103. Kasch H, Hjorth T, Svensson P, Nyhuus L, Jensen TS. Temporomandibular disorders after whiplash injury: A controlled, prospective study. J Orofac Pain 2002;16:118–128.

104. Burgess J, Kolbinson DA, Lee PT, Epstein JB. Motor vehicle accidents and TMDs: Assessing the relationship. J Am Dent Assoc 1996;127:1767–1772.

105. Howard RP, Benedict JV, Raddin JH, Smith HL. Assessing neck extension-flexion as a basis for temporomandibular joint dysfunction. J Oral Maxillofac Surg 1991;39:1210–1213.

106. Szabo TJ, Welcher J, Anderson RD. Human occupant kinematic response to low speed rear-end impacts. In: Proceedings of the Thirty Eighth Stapp Car Crash Conference. Warrendale, Pennsylvania: Society of Automotive Engineers, 1994:23–35. SAE 940532.

107. Wright EF. Referred craniofacial pain patterns in patients with temporomandibular disorders. J Am Dent Assoc 2000;131:1307–1315.

108. Wright EF. Manual of Temporomandibular Disorders. Ames, IA: Blackwell Publishing, 2005.

109. Simons DG, Travell JG, Simons LS. Apropos of all muscles. In: Simons DG, Travell JG, Simons LS. Myofascial Pain and Dysfunction: The Trigger Point Manual, ed 2. Baltimore: Lipincott Williams & Wilkins, 1999:94–177.

110. Marbach JJ, Raphael KG, Dohrenwend BP, Lennon MC. The validity of tooth grinding measures: Etiology of pain dysfunction syndrome revisited. J Am Dent Assoc 1990;120:327–333.

111. Marbach JJ. The 'temporomandibular pain dysfunction syndrome' personality: Fact or fiction? J Oral Rehabil 1992;19:545–660.

112. Scholte AM, Steenks MH, Bosman F. Characteristics and treatment outcome of diagnostic subgroups of CMD patients: A retrospective study. Community Dent Oral Epidemiol 1993;21:215–220.

113. Nilner M. Relationships between oral parafunctions and functional disturbances in the stomatognathic system among 15 to 18 year olds. Acta Odontol Scand 1983;41:197–201.

114. Schiffman E, Fricton JR, Harley D. The relationship of occlusion, parafunctional habits and recent life events to mandibular dysfunction in a non-patient population. J Oral Rehabil 1992;19:201–223.

115. Dao TT, Lund JP, Lavigne GJ. Comparison of pain and quality of life in bruxers and patients with myofascial pain of the masticatory muscles. J Orofac Pain 1994;8:350–356.

116. Attanasio R. An overview of bruxism and its management. Dent Clin North Am 1997;41:229–241.

117. Faulkner KD. Bruxism: A review of the literature. Part I. Aust Dent J 1990;35:266–276.

118. Faulkner KD. Bruxism: A review of the literature. Part II. Aust Dent J 1990;35:355–361.

119. Glaros AG, Forbes D, Shanker J, Glass EG. Effect of parafunctional clenching on temporomandibular disorder pain and proprioceptive awareness. Cranio 2000;18:198–204.

120. Nitzan DW. 'Friction and adhesive forces'–Possible underlying causes for temporomandibular joint internal derangement. Cells Tissues Organs 2003;174:6–16.

121. Glaros AG, Burton E. Parafunctional clenching, pain, and effort in temporomandibular disorders. J Behav Med 2004;27:91–100.

122. Castelo PM, Gaviao MB, Pereira LJ, Bonjardim LR. Relationship between oral parafunctional/nutritive sucking habits and temporomandibular joint dysfunction in primary dentition. Int J Paediatr Dent 2005;15:29–36.

123. Pullinger A, Seligman DA. The degree to which attrition characterizes differentiated patient groups of temporomandibular disorders. J Orofac Pain 1993;7:196–208.

124. Rugh JD. Association between bruxism and TMD. In: McNeill C (ed). Current Controversies in Temporomandibular Disorders. Chicago: Quintessence, 1992:29–31.

125. De Leeuw JRJ, Steenks MH, Ros WJG, Lobbezoo-Scholte AM, Bosman F, Winnubst JA. Multidimensional evaluation of craniomandibular dysfunction. I. Symptoms and correlates. J Oral Rehabil 1994;21:504–514.

126. Junge D, Clark GT. Electromyographic turns analysis of sustained contraction in human masseter muscles at various isometric force levels. Arch Oral Biol 1993;38:583–588.

127. Kamisaka M, Yatani H, Kuboki T, Matsuka Y, Minakuchi H. Four-year longitudinal course of TMD symptoms in an adult population and the estimation of risk factors in relation to symptoms. J Orofac Pain 2000;14:224–232.

128. Arima T, Svensson P, Arendt-Nielsen L. Experimental grinding in healthy subjects: A model for postexercise jaw muscle soreness? J Orofac Pain 1999;13:104–114.

129. Pierce CJ, Chrisman K, Bennett ME, Close JM. Stress, anticipatory stress, and psychologic measures related to sleep bruxism. J Orofac Pain 1995;9:51–56.

130. Lobbezoo F, Naeije M. Bruxism is mainly regulated centrally, not peripherally. J Oral Rehabil 2001;28:1085–1091.

131. Weiner S, Shaikh MB, Siegel A. Electromyographic activity in the masseter muscle resulting from stimulation of hypothalamic behavioral sites in the cat. J Orofac Pain 1993;7:370–377.

132. Fahn S. The extrapyramidal disorders. In: Wyngaarden JB, Smith LH (eds). Cecil Textbook of Medicine. Philadelphia: Saunders, 1985:2068–2079.

133. Menapace SE, Rinchuse DJ, Zullo T, Pierce CJ, Shnorhokian H. The dentofacial morphology of bruxers versus non-bruxers. Angle Orthod 1994;64:43–52.

134. Holmgren K, Sheikholeslam A, Riise C. Effect of a full-arch maxillary occlusal splint on parafunctional activity during sleep in patients with nocturnal bruxism and signs and symptoms of craniomandibular disorders. J Prosthet Dent 1993;69:293–297.

135. Silness J, Johannessen G, Roystrand T. Longitudinal relationship between incisal occlusion and incisal tooth wear. Acta Odontol Scand 1993;51:15–21.

136. Hugoson A, Bergendal T, Ekfeldt A, Helkimo M. Prevalence and severity of incisal and occlusal tooth wear in an adult Swedish population. Acta Odontol Scand 1988;46:255–265.

137. Bernhardt O, Gesch D, Splieth C, et al. Risk factors for high occlusal wear scores in a population-based sample: Results of the Study of Health in Pomerania (SHIP). Int J Prosthodont 2004;17:333–339.

138. Johansson A, Fareed K, Omar R. Lateral and protrusive contact schemes and occlusal wear: A correlational study in a young adult Saudi population. J Prosthet Dent 1994;7:159–164.

139. Waltimo A, Nystrom M, Kononen M. Bite force and dentofacial morphology in men with severe dental attrition. Scand J Dent Res 1994;102:92–96.

140. Krogstad O, Dahl BL. Dento-facial morphology in patients with advanced attrition. Eur J Orthod 1985;7:57–62.

141. Varrela J. Effects of attritive diet on craniofacial morphology: A cephalometric analysis of a Finnish skull sample. Eur J Orthod 1990;12:219–223.

142. Helkimo E, Ingergvall B. Bite force and functional state of the masticatory system in young men. Swed Dent J 1978;2:167–175.

143. Johansson A, Omar R, Fareed K, Haraldson T, Kiliaridis S, Carlsson GE. Comparison of the prevalence, severity and possible causes of occlusal tooth wear in two young adult populations. J Oral Rehabil 1993;20:463–471.

144. Ekfeldt A. Incisal and occlusal tooth wear and wear of some prosthodontic materials. An epidemiological and clinical study. Swed Dent J 1989;65(suppl): 1–62.

145. Kaidonis JA, Richards LC, Townsend GC. Nature and frequency of dental wear facets in an Australian aboriginal population. J Oral Rehabil 1993;20:333–340.

146. Wilding RJ. The association between chewing efficiency and occlusal contact area in man. Arch Oral Biol 1993;38:589–596.

147. Johansson A, Haraldson T, Omar R, Kiliaridis S, Carlsson GE. A system for assessing the severity and progression of occlusal tooth wear. J Oral Rehabil 1993;20:125–131.

148. Boldsen JL. Analysis of dental attrition and mortality in the medieval village of Tirup, Denmark. Am J Phys Anthropol 2005;126:169–176.

149. Bartlett D. The implication of laboratory research on tooth wear and erosion. Oral Dis 2005;11:2–6.

150. Haketa T, Baba K, Akishige S, Fueki K, Kino K, Ohyama T. Accuracy and precision of a system for assessing severity of tooth wear. Int J Prosthodont 2004;17:581–584.

151. Schellhas KP, Pollei SR, Wilkes CH. Pediatric internal derangements of the temporomandibular joint: Effect on facial development. Am J Orthod Dentofac Orthop 1993;104:51–59.

152. Hackney J, Bade D, Clawson A. Relationship between forward head posture and diagnosed internal derangement of the temporomandibular joint. J Orofac Pain 1993;7:386–390.

153. Isberg A, Westesson PL. Steepness of articular eminence and movement of the condyle and disk in asymptomatic temporomandibular joints. Oral Surg Oral Med Oral Pathol Oral Radiol Endod 1998;86:152–157.

154. Panmekiate S, Petersson A, Akerman S. Angulation and prominence of the posterior slope of the eminence of the temporomandibular joint in relation to disc position. Dentomaxillofac Radiol 1991; 20:205–208.

155. Ren YF, Isberg A, Westesson PL. Steepness of the articular eminence in the temporomandibular joint. Tomographic comparison between asymptomatic volunteers with normal disk position and patients with disk displacement. Oral Surg Oral Med Oral Pathol Oral Radiol Endod 1995;80:258–266.

156. Yamada K, Tsuruta A, Hanada K, Hayashi T. Morphology of the articular eminence in temporomandibular joints and condylar bone change. J Oral Rehabil 2004;31:438–444.

157. Seligman DA, Pullinger A. The role of functional occlusal relationships in temporomandibular disorders: A review. J Craniomandib Disord Facial Oral Pain 1991;5:265–279.

158. Wanman A, Agerberg G. Etiology of craniomandibular disorders: Evaluation of some occlusal and psychosocial factors in 19-year-olds. J Craniomandib Disord Facial Oral Pain 1991;5:35–44.

159. Seligman DA, Pullinger A. The role of intercuspal occlusal relationships on temporomandibular disorders: A review. J Craniomandib Disord Facial Oral Pain 1991;5:96–106.

160. Pullinger A, Seligman DA, Gornbein JA. A multiple logistic regression analysis of the risk and relative odds of temporomandibular disorders as a function of common occlusal features. J Dent Res 1993;72: 968–979.

161. Smith V, Williams B, Stapleford R. Rigid internal fixation and the effects on the temporomandibular joint and masticatory system: A prospective study. Am J Orthod Dentofac Orthop 1992;102:491–500.

162. Vanderas AP. Relationship between craniomandibular dysfunction and malocclusion in white children with and without unpleasant life events. J Oral Rehabil 1994;21:177–183.

163. Lobbezoo-Scholte AM, Lobbezoo F, Steenks MH, de Leeuw JR, Bosman F. Diagnostic subgroups of craniomandibular disorders. Part II. Symptom profiles. J Orofac Pain 1995;9:37–43.

164. McNamara JA Jr, Seligman DA, Okeson JP. Occlusion, Orthodontic treatment, and temporomandibular disorders: A review. J Orofac Pain 1995;9:73–90.

165. Seligman DA, Pullinger A. A multiple stepwise logistic regression analysis of trauma history and 16 other history and dental cofactors in females with temporomandibular disorders. J Orofac Pain 1996; 10:351–361.

166. Seligman DA, Pullinger A. Analysis of occlusal variables, dental attrition, and age for distinguishing healthy controls from female patients with intracapsular temporomandibular disorders. J Prosthet Dent 2000;83:76–82.

167. Pullinger A, Seligman DA. Quantification and validation of predictive values of occlusal variables in temporomandibular disorders using a multifactoral analysis. J Prosthet Dent 2000;83:66–75.

168. De Boever JA, Carlsson GE, Klineberg IJ. Need for occlusal therapy and prosthodontic treatment in the management of temporomandibular disorders. Part I. Occlusal interferences and occlusal adjustment. J Oral Rehabil 2000;27:367–379.

169. Whittaker DK, Jones JW, Edwards PW, Molleson T. Studies on the temporomandibular joints of an eighteenth-century London population (Spitalfields). J Oral Rehabil 1990;17(1):89–97.

170. De Boever JA, Adriaens PA. Occlusal relationship in patients with pain-dysfunction symptoms in the temporomandibular joints. J Oral Rehabil 1983; 10:1–7.

171. Holmlund A, Axelsson S. Temporomandibular joint osteoarthrosis. Correlation of clinical and arthroscopic findings with degree of molar support. Acta Odontol Scand 1994;52:214–218.

172. Leake JL, Hawkins R, Locker D. Social and functional impact of reduced posterior dental units in older adults. J Oral Rehabil 1994;21:1–10.

173. Lundeen TF, Scruggs RR, McKinney MW, Daniel SJ, Levitt SR. TMD symptomology among denture patients. J Craniomandib Disord Facial Oral Pain 1990;4(1):40–46.

174. Muir CB, Goss AN. The radiologic morphology of asymptomatic temporomandibular joints. Oral Surg Oral Med Oral Pathol 1990;70:349–354.

175. Pekkarinen V, Yli-Urpo A. Helkimo's indices before and after prosthodontic treatment in selected cases. J Oral Rehabil 1987;14:35–42.

176. Pullinger A, Baldioceda R, Bibb CA. Relationship of TMJ articular soft tissue to underlying bone in young adult condyles. J Dent Res 1990;69:1512–1518.

177. Wilding RJ, Owen CP. The prevalence of temporomandibular joint dysfunction in edentulous non-denture wearing individuals. J Oral Rehabil 1987;14: 175–182.

178. Wittter DJ, De Haan AF, Kayser AF, Van Rossum GM. A 6-year following-up study of oral function in shortened dental arches. Part II. Craniomandibular dysfunction and oral comfort. J Oral Rehabil 1994;21:353–366.

179. Rivera-Morales WC, Mohl ND. Relationship of occlusal vertical dimension to the health of the masticatory system. J Prosthet Dent 1991;65:547–553.

180. Rashed MZ, Sharaway MM. Histopathological and immunocytochemical studies of the effect of raised occlusal vertical dimension on the condylar cartilage of the rabbit. Cranio 1993;11:291–296.

181. Ingervall B, Mohlin B, Thilander B. Prevalence of symptoms of functional disturbances of the masticatory system in Swedish men. J Oral Rehabil 1980;7:185–197.

182. Selaimen CM, Jeronymo JC, Brilhante DP, Lima EM, Grossi PK, Grossi ML. Occlusal risk factors for temporomandibular disorders. Angle Orthod 2007;77: 471–477.

183. Bush FM. Malocclusion, masticatory muscle, and temporomandibular joint tenderness. J Dent Res 1985;64:129–133.

184. Roberts CA, Tallents RH, Katzberg RW, Sanchez-Woodworth RE, Espeland MA, Handelman SL. Comparison of internal derangements of the TMJ with occlusal findings. Oral Surg Oral Med Oral Pathol 1987;63:645–650.

185. Runge ME, Sadowsky C, Sakols EI, BeGole EA. The relationship between temporomandibular joint sounds and malocclusion. Am J Orthod Dentofac Orthop 1989;96(1):36–42.

186. Solberg W, Flint RT, Brantner JP. Temporomandibular joint pain and dysfunction: A clinical study of emotional and occlusal components. J Prosthet Dent 1972;28:412–422.

187. Kahn J, Tallents RH, Katzberg RW, Ross ME, Murphy WC. Prevalence of dental occlusal variables and intraarticular temporomandibular disorders: Molar relationship, lateral guidance, and nonworking side contacts. J Prosthet Dent 1999;82:410–415.

188. Seligman DA, Pullinger A, Solberg W. Temporomandibular disorders. Part III: Occlusal and articular factors associated with muscle tenderness. J Prosthet Dent 1988;59:483–489.

189. Williamson EH, Hall JT, Zwemer JD. Swallowing patterns in human subjects with and without temporomandibular dysfunction. Am J Orthod Dentofac Orthop 1990;98:507–511.

190. Tegelberg A, Kopp S. Clinical findings in the stomatognathic system for individuals with rheumatoid arthritis and osteoarthrosis. Acta Odontol Scand 1987;45:65–75.

191. Akerman S, Kopp S, Nilner M, Petersson A, Rohlin M. Relationship between clinical and radiologic findings of the temporomandibular joint in rheumatoid arthritis. Oral Surg Oral Med Oral Pathol 1988;66:639–643.

192. Riolo ML, Brandt D, TenHave TR. Associations between occlusal characteristics and signs and symptoms of TMJ dysfunction in children and young adults. Am J Orthod Dentofac Orthop 1987;92: 467–477.

193. Heloe B, Heiberg AN. A multiprofessional study of patients with myofascial pain-dysfunction syndrome. II. Acta Odontol Scand 1980;38(2):119–128.

194. Tsolka P, Fenlon MR, McCullock AJ, Preiskel HW. A controlled clinical, electromyographic, and kinesiographic assessment of craniomandibular disorders in women. J Orofac Pain 1994;8(1):80–89.

195. Cachiotti DA, Plesh O, Bianchi P, McNeill C. Signs and symptoms in samples with and without temporomandibular disorders. J Craniomandib Disord Facial Oral Pain 1991;5:167–172.

196. Castaneda R, McNeill C, Noble W. Biomechanics in TMJ osteoarthritis [abstract]. J Dent Res 1988;67 (special issue).

197. Gunn SM, Woolfolk MW, Faja BW. Malocclusion and TMJ symptoms in migrant children. J Craniomandib Disord Facial Oral Pain 1988;2:196–200.

198. Lieberman MA, Gazot E, Fuchs C, Lilos P. Mandibular dysfunction in 10-18 year old school children as related to morphological malocclusion. J Oral Rehabil 1985;12:209–214.

199. Seligman DA, Pullinger A. Association of occlusal variables among refined TM patient diagnostic groups. J Craniomandib Disord Facial Oral Pain 1989;3:227–236.

200. Heloe B, Heloe LA. Characteristics of a group of patients with temporomandibular joint disorders. Community Dent Oral Epidemiol 1975;3(2):72–79.

201. De Boever JA, Van den Berghe LI. Longitudinal study of functional conditions in the masticatory system in Flemish children. Community Dent Oral Epidemiol 1989;15:100–103.

202. Mohlin B, Kopp S. A clinical study on the relationship between malocclusion, occlusal interferences and mandibular pain and dysfunction. Swed Dent J 1978;2:105–112.

203. Juniper RP. The shape of the condyle and position of the meniscus in temporomandibular joint dysfunction. Br J Oral Maxillofac Surg 1994;32(2):71–76.

204. Demisch A, Ingervall B, Thuer U. Mandibular displacement in Angle Class II, division 2 malocclusion. Am J Orthod Dentofac Orthop 1992;102:509–518.

205. Visser A, McCarroll RS, Oosting J, Naeije M. Masticatory electromyographic activity in healthy young adults and myogenous craniomandibular disorder patients. J Oral Rehabil 1994;21(1):67–76.

206. Byrd KE, Stein ST. Effects of lesions to the trigeminal motor nucleus on temporomandibular disc morphology. J Oral Rehabil 1990;17:529–540.

207. Hagberg C, Hellsing G, Hagberg M. Perception of cutaneous electrical stimulation in patients with craniomandibular disorders. J Craniomandib Disord Facial Oral Pain 1990;4:120–125.

208. El-Labben NG, Harris M, Hopper C, Barber P. Degenerative changes in masseter and temporalis muscles in limited mouth opening and TMJ ankylosis. J Oral Pathol Med 1990;19:423–425.

209. Hesse JR, Naeije M, Hansson TL. Craniomandibular stiffness toward maximum mouth opening in healthy subjects: A clinical and experimental investigation. J Craniomandib Disord Facial Oral Pain 1990;4:257–266.

210. Buckingham RB, Braun T, Harinstein DA, et al. Temporomandibular joint dysfunction syndrome: A close association with systemic joint laxity (the hypermobile joint syndrome). Oral Surg Oral Med Oral Pathol 1991;72:514–519.

211. Westling L. Temporomandibular joint dysfunction and systemic joint laxity. Swed Dent J 1992;81 (suppl):1–79.

212. De Coster PJ, Van den Berghe LI, Martens LC. Generalized joint hypermobility and temporomandibular disorders: Inherited connective tissue disease as a model with maximum expression. J Orofac Pain 2005;19:47–57.

213. Kavuncu V, Sahin S, Kamanli A, Karan A, Aksoy C. The role of systemic hypermobility and condylar hypermobility in temporomandibular joint dysfunction syndrome. Rheumatol Int 2006;26:257–260.

214. Pereira FJ, Lundh H, Eriksson L, Westesson PL. Microscopic changes in the retrodiscal tissues of painful temporomandibular joints. J Oral Maxillofac Surg 1996;54(4):461–468; discussion 469.

215. Perrini F, Tallents RH, Katzberg RW, Ribeiro RF, Kyrkanides S, Moss ME. Generalized joint laxity and temporomandibular disorders. J Orofac Pain 1997; 11:215–221.

216. Dijkstra PU, De Bont LGM, van der Weele LT, Boering G. The relationship between temporomandibular joint mobility and peripheral joint mobility reconsidered. Cranio 1994;12:149–155.

217. Dijkstra PU. Temporomandibular Joint Osteoarthrosis and Joint Mobility [thesis]. Groningen, The Netherlands: Univ of Groningen, 1993.

218. Dijkstra PU, Kropmans TJ, Stegenga B. The association between generalized joint hypermobility and temporomandibular joint disorders: A systematic review. J Dent Res 2002;81:158–163.

219. Akeel R, Nilner M, Nilner K. Masticatory efficiency in individuals with natural dentitions. Swed Dent J 1993;17:191–198.

220. Wilding RJ, Lewin A. The determination of optimal human jaw movements based on their association with chewing performance. Arch Oral Biol 1994; 39:333–343.

221. van der Bilt A, Olthoff LW, Bosman F, et al. The effect of missing postcanine teeth on chewing performance in man. Arch Oral Biol 1993;38:423–429.

222. Kiliaridis S, Kjellberg H, Wenneberg B, Engström C. The relationship between maximal bite force, bite force endurance, and facial morphology during growth. Acta Odontol Scand 1993;51:323–331.

223. Ahlberg JP, Kovero OA, Hurmerinta KA, Zepa I, Nissinen MJ, Konomen MH. Maximal bite force and its association with signs and symptoms of TMD, occlusion, and body mass index in a cohort of young adults. Cranio 2003;21:248-252.

224. Kohyama K, Mioche L, Bourdiol P. Influence of age and dental status on chewing behavior studied by EMG recordings during consumption of various food samples. Gerodontology 2003;20:15-23.

225. Stegenga B, De Bont LGM, De Leeuw R, Boering G. Assessment of mandibular function impairment associated with temporomandibular joint osteoarthrosis and internal derangement. J Orofac Pain 1993; 7:193-195.

226. Wang K, Arima T, Arendt-Nielsen L, Svensson P. EMG-force relationships are influenced by experimental jaw-muscle pain. J Oral Rehabil 2000;27: 394-402.

227. Shiau YY, Peng CC, Wen SC, Lin LD, Wang JS, Lou KL. The effects of masseter muscle pain on biting performance. J Oral Rehabil 2003;30:978-984.

228. Mioche L, Bourdiol P, Monier S, Martin JF, Cormier D. Changes in jaw muscles activity with age: Effects on food bolus properties. Physiol Behav 2004;82: 621-627.

229. Hansdottir R, Bakke M. Joint tenderness, jaw opening, chewing velocity, and bite force in patients with temporomandibular joint pain and matched healthy control subjects. J Orofac Pain 2004;18:108-113.

230. Dolan EA, Keefe FJ. Muscle activity in myofascial pain-dysfunction syndrome patients: A structured clinical evaluation. J Craniomandib Disord Facial Oral Pain 1988;2:101-105.

231. Reid KI, Gracely RH, Dubner RA. The influence of time, facial side, and location on pain-pressure thresholds in chronic myogenous temporomandibular disorder. J Orofac Pain 1994;8:258-265.

232. Browne PA, Clark GT, Yang Q, Nakano M. Sternocleidomastoid muscle inhibition induced by trigeminal stimulation. J Dent Educ 1993;72:1503-1508.

233. Clark GT, Browne PA, Nakano M, Yang Q. Co-activation of sternocleidomastoid muscles during maximum clenching. J Dent Res 1993;72:1499-1502.

234. Hu JW, Yu XM, Vernon H, Sessle BJ. Excitatory effects on the neck and jaw muscle activity of inflammatory irritant applied to cervical paraspinal tissues. Pain 1993;55:243-250.

235. Okuda-Akabane K. Hyperalgesic change over the craniofacial area following urate crystal injection in the rabbit's temporomandibular joint. J Oral Rehabil 1994;21:311-322.

236. Hansson T, Oberg T, Carlsson GE, Kopp S. Thickness of the soft tissue layers and the articular disk in the temporomandibular joint. Acta Odontol Scand 1977;35(2):77-83.

237. Lubsen CC, Hansson TL, Nordstrom BB, Solberg WK. Histomorphometric analysis of cartilage and subchondral bone in mandibular condyles of young human adults at autopsy. Arch Oral Biol 1985;30: 129-136.

238. Bibb CA, Pullinger A, Baldioceda R. The relationship of undifferentiated mesenchymal cells to TMJ articular tissue thickness. J Dent Res 1992;71:1816-1821.

239. Flygare L, Klinge B, Rohlin M, Akerman S, Lanke J. Calcified cartilage zone and its dimensional relationship to the articular cartilage in the human temporomandibular joint of elderly individuals. Acta Odontol Scand 1993;51:183-191.

240. De Bont LG, Boering G, Liem RS, Havinga P. Osteoarthritis of the temporomandibular joint: A light microscopic and scanning electron microscopic study of the articular cartilage of the mandibular condyle. J Oral Maxillofac Surg 1985;43:481-488.

241. Stegenga B, De Bont LGM. TMJ growth, adaptive modeling and remodeling, and compensatory mechanisms. In: Laskin DM, Greene CS, Hylander WL (eds). Temporomandibular Disorders: An evidence-Based Approach to Diagnosis and Treatment. Chicago: Quintessence, 2006:53-64.

242. Luder HU. Articular degeneration and remodeling in human temporomandibular joints with normal and abnormal disc position. J Orofac Pain 1993;7: 391-402.

243. Bade DM, Lovasko JH, Dimitroff M, Jones TD, Hirsch M. Clinical comparison of temporomandibular joint sound auscultation and emission imaging studies. J Orofac Pain 1994;8(1):55-60.

244. Dijkstra PU, De Bont LGM, De Leeuw R, Stegenga B, Boering G. Temporomandibular joint osteoarthrosis and temporomandibular joint hypermobility. Cranio 1993;11:268-275.

245. Holmlund AB, Gynther G, Reinholt FP. Rheumatoid arthritis and disk derangement of the temporomandibular joint. A comparative arthroscopic study. Oral Surg Oral Med Oral Pathol 1993;73:273-277.

246. Anderson GC, Schiffman EL, Schellhas KP, Fricton JR. Clinical vs arthrographic diagnosis of TMJ internal derangement. J Dent Res 1989;68:826-829.

247. Fishima K, Sato S, Suzuki Y, Kashima I. Horizontal condylar path in patients with disk displacement with reduction. Cranio 1994;12:78-86.

248. Toller PA. The synovial apparatus and temporomandibular joint function. Br Dent J 1961;40:347-353.

249. Nitzan DW. The process of lubrication impairment and its involvement in temporomandibular joint disc displacement: A theoretical concept. J Oral Maxillofac Surg 2001;59:35-45.

250. Kopp S, Wenneberg B, Clemensson E. Clinical, microscopical and biochemical investigation of synovial fluid from temporomandibular joints. Scand J Dent Res 1983;91(1):33-41.

251. Israel HA. Synovial fluid analysis. Oral Maxillofac Surg Clin North Am 1989;1:85–92.

252. Fujimura K, Segami N, Yoshitake Y, et al. Electrophoretic separation of the synovial fluid proteins in patients with temporomandibular joint disorders. Oral Surg Oral Med Oral Pathol 2006;101:463–468.

253. Shafer DM, Assael L, White LB, Rossomando EF. Tumor necrosis factor-α as a biochemical marker of pain and outcome in temporomandibular joints with internal derangements. J Oral Maxillofac Surg 1994;52:786–791.

254. Uehara J, Kuboki T, Fujisawa T, Kojima S, Maekawa K, Yatani H. Soluble tumour necrosis factor receptors in synovial fluids from temporomandibular joint with painful anterior disc displacement without reduction and osteoarthritis. Arch Oral Biol 2004;49:133–142.

255. Kaneyama K, Segami N, Nishimura M, Suzuki T, Sato J. Importance of proinflammatory cytokines in synovial fluid from 121 joints with temporomandibular disorders. Br J Oral Maxillofac Surg 2002;40:418–423.

256. Kaneyama K, Segami N, Sun W, Sato J, Fujimura K. Analysis of tumor necrosis factor-α, interleukin-6, interleukin-1β, soluble tumor necrosis factor receptors I and II, interleukin-6 soluble receptor, interleukin-1 soluble receptor type II, interleukin-1 receptor antagonist, and protein in the synovial fluid of patients with temporomandibular joint disorders. Oral Surg Oral Med Oral Pathol Oral Radiol Endod 2005;99:276–284.

257. Quinn JH, Bazan NG. Identification of prostaglandin $E_2$ and leukotriene $B_4$ in the synovial fluid of painful, dysfunctional temporomandibular joints. J Oral Maxillofac Surg 1990;48:968–971.

258. Appelgren A, Appelgren B, Kopp S, Lundeberg T, Theodorsson E. Neuropeptides in the arthritic TMJ and symptoms and signs from the stomatognathic system with special consideration to rheumatoid arthritis. J Orofac Pain 1995;9:215–225.

259. Appelgren A, Appelgren B, Kopp S, Lundeberg T, Theodorsson E. Substance P-associated increase of intra-articular temperature and pain threshold in the arthritic TMJ. J Orofac Pain 1998;12:101–107.

260. Takahashi T, Konodoh T, Ohtahni M, Homma H, Fukuda M. Association between arthroscopic diagnosis of temporomandibular joint osteoarthritis and synovial fluid nitric oxide levels. Oral Surg Oral Med Oral Pathol 1999;88:129–136.

261. Kubota T, Kubota E, Matsumoto A, et al. Identification of matrix metalloproteinases (MMPs) in synovial fluid from patients with temporomandibular disorder. Eur J Oral Sci 1998;106:992–998.

262. Quinn JH, Kent JH, Moise A, Lukiw WJ. Cyclo-oxygenase-2 in synovial tissue and fluid of dysfunctional temporomandibular joints with internal derangement. J Oral Maxillofac Surg 2000;58:1229–1232.

263. Srinivas R, Sorsa T, Tjaderhane L, et al. Matrix metalloproteinases in mild and severe temporomandibular joint internal derangement synovial fluid. Oral Surg Oral Med Oral Pathol 2001;91:517–525.

264. Mizui T, Ishimaru J, Miyamoto K, Kurita K. Matrix metalloproteinase-2 in synovial lavage fluid of patients with disorders of the temporomandibular joint. Br J Oral Maxillofac Surg 2001;39:310–314.

265. Suenaga S, Abeyama K, Hamasaki A, Mimura T, Noikura T. Temporomandibular disorders: Relationship between joint pain and effusion and nitric oxide concentration in the joint fluid. Dentomaxillofac Radiol 2001;30:214–218.

266. Tanaka A, Kumagai S, Kawashiri S, et al. Expression of matrix metalloproteinase-2 and -9 in synovial fluid of the temporomandibular joint accompanied by anterior disc displacement. J Oral Pathol Med 2001;30:59–64.

267. Suzuki T, Segami N, Nishimura M, Sato J, Noijima T. Bradykinin expression in synovial tissues and synovial fluids obtained from patients with internal derangement of the temporomandibular joint. Cranio 2003;21:265–270.

268. Arinci A, Ademoglu E, Asian A, Mutlu-Turkoglu U, Karabulut AB, Karan A. Molecular correlates of temporomandibular joint disease. Oral Surg Oral Med Oral Pathol 2005;99:666–670.

269. Yoshida K, Takatsuka S, Hatada E, et al. Expression of matrix metalloproteinases and aggrecanase in the synovial fluids of patients with symptomatic temporomandibular disorders. Oral Surg Oral Med Oral Pathol 2006;102:22–27.

270. Erhardson S, Sheikiholeslam A, Forsberg CM, Lockowandt P. Vertical forces developed by the jaw elevator muscles during unilateral maximal clenching and their distribution on teeth and condyles. Swed Dent J 1993;17:23–34.

271. Korioth TW, Hannam AG. Mandibular forces during simulated tooth clenching. J Orofac Pain 1994;8:178–189.

272. Nickel JC, McLachlan KR. An analysis of surface congruity in the growing human temporomandibular joint. Arch Oral Biol 1994;39:315–321.

273. Nickel JC, McLachlan KR. In vitro measurement of the frictional properties of the temporomandibular joint disc. Arch Oral Biol 1994;39:323–331.

274. Nickel JC, McLachlan KR. In vitro measurement of the stress-distribution properties of the pig temporomandibular joint. Arch Oral Biol 1994;39:439–448.

275. Scapino RP, Canham PB, Finlay HM, Mills DK. The behaviour of collagen fibers in stress relaxation and stress distribution in the jaw-joint disc of rabbits. Arch Oral Biol 1996;41:1039–1052.

276. Korioth TW, Hannam AG. Deformation of the human mandible during simulated tooth clenching. J Dent Res 1994;73(1):56–66.

277. Bell WE. Temporomandibular Disorders: Classification, Diagnosis, Management. Chicago: Year Book, 1990.

278. Nitzan DW. Intraarticular pressure in the functioning human temporomandibular joint and its alteration by uniform elevation of the occlusal plane. J Oral Maxillofac Surg 1994;52:671–679.

279. Ogasawara T, Kitagawa Y, Ogawa T, Yamada T, Kawamura Y, Sano K. Inflammatory change in the upper joint space in temporomandibular joint with internal derangement on gadolinium-enhanced MR imaging. Int J Oral Maxillofac Surg 2002;31:252–256.

280. Schiffman EL, Anderson GC, Fricton JR, Lindgren BR. The relationship between level of mandibular pain and dysfunction and stage of temporomandibular joint internal derangement. J Dent Res 1992;71:1812–1815.

281. Abubaker AO, Raslan WF, Sotereanos GC. Estrogen and progesterone receptors in temporomandibular joint discs of symptomatic and asymptomatic persons: A preliminary study. J Oral Maxillofac Surg 1993;51:1096–1100.

282. Campbell JH, Courey MS, Bourne P, Odziemiec C. Estrogen receptor analysis of human temporomandibular disc. J Oral Maxillofac Surg 1993;51:1101–1105.

283. Glaros AG, Baharloo L, Glass EG. Effect of parafunctional clenching and estrogen on temporomandibular disorder pain. Cranio 1998;16(2):78–83.

284. Nappi RE, Cagnacci A, Granella F, Piccinini F, Polatti F, Facchinetti F. Course of primary headaches during hormone replacement therapy. Maturitas 2001;38:157–163.

285. LeResche L, Saunders K, Von Korff MR, Barlow W, Dworkin SF. Use of exogenous hormones and risk of temporomandibular disorder pain. Pain 1997;69(1–2):153–160.

286. Dao TT, Knight K, Ton-That V. Modulation of myofascial pain by the reproductive hormones: A preliminary report. J Prosthet Dent 1998;79:663–670.

287. Stegenga B. Temporomandibular Joint Osteoarthrosis and Internal Derangement: Diagnostic and Therapeutic Outcome Assessment [thesis].Groningen, The Netherlands: Univ of Groningen, 1991.

288. Stegenga B. Osteoarthritis of the temporomandibular joint organ and its relationship to disc displacement. J Orofac Pain 2001;15:193–205.

289. Wonwatana S, Kronman JH, Clark RE, Kabani S, Mehta N. Anatomic basis for disk displacement in temporomandibular joint (TMJ) dysfunction. Am J Orthod Dentofacial Orthop 1994;105:257–264.

290. Lang TC, Zimmy ML, Vijayagopal P. Experimental temporomandibular joint disc perforation in the rabbit: A gross morphological, biochemical, and ultrastructural analysis. J Oral Maxillofac Surg 1993;51:1115–1128.

291. Milam SB, Zardeneta G, Schmitz JP. Oxidative stress and degenerative temporomandibular joint disease: A proposed hypothesis. J Oral Maxillofac Surg 1998; 56:214–223.

292. Dijkgraaf LC, Zardeneta G, Cordewener FW, et al. Crosslinking of fibrinogen and fibronectin by free radicals: A possible initial step in adhesion formation in osteoarthritis of the temporomandibular joint. J Oral Maxillofac Surg 2003;61:101–111.

293. Diatchenko L, Slade GD, Nackley AG, et al. Genetic basis for individual variations in pain perception and the development of a chronic pain condition. Hum Mol Genet 2005;14:135–143.

294. Rugh JD, Solberg W. Psychological implications in temporomandibular pain and dysfunction. In: Zarb GA, Carlsson GE (eds). Temporomandibular Joint Function and Dysfunction. Copenhagen: Munksgaard, 1979:239–258.

295. Eversole LR, Stone CE, Matheson D, Kaplan H. Psychometric profiles and facial pain. Oral Surg Oral Med Oral Pathol 1985;60:269–274.

296. Southwell J, Deary IJ, Geissler P. Personality and anxiety in temporomandibular joint syndrome patients. J Oral Rehabil 1990;17:239–243.

297. Flor H, Birbaumer N, Schulte W, Roos R. Stress related electromyographic responses in patients with chronic temporomandibular pain. Pain 1991;46:145–182.

298. McCreary CP, Clark GT, Merrill RL, et al. Psychological distress and diagnostic subgroups of temporomandibular disorder patients. Pain 1991;44:29–34.

299. List T, Wahlund K, Larsson B. Psychosocial functioning and dental factors in adolescents with temporomandibular disorders: A case-control study. J Orofac Pain 2001;15:218–227.

300. Wright AR, Gatchel RJ, Wildenstein L, Riggs R, Buschang P, Ellis E. Biopsychosocial differences between high-risk and low-risk patients with acute TMD-related pain. J Am Dent Assoc 2004;135:474–483.

301. Manfredini D, Bandettini di Poggio A, Cantini E, Dell'Osso L, Bosco M. Mood and anxiety psychopathology and temporomandibular disorder: A spectrum approach. J Oral Rehabil 2004;31:933–940.

302. De Leeuw R, Bertoli E, Schmidt JE, Carlson CR. Prevalence of post-traumatic stress disorder symptoms in orofacial pain patients. Oral Surg Oral Med Oral Pathol 2005;99:558–568.

303. Carlson N, Moline D, Huber L, et al. Comparison of muscle activity between conventional and neuromuscular splints. J Prosthet Dent 1993;70:39–43.

304. Arntz A, Dreesen L, de Jong HP. The influence of anxiety on pain: Attentional and attributional mediators. Pain 1994;56:307–314.

305. Jones DA, Rollman GB, Brooke RI. The cortisol response to psychological stress in temporomandibular dysfunction. Pain 1997;72:171–182.

306. Turner JA, Dworkin SF, Mancl L, Huggins KH, Truelove EL. The roles of beliefs, catastrophizing, and coping in the functioning of patients with temporomandibular disorders. Pain 2001;92:41–51.

307. Gold S, Lipton JA, Marbach JJ, et al. Sites of psychophysiological complaints in MPD patients. II. Areas remote from the orofacial region [abstract]. J Dent Res 1975;54(special issue):165.

308. Malow RM, Olson RE, Greene CS. Myofascial pain dysfunction syndrome: A psychophysiological disorder. In: Golden C, Alcaparras S, Strider F, Graber B (eds). Applied Techniques in Behavioral Medicine. New York: Grune and Stratton, 1981:101–133.

309. Magni G, Moreschi C, Rigatti-Luchini S, Merskey H. Prospective study on the relationship between depressive symptoms and chronic musculoskeletal pain. Pain 1994;56:289–297.

310. Turk DC, Rudy TE. The robustness of an empirically derived taxonomy of chronic pain patients. Pain 1990;43:27–35.

311. Aghabeigi B, Feinmann C, Glover V, et al. Tyramine conjugation deficit in patients with chronic idiopathic temporomandibular joint and orofacial pain. Pain 1993;54:159–163.

312. Schurr RF, Brooke RI, Rollman GB. Psychological correlates of temporomandibular joint pain and dysfunction. Pain 1990;42:153–165.

313. Schulte JK, Anderson GC, Hathaway KM, Will TE. Psychometric profiles and related pain characteristics of temporomandibular disorders patients. J Orofac Pain 1993;7:247–253.

314. Pankhurst CL. Controversies in the aetiology of temporomandibular disorders. Part 1. Temporomandibular disorders: All in the mind? Prim Dent Care 1997;4:25–30.

315. Manfredini D, di Poggio A, Romagnoli M, Dell'Osso L, Bosco M. Mood spectrum in patients with different painful temporomandibular disorders. Cranio 2004;22:234–240.

316. Reisine ST, Weber J. The effects of temporomandibular joint disorders on patients' quality of life. Community Dent Health 1987;6:257–270.

317. Parker MW, Holmes EK, Terezhalmy GT. Personality characteristics of patients with temporomandibular disorders: Diagnostic and therapeutic implications. J Orofac Pain 1993;7:337–344.

318. Gamsa A. Is emotional disturbance a precipitator or a consequence of chronic pain? Pain 1990;42:183–195.

319. Dworkin SF, Wilson L, Massoth DL. Somatizing as a risk factor for chronic pain. In: Grezesiak RC, Ciccone DS (eds). Psychologic Vulnerability to Chronic Pain. New York: Springer, 1994:28–54.

320. American Psychiatric Association. Diagnostic and Statistical Manual of Mental Disorders, ed 4. Washington, DC: American Psychiatric Association Press, 1994.

321. Bridges RN, Goldberg DP. Somatic presentation of DSM-III psychiatric disorders in primary care. J Psychosom Res 1985;29:563–569.

322. Lipowski ZJ. Somatization: The concept and its clinical application. Am J Psychiatry 1988;145:1358–1368.

323. Morrison J, Herbstein J. Secondary affective disorder in women with somatization disorder. Compr Psychiatry 1988;29:433–440.

324. McWilliams LA, Cox B, Enns MW. Mood and anxiety disorders associated with chronic pain: An examination in a nationally representative sample. Pain 2003;106:127–133.

325. Mechanic D. The concept of illness behavior: Culture, situation and personal predisposition. Psychol Med 1986;16:1–7.

326. Pilowsky I, Smith QP, Katsikitis M. Illness behavior and general practice utilization: A prospective study. J Psychosom Res 1987;31:177–183.

327. Pearce JM. Psychosocial factors in chronic disability. Med Sci Monit 2002;8:RA275–RA281.

328. Fordyce WE. Behavioral Methods for Chronic Pain and Illness. St Louis: Mosby, 1976.

329. Dworkin SF, Le Resche L. Research Diagnostic Criteria for Temporomandibular Disorders: Review, criteria, examination and specifications critique. J Craniomandib Disord Facial Oral Pain 1992;4:301–355.

330. Fries JF, Hochberg MC, Medsger TA Jr, Hunder GG, Bombardier C. Criteria for rheumatic disease: Different types and different functions. Arthritis Rheum 1994;37:454–462.

331. Altman RD. Criteria for classification of clinical osteoarthritis. J Rheumatol 1991;18(suppl 27):10–12.

332. Headache Classification Committee of the International Headache Society. The International Classification of Headache Disorders, ed 2. Cephalalgia 2004;24(suppl):S1–S151.

333. US Department of Health and Human Services. International Classification of Diseases, Ninth Revision, Clinical Modification, ed 6. Washington, DC: US Dept of Health and Human Services, 2006.

334. Poswillo D. The pathogenesis of first and second branchial arch syndrome. Oral Surg Oral Med Oral Pathol 1973;35:302–328.

335. Kaban LB. Congenital abnormalities of the temporomandibular joint. In: Kaban LB, Troulis MJ (eds). Pediatric Oral and Maxillofacial Surgery. Philadelphia: Saunders, 2004:302–339.

336. Vargervik K, Kaban LB. Management of hemifacial microsomia in the growing child. In: Shelton DW, Irby WB (eds). Modern Practice in Orthognathic and Reconstructive Surgery. Philadelphia: Saunders, 1991:1533–1560.

337. Stelnicki EJ, Boyd JB, Nott RL, Barnavon Y, Uecker C, Henson T. Early treatment of severe mandibular hypoplasia with distraction mesenchymogenesis and bilateral free fibula flaps. J Craniofac Surg 2001; 12:337–348.

338. Steinbacher DM, Kaban LB, Troulis MJ. Mandibular advancement by distraction osteogenesis for tracheostomy-dependent children with severe micrognathia. J Oral Maxillofac Surg 2005;63:1072–1079.

339. Ricketts RM. Cephalometric synthesis. Am J Orthod 1960;46:647–673.

340. Gray RJ, Sloan P, Quayle AA, Carter DH. Histopathological and scintigraphic features of condylar hyperplasia. Int J Oral Maxillofac Surg 1990;19:65–71.

341. Poswillo D. Congenital malformations: Prenatal experimental studies. In: Sarnat BG, Laskin DM (eds). The Temporomandibular Joint, ed 3. Springfield, IL: Charles C. Thomas, 1979:127–150.

342. Schajowicz F, Ackerman LV, Sissons AA, et al. Histological Typing of Bone Tumors. Geneva: World Health Organization, 1972.

343. Trumpy IG, Lyberg T. Temporomandibular joint dysfunction and facial pain caused by neoplasms: Report of three cases. Oral Surg Oral Med Oral Pathol 1993;76:149–152.

344. Warner BF, Luna MA, Robert NT. Temporomandibular joint neoplasms and pseudotumors. Adv Anat Pathol 2000;7:365–381.

345. Butler JH. Myofascial pain dysfunction syndrome involving tumor metastasis. Case report. J Periodontol 1975;46:309–311.

346. Stypulkowsda J, Bartkowski S, Panas M, Zaleska M. Metastatic tumors of the jaws and oral cavity. J Oral Surg 1979;37:805–889.

347. Rubin MM, Jui V, Cozzi GM. Metastatic carcinoma of the mandibular condyle presenting as temporomandibular joint syndrome. J Oral Maxillofac Surg 1989;47:507–510.

348. Sanchez-Aniceto G, Garcia-Penin A, de la Mata-Pages R, Montalvo-Moreno JJ. Tumors metastatic to the mandible: Analysis of nine cases and review of the literature. J Oral Maxillofac Surg 1990;48:246–251.

349. Nortje CJ, van Rensburg LJ, Thompson IOC. Magnetic resonance features of metastatic melanoma of the temporomandibular joint and mandible. Dentomaxillofac Radiol 1996;25:292–297.

350. Orlean SL, Robinson NR, Ahern JP, et al. Carcinoma of the maxillary sinus manifested by temporomandibular joint pain dysfunction syndrome. J Oral Med 1966;21:127–131.

351. Shapshay SM, Elber E, Strong MS. Occult tumors of the infratemporal fossa. Arch Otolaryngol 1976; 102:535–538.

352. Sharav Y, Feinsod M. Nasopharyngeal tumor initially manifested as myofascial pain dysfunction syndrome. Oral Surg Oral Med Oral Pathol 1977;44(1): 54–57.

353. DelBalso AM, Pyatt RS, Busch RF, Hirokawa R, Fink CS. Synovial cell sarcoma of the temporomandibular joint. Arch Otolaryngol 1982;108:520–522.

354. Owen GO, Stelling CB. Condylar metastasis with initial presentation of TMJ syndrome. J Oral Med 1985;40:198–201.

355. Roistacher SL, Tanenbaum D. Myofascial pain associated with oropharyngeal cancer. Oral Surg Oral Med Oral Pathol 1986;61:459–462.

356. Christiansen EL, Thompson JR, Appleton SS. Temporomandibular joint pain/dysfunction overlying more insidious diseases: Report of two cases. J Oral Maxillofac Surg 1987;45:335–337.

357. Cohen SG, Quinn PD. Facial trismus and myofascial pain associated with infections and malignant disease: Report of five cases. Oral Surg Oral Med Oral Pathol 1988;65:538–544.

358. Epstein JB, Jones CK. Presenting signs and symptoms of nasopharyngeal carcinoma. Oral Surg Oral Med Oral Pathol Oral Radiol Endod 1993;75:31–36.

359. Grace EG, North AF. Temporomandibular joint dysfunction and orofacial pain caused by parotid gland malignancy: Report of case. J Am Dent Assoc 1988;116:348–350.

360. Malins TJ, Farrow A. Facial pain due to occult parotid adenoid cystic carcinoma. J Oral Maxillofac Surg 1991;49:1127–1129.

361. Raustia AM, Oikarinen KS, Luotonen J, Salo T, Pyhtinen J. Parotid gland carcinoma simulating signs and symptoms of craniomandibular disorders—A case report. Cranio 1993;11:153–156.

362. Halfpenny W, Verey A, Bardsley V. Myxoma of the mandibular condyle. A case report and review of the literature. Oral Surg Oral Med Oral Pathol Oral Radiol Endod 2000;90:348–353.

363. Kondoh T, Seto K, Kobayashi K. Osteoma of the mandibular condyle: Report of a case with a review of the literature. J Oral Maxillofac Surg 1998;56: 972–979.

364. Blankestijn J, Boering G. Posterior dislocation of the temporomandibular joint. Int J Oral Surg 1985;14: 437–443.

365. Westesson PL, Larheim TA, Tanaka H. Posterior disc displacement in the temporomandibular joint. J Oral Maxillofac Surg 1998;56:1266–1273.

366. Khoury MD, Dolan EA. Sideways dislocation of the temporomandibular joint meniscus: The edge sign. Am J Nucl Radiol 1986;7:869–872.

367. Westesson PL, Kurita K, Ericksson L, et al. Cryosectional observations of functional anatomy of the temporomandibular joint. Oral Surg Oral Med Oral Pathol 1989;68:247–251.

368. Liedberg J, Westesson PL, Kurita K. Side-ways and rotational displacement of the temporomandibular joint disc: Diagnosis by arthrography and correlation to cryosectional morphology. Oral Surg Oral Med Oral Pathol 1990;69:757–753.

369. Kurita K, Westesson PL, Tasaki MM, Liedberg J. Temporomandibular joint: Diagnosis of medial and lateral disc displacement with anterioposterior arthrography. Correlation with cryosections. Oral Surg Oral Med Oral Pathol Oral Radiol Endod 1992;73:364–368.

370. Isberg-Holm AM, Westesson PL. Movement of the disc and condyle in temporomandibular joints with clicking: An arthrographic and cineradiographic study on autopsy specimens. Acta Odontol Scand 1982;40:151–164.

371. Farrar WB, McCarty VL Jr. A Clinical Outline of Temporomandibular Joint Diagnosis and Treatment, ed 7. Montgomery, AL: Normandy, 1983.

372. Tallents RH, Hatala M, Katzberg RW, Westesson PL. Temporomandibular joint sounds in asymptomatic volunteers. J Prosthet Dent 1993;69:298–304.

373. Davant TSI, Greene CS, Perry HT, Lautenschlager EP. A quantitative computer-assisted analysis of the disc displacement in patients with internal derangement using sagittal view and magnetic resonance imaging. J Oral Maxillofac Surg 1993;51:974–979.

374. Stegenga B, De Bont LGM, Boering G, van Willigen JD. Tissue responses to degenerative changes in the temporomandibular joint: A review. J Oral Maxillofac Surg 1991;49:1079–1088.

375. Westesson PL, Bifano JA, Tallents RH, et al. Increased horizontal angle of the mandibular condyle in abnormal temporomandibular joints: A magnetic resonance imaging study. Oral Surg Oral Med Oral Pathol 1991;72:359–363.

376. Nilner K, Petersson A. Clinical and radiological findings related to treatment outcome in patients with temporomandibular disorders. J Dentomaxillofac Radiol 1995;24:128–131.

377. Stegenga B, De Bont LGM, van der Kujil B, Boering G. Classification of temporomandibular joint osteoarthrosis and internal derangement. 1. Diagnostic significance of clinical and radiographic symptoms and signs. Cranio 1992;10:96–106.

378. Rohlin M, Akerman S, Kopp S. Tomography as an aid to detect macroscopic changes of the temporomandibular joint. An autopsy study of the aged. Acta Odontol Scand 1986;44:131–140.

379. Scapino RP. Histopathology associated with malposition of the human temporomandibular joint disc. Oral Surg Oral Med Oral Pathol 1983;55:382–397.

380. Blaustein D, Scapino RP. Remodeling of the temporomandibular joint disc and posterior attachments in disc displacement specimens in relation to glycosaminoglycan content. Plast Reconstr Surg 1986;78:756–764.

381. Greene CS, Laskin DM. Long-term status of TMJ clicking in patients with myofascial pain dysfunction. J Am Dent Assoc 1988;117:461–465.

382. Sato J, Goto S, Nasu F, Motegi K. The natural course of disc displacement with reduction of the temporomandibular joint: Changes in clinical signs and symptoms. J Oral Maxillofac Surg 2003;61:32–34.

383. Stegenga B, De Bont LGM, Boering G. A proposed classification of temporomandibular disorders based on synovial joint pathology. Cranio 1989;7:107–118.

384. Stegenga B, De Bont LGM, Boering G. Temporomandibular joint pain assessment. J Orofac Pain 1993;7:23–37.

385. Stegenga B, De Bont LGM, Dijkstra PU, Boering G. Short-term outcome of arthroscopic surgery of the temporomandibular joint osteoarthrosis and internal derangement: A randomized controlled clinical trial. Br J Oral Maxillofac Surg 1993;31:3–14.

386. Sato S, Takahashi K, Kawamura H, Motegi K. The natural course of nonreducing disk displacement of the temporomandibular joint: Changes in condylar mobility and radiographic alterations of one-year follow-up. Int J Oral Maxillofac Surg 1998;27:173–177.

387. Choi BH, Yoo JH, Lee WY. Comparison of magnetic resonance imaging before and after nonsurgical treatment of closed lock. Oral Surg Oral Med Oral Pathol 1994;78:301–305.

388. Kurita K, Westesson PL, Yuasa H, Toyoma M, Machida J, Ogi N. Natural course of untreated symptomatic temporomandibular joint disc displacement without reduction. J Dent Res 1998;77:361–365.

389. Minakuchi H, Kuboki T, Matsuka Y, Maekawa K, Yatani H, Yamashita A. Randomized controlled evaluation of non-surgical treatments for temporomandibular joint anterior disc displacement without reduction. J Dent Res 2001;80:924–928.

390. Eversole LR, Machado L. Temporomandibular joint internal derangements and associated neuromuscular disorders. J Am Dent Assoc 1985;110:69–79.

189

391. Schille H. Injuries of the temporomandibular joint: Classification, diagnosis and fundamentals of treatment. In: Kruger E, Schilli W (eds). Oral and Maxillofacial Traumatology, vol 1. Chicago: Quintessence, 1986:45–106.

392. Gynther GW, Holmlund AB, Reinholt FP. Synovitis in internal derangement of the temporomandibular joint: Correlations between arthroscopic and histologic findings. J Oral Maxillofac Surg 1994;52:913–917.

393. Yoshida H, Fujita S, Nishida M, Iizuka T. Immunohistochemical distribution of lymph capillaries and blood capillaries in the synovial membrane in cases of internal derangement of the temporomandibular joint. J Oral Pathol Med 1997;26:356–361.

394. Dijkgraaf LC, Liem RS, De Bont LGM. Ultrastructural characteristics of the synovial membrane in osteoarthritic temporomandibular joints. J Oral Maxillofac Surg 1997;55:1269–1279; discussion 1279–1280.

395. Takahashi T, Kondoh T, Fukuda M, Yamazaki Y, Toyosaki T, Suzuki R. Proinflammatory cytokines detectable in synovial fluids from patients with temporomandibular disorders. Oral Surg Oral Med Oral Pathol Oral Radiol Endod 1998;85:135–141.

396. Yoshida H, Yoshida T, Iizuka T, Sakakura T, Fujita S. The localization of matrix metalloproteinase-3 and tenascin in synovial membrane of the temporomandibular joint with internal derangement. Oral Dis 1999;5(1):50–54.

397. Ishimaru JI, Oguma Y, Goss AN. Matrix metalloproteinase and tissue inhibitor of metalloproteinase in serum and lavage synovial fluid of patients with temporomandibular joint disorders. Br J Oral Maxillofac Surg 2000;38:354–359.

398. Yoshida H, Fujita S, Iizuka T, Yoshida T, Sakakura T. The specific expression of tenascin in the synovial membrane of the temporomandibular joint with internal derangement: An immunohistochemical study. Histochem Cell Biol 1997;107:479–484.

399. Yoshida H, Yoshida T, Iizuka T, Sakakura T, Fujita S. The expression of transforming growth factor beta (TGF-beta) in the synovial membrane of human temporomandibular joint with internal derangement: A comparison with tenascin expression. J Oral Rehabil 1999;26:814–820.

400. Emshoff R, Puffer P, Rudisch A, Gassner R. Temporomandibular joint pain: Relationship to internal derangement type, osteoarthrosis, and synovial fluid mediator level of tumor necrosis factor-α. Oral Surg Oral Med Oral Pathol Oral Radiol Endod 2000;90:442–449.

401. Alstergren P, Kopp S, Theodorsson E. Synovial fluid sampling from the temporomandibular joint: Sample quality criteria and levels of interleukin-1β and serotonin. Acta Odontol Scand 1999;57(1):16–22.

402. Sandler NA, Buckley MJ, Cillo JE, Braun TW. Correlation of inflammatory cytokines with arthroscopic findings in patients with temporomandibular joint internal derangements. J Oral Maxillofac Surg 1998;56:534–543; discussion 543–544.

403. Yoshida H, Fujita S, Nishida M, Iizuka T. The expression of substance P in human temporomandibular joint samples: An immunohistochemical study. J Oral Rehabil 1999;26:338–344.

404. Kopp S. Clinical findings in temporomandibular joint osteoarthrosis. Scand J Dent Res 1977;85:434–443.

405. Bland JH, Stulberg SD. Osteoarthritis: Pathology and clinical patterns. In: Kelley WN, Harris ED Jr, Ruddy S, Sledge CB (eds). Textbook of Rheumatology, ed 2. Philadelphia: Saunders, 1985.

406. Castelli WA, Nasjleti CE, Diaz-Perez R, Caffesse RG. Histopathologic findings in temporomandibular joints of aged individuals. J Prosthet Dent 1985;53:415–419.

407. Shinoda C, Takaku S. Interleukin-1β, interleukin-6, and tissue inhibitor of metalloproteinase-1 in the synovial fluid of the temporomandibular joint with respect to cartilage destruction. Oral Dis 2000;6:383–390.

408. Nordahl S, Alstergren P, Eliasson S, Kopp S. Interleukin-1β in plasma and synovial fluid in relation to radiographic changes in arthritic temporomandibular joints. Eur J Oral Sci 1998;106(1):559–563.

409. Kanyama M, Kuboki T, Kojima S, et al. Matrix metalloproteinases and tissue inhibitors of metalloproteinases in synovial fluids of patients with temporomandibular joint osteoarthritis. J Orofac Pain 2000;14:20–30.

410. Suzuki T, Segami N, Nishimura M, Hattori H, Nojima T. Analysis of 70Kd heat shock protein expression in patients with internal derangement of the temporomandibular joint. Int J Oral Maxillofac Surg 2000;29:301–304.

411. Fang PK, Ma XC, Ma DL, Fu KY. Determination of interleukin-1 receptor antagonist, interleukin-10, and transforming growth factor-β1 in synovial fluid aspirates of patients with temporomandibular disorders. J Oral Maxillofac Surg 1999;57:922–928; discussion 928–929.

412. Suzuki T, Bessho K, Segami N, Nojima T, Iizuka T. Bone morphogenetic protein-2 in temporomandibular joints with internal derangement. Oral Surg Oral Med Oral Pathol Oral Radiol Endod 1999;88:670–673.

413. Murakami KI, Shibata T, Kubota E, Maeda H. Intraarticular levels of prostaglandin E2, hyaluronic acid, and chondroitin-4 and -6 sulfates in the temporomandibular joint synovial fluid of patients with internal derangement. J Oral Maxillofac Surg 1998;56:199–203.

414. Ratcliffe A, Israel HA, Saed-Nejad F, Diamond B. Proteoglycans in the synovial fluid of the temporomandibular joint as an indicator of changes in cartilage metabolism during primary and secondary osteoarthritis. J Oral Maxillofac Surg 1998;56: 204–208.

415. Fu K, Ma X, Zhang Z, Pang X, Chen W. Interleukin-6 in synovial fluid and HLA-DR expression in synovium from patients with temporomandibular disorders. J Orofac Pain 1995;9:131–137.

416. Carlsson GE. Mandibular dysfunction and temporomandibular joint pathology. J Prosthet Dent 1980;43:658–662.

417. Dijkgraaf LC, Spijkervet FK, De Bont LGM. Arthroscopic findings in osteoarthritic temporomandibular joints. J Oral Maxillofac Surg 1999;57:255–268; discussion 269–270.

418. Israel HA, Diamond B, Saed-Nejad F, Ratcliffe A. Osteoarthritis and synovitis as major pathoses of the temporomandibular joint: Comparison of clinical diagnosis with arthroscopic morphology. J Oral Maxillofac Surg 1998;56:1023–1027; discussion 1028.

419. Brandt KD, Slemenda CW. Osteoarthritis: Epidemiology, pathology, and pathogenesis. In: Schumacher HR (ed). Primer on the Rheumatic Diseases, ed 10. Atlanta: Arthritis Foundation, 1993:184–188.

420. Rasmussen CO. Clinical findings during the course of temporomandibular arthropathy. Scand J Dent Res 1981;89:283–288.

421. Boering G. Temporomandibular Joint Arthrosis: A Clinical and Radiographic Investigation [thesis]. The Netherlands: Univ of Groningen, 1966.

422. Toller PA. Osteoarthrosis of the mandibular condyle. Br Dent J 1973;134:223–231.

423. De Leeuw R, Boering G, Stegenga B, de Bont LG. Clinical signs of TMJ osteoarthrosis and internal derangement 30 years after nonsurgical treatment. J Orofac Pain 1994;8:18–24.

424. Westesson PL, Rohlin M. Internal derangement related to osteoarthrosis in temporomandibular joint autopsy specimens. Oral Surg Oral Med Oral Pathol 1984;57:17–22.

425. Rabey GB. Bilateral mandibular condylysis—A morphanalytic diagnosis. Br J Oral Surg 1977;15:121–134.

426. Caplan HI, Benny RA. Total osteolysis of the mandibular condyle in progressive systemic sclerosis. Oral Surg 1978;46:362–366.

427. Lanigan DT, Myall RWT, West RA, et al. Condylsis in a patient with a mixed collagen vascular disease. Oral Surg 1979;48:198–204.

428. Huang YL, Pogrel MA, Kaban LB. Diagnosis and management of condylar resorption. J Oral Maxillofac Surg 1997;55:114–119; discussion 119–120.

429. Wolford LM, Cardenas L. Idiopathic condylar resorption: Diagnosis, treatment protocol, and outcomes. Am J Orthod Dentofac Orthop 1999;116: 667–677.

430. Block MS, Provenzano J, Neary JP. Complications of mandibular fractures. Oral Maxillofac Surg Clin North Am 1990;2:525–550.

431. Nitzan DW, Bar-Ziv J, Shteyer A. Surgical management of temporomandibular joint ankylosis type III by retaining the displaced condyle and disc. J Oral Maxillofac Surg 1998;56:1133–1138; discussion 1139.

432. Guven O. A clinical study on temporomandibular joint ankylosis. Auris Nasus Larynx 2000;27(1): 27–33.

433. Silvennoinen U, Raustia AM, Lindqvist C, Ojkiarinen K. Occlusal and temporomandibular joint disorders in patients with unilateral condylar fracture. A prospective one-year study. Int J Oral Maxillofac Surg 1998;27:280–285.

434. Ellis E III, Throckmorton G. Facial symmetry after closed and open treatment of fractures of the mandibular condylar process. J Oral Maxillofac Surg 2000;58:719–728; discussion 729–730.

435. Mense S. Physiology of nociception in muscles. In: Fricton JR, Awad E (eds). Advances in Pain Research and Therapy. New York: Raven, 1990:67–85.

436. Mense S. Considerations concerning the neurobiological basis of muscle pain. Can J Physiol Pharmacol 1991;69:610–616.

437. Mense S. Nociception from skeletal muscle in relation to clinical muscle pain. Pain 1993;54:241–290.

438. Layzer RB. Muscle pain, cramps and fatigue. In: Engle AG, Franzini-Armstrong C (eds). Myology. New York: McGraw-Hill, 1994:1754–1786.

439. Grassi C, Passatore M. Action of the sympathetic system on skeletal muscle. Ital J Neurol Sci 1988;9: 23–28.

440. Passatore M, Grassi C, Philippi GM. Sympathetically induced development of tension in jaw muscles: The possible contraction of intrafusal muscle fibers. Pflugers Arch 1985;405:297–304.

441. Carlson CR, Okeson JP, Falace DA, Nitz AJ, Curran SL, Anderson D. Comparison of psychologic and physiologic functioning between patients with masticatory muscle pain and matched controls. J Orofac Pain 1993;7:15–22.

442. McNulty WH, Gevirtz RN, Hubbard DR, Berkoff GM. Needle electromyographic evaluation of trigger point response to a psychological stressor. Psychophysiology 1994;31:313–316.

443. Dworkin SF, Le Resche L, Van Korff M, Truelove E, Sommers E. Epidemiology of signs and symptoms in temporomandibular disorders. I. Clinical signs in cases and controls. J Am Dent Assoc 1990;120:273–281.

444. Gonzales R, Coderre TJ, Sherbourne CD, Levine JD. Postnatal development of neurogenic inflammation in the rat. Neurosci Lett 1991;127:25–27.

445. Mense S. The pathogenesis of muscle pain. Curr Pain Headache Rep 2003;7:419–425.

446. Dahlstrom L, Carlsson SG, Gale EN, Jansson TG. Stress induced muscular activity in mandibular dysfunction: Effect of biofeedback training. J Behav Med 1985;8:191–200.

447. Lund JP, Donga R, Widmer CG, Stohler CS. The pain adaptation model: A discussion of the relationship between chronic musculoskeletal pain and motor activity. Can J Physiol Pharmacol 1991;69:683–694.

448. Lund JP, Stohler CS, Widmer CG. The relationship between pain and muscle activity in fibromyalgia and similar conditions. In: Vaeroy H, Merskey H (eds). Progress in Fibromyalgia and Myofascial Pain. Amsterdam: Elsevier, 1993:311–327.

449. Gay T, Maton B, Rendell J, Majourau A. Characteristics of muscle fatigue in patients with myofascial pain dysfunction syndrome. Arch Oral Biol 1994;39:847–852.

450. Lund JP. Pain and movement. In: Lund JP, Lavigne GJ, Dubner RA, Sessle B (eds). Orofacial Pain: From Basic Science to Clinical Management. Chicago: Quintessence, 2001:151–163.

451. de Abreu TC, Nilner M, Thulin T, Vallon D. Office and ambulatory blood pressure in patients with craniomandibular disorders. Acta Odontol Scand 1993;51:161–170.

452. Rogers EJ, Rogers RJ. Tension-type headaches, fibromyalgia, or myofasical pain. Headache Q 1991;2:273–277.

453. Gerwin RD. A review of myofascial pain and fibromyalgia—Factors that promote their persistence. Acupunct Med 2005;23:121–134.

454. Waylonis GW, Heck W. Fibromyalgia syndrome. New associations. Am J Phys Med Rehabil 1992;71:343–348.

455. Baumstark KE, Buckelew SP, Sher KJ, et al. Pain behavior predictors among fibromyalgia patients. Pain 1993;55:339–346.

456. Goldenberg DL. Clinical features of fibromyalgia. In: Fricton JR, Awad E (eds). Advances in Pain Research and Therapy, vol 17: Myofasical Pain and Fibromyalgia. New York: Raven, 1990:139–163.

457. Wolfe F, Smythe HA, Yunus MB, et al. The American College of Rheumatology, 1990: Criteria for the classification of fibromyalgia. Report of the Multicenter Criteria Committee. Arthritis Rheum 1990;33:160–172.

458. Bennett RM, Smyth HA, Wolfe F. Recognizing fibromyalgia. Patient Care 1989;23:60–83.

459. Bennett RM. Etiology of the fibromyalgia syndrome: A contemporary hypothesis. Intern Med Specialist 1990;11:48–61.

460. Henriksson C, Gundmark I, Bengtsson A, Ek AC. Living with fibromyalgia. Consequences for everyday life. Clin J Pain 1992;8:138–144.

461. Schochat T, Raspe H. Elements of fibromyalgia in an open population. Rheumatology 2003;42:829–835.

462. Sahlin K, Edstrom L, Sjoholm H, Hultman E. Effects of lactic acid accumulation and ATP decrease on muscle tension and relaxation. Am J Physiol 1981;240:C121–C126.

463. Lieber RL, Friden J. Morphologic and mechanical basis of delayed-onset muscle soreness. J Am Acad Orthop Surg 2002;10(1):67–73.

464. Lieber RL, Shah S, Friden J. Cytoskeletal disruption after eccentric contraction-induced muscle injury. Clin Orthop Relat Res 2002;(403 suppl):S90–S99.

465. Yu JG, Thornell LE. Desmin and actin alterations in human muscles affected by delayed onset muscle soreness: A high resolution immunocytochemical study. Histochem Cell Biol 2002;118:171–179.

466. Yu JG, Carlsson L, Thornell LE. Evidence for myofibril remodeling as opposed to myofibril damage in human muscles with DOMS: An ultrastructural and immunoelectron microscopic study. Histochem Cell Biol 2004;121:219–227.

467. Close GL, Ashton T, McArdle A, Maclaren DP. The emerging role of free radicals in delayed onset muscle soreness and contraction-induced muscle injury. Comp Biochem Physiol A Mol Integr Physiol 2005;142:257–266.

468. Gerwin RD. Classification, epidemiology, and natural history of myofascial pain syndrome. Curr Pain Headache Rep 2001;5:412–420.

469. Schiffman A. Myofascial pain associated with unilateral masseteric hypertrophy in a condylectomy patient. Cranio 1984;2:373–376.

470. Clark GT. Muscle hyperactivity, pain and dysfunction. In: Klineberg I, Sessle BJ (eds). Orofacial Pain and Neuromuscular Dysfunction Mechanisms and Clinical Correlates. Sydney: Pergamon, 1985:103–111.

471. Solberg W. Temporomandibular disorders: Masticatory myalgia and its management. Br Dent J 1986;160:351–356.

472. Fricton JR. Myofascial pain syndrome: Characteristics and epidemiology. In: Fricton JR, Awad E (eds). Advances in Pain Research and Therapy, vol 17: Myofasical Pain and Fibromyalgia. New York: Raven, 1990:107–127.

473. Dao TT, Lavigne GJ, Charbonneau A, Feine JS, Lund JP. The efficacy of oral splints in the treatment of myofascial pain of the jaw muscles. A controlled clinical trial. Pain 1994;56:85–94.

474. Svensson P. Muscle pain in the head: Overlap between temporomandibular disorders and tension-type headaches. Curr Opin Neurol 2007;20:320–325.

475. Fricton JR. Masticatory myofascial pain: An explanatory model integrating clinical, epidemiological and basic science research. Bull Group Int Rech Sci Stomatol Odontol 1999;41:14–25.

476. McMillan AS, Blasberg B. Pain-pressure threshold in painful jaw muscles following trigger point injection. J Orofac Pain 1994;8:384–390.

477. Gerwin RD, Dommerholt J, Shah JP. An expansion of Simons' integrated hypothesis of trigger point formation. Curr Pain Headache Rep 2004;8:468–475.

478. Shah JP, Phillips TM, Danoff JV, Gerber LH. An in vivo microanalytical technique for measuring the local biochemical milieu of human skeletal muscle. J Appl Physiol 2005;99:1977–1984.

479. Bowsher D. Neurogenic pain syndromes and their management. Br Med Bull 1991;47:644–666.

480. LaMotte RH, Shain CN, Simone DA, Tsai EF. Neurogenic hyperalgesia: Psychophysical studies of underlying mechanisms. J Neurophysiol 1991;66(1):190–211.

481. Simone DA, Sorkin LS, Oh U, et al. Neurogenic hyperalgesia: Central neural correlates in responses of spinothalamic tract neurons. J Neurophysiol 1991;66(1):228–246.

482. Sessle BJ. The neural basis of temporomandibular joint and masticatory muscle pain. J Orofac Pain 1999;13:238–245.

483. Lazer RB. Diagnostic implications of clinical fasciculations and cramps. In: Rowland LP (ed). Human Motor Neuron Diseases. New York: Raven, 1982:23–27.

484. Roth G. The origin of fasciculations. Ann Neurol 1982;12:542–547.

485. Tong KA, Christiansen EL, Heisler W, Hinshaw DB, Hasso AN. Asymptomatic myositis ossificans of the medial pterygoid muscles: A case report. J Orofac Pain 1994;8:223–226.

486. Kim DD, Lazow SK, Har-El G, Berger JR. Myositis ossificans traumatica of masticatory musculature: A case report and literature review. J Oral Maxillofac Surg 2002;60:1072–1076.

487. Baude Brogniez A, Ferri J, Vandenhaute B, Lecomte Houcke M, Donazzan M. Intra-masseter metastasis of a gastric adenocarcinoma. Rev Stomatol Chir Maxillofac 1997;98:303–305.

488. Mehra P, Cottrell DA, Booth DF, Jamil S. An unusual presentation of metastatic prostate cancer. J Oral Maxillofac Surg 1998;56:517–521.

489. Ahuja AT, King AD, Bradley MJ, Yeo WW, Mok TS, Metreweli C. Sonographic findings in masseter-muscle metastases. J Clin Ultrasound 2000;28:299–302.

490. Hashizume A, Nakagawa Y, Nagashima H, Ishibashi K. Rectal adenocarcinoma metastatic to the masseter muscle. J Oral Maxillofac Surg 2000;58:324–327.

491. Mizen KD, Loukota RA, Addante RR. Mass in the masseter muscle. J Oral Maxillofac Surg 2004;62:607–610.

492. Greene CS, Laskin DM. Long term evaluation of treatment for myofascial pain-dysfunction syndrome: A comparative analysis. J Am Dent Assoc 1983;107:235–238.

493. Mejersjo C, Carlsson GE. Long term results of treatment of temporomandibular pain-dysfunction. J Prosthet Dent 1983;49:809–815.

494. Fricton JR. Recent advances in temporomandibular disorders and orofacial pain. J Am Dent Assoc 1991;122:25–32.

495. Yatani H, Kaneshima T, Kuboki T, Yoshimoto A, Matsuka Y, Yamashita A. Long-term follow-up study on drop-out TMD patients with self-administered questionnaires. J Orofac Pain 1997;11:258–269.

496. Laskin DM, Greenfield W, Gale E, et al (eds). The President's Conference on the Examination, Diagnosis and Management of Temporomandibular Disorders. Chicago: American Dental Association, 1983.

497. Dahlstrom L. Conservative treatment methods in craniomandibular disorder. Swed Dent J 1992;16:217–230.

498. Clark GT. A diagnosis and treatment algorithm for common TM disorders. J Jpn Prosthodont Soc 1996;40:1029–1043.

499. Stohler CS, Zarb GA. On the management of temporomandibular disorders: A plea for a low-tech, high-prudence therapeutic approach. J Orofac Pain 1999;13:255–261.

500. Syrop SB. Initial management of temporomandibular disorders. Dent Today 2002;21:52–57.

501. Carlsson GE. Long-term effects of treatment of craniomandibular disorders. Cranio 1985;3:337–342.

502. Brown DT, Gaudet EL. Outcome measurement for treated and untreated TMD patients using the TMJ scale. Cranio 1994;12:216–221.

503. Apfelberg DB, Lavey E, Janetos G, Maser MR, Lash H. Temporomandibular joint diseases. Results of a ten-year study. Postgrad Med J 1979;65:167–172.

504. Okeson JP, Hayes DK. Long-term results of treatment for temporomandibular disorders: An evaluation by patients. J Am Dent Assoc 1986;112:473–478.

505. Garefis P, Grigoriadou E, Zarifi A, Koidis PT. Effectiveness of conservative treatment for craniomandibular disorders: A 2-year longitudinal study. J Orofac Pain 1994;8:309–314.

506. Helkimo E, Westling L. History, clinical findings, and outcome of treatment of patients with anterior disc displacement. Cranio 1987;5:269–276.

507. Murakami K, Kaneshita S, Kanoh C, Yamamura I. Ten-year outcome of nonsurgical treatment for the internal derangement of the temporomandibular joint with closed lock. Oral Surg Oral Med Oral Pathol Oral Radiol Endod 2002;94:572–575.

508. Schmitter M, Zahran M, Duc JM, Henschel V, Rammelsberg P. Conservative therapy in patients with anterior disc displacement without reduction using 2 common splints: A randomized clinical trial. J Oral Maxillofac Surg 2005;63:1295–1303.

509. Rasmussen OC. Temporomandibular arthropathy. Int J Oral Surg 1983;12:365–397.

510. De Leeuw R, Boering G, van der Kuijl B, Stegenga B. Hard and soft tissue imaging of the temporomandibular joint 30 years after diagnosis of osteoarthrosis and internal derangement. J Oral Maxillofac Surg 1996;54:1270–1280; discussion 1280–1281.

511. Rammelsberg P, LeResche L, Dworkin SF, Mancl L. Longitudinal outcome of temporomandibular disorders: A 5-year epidemiological study of muscle disorders defined by Research Diagnostic Criteria for Temporomandibular Disorders. J Orofac Pain 2003; 17:9–20.

512. Linton SJ, Hellsing AL, Andersson D. A controlled study of the effects of an early intervention on acute musculoskeletal pain problems. Pain 1993;54:353–359.

513. List T, Helkimo M. Acupuncture and occlusal splint therapy in the treatment of craniomandibular disorders. II. A 1-year follow-up study. Acta Odontol Scand 1992;50:375–385.

514. Roberts AH, Kewman DG, Mercier L, Hovell M. The power of nonspecific effects in healing: Implications for psychosocial and biological treatments. Clin Psych Rev 1993;13:375–391.

515. Greene CS, Laskin DM. Splint therapy for the myofascial pain-dysfunction (MPD) syndrome: A comparative study. J Am Dent Assoc 1972;624–628.

516. Flor H, Fydrich T, Turk DC. Efficacy of multidisciplinary pain treatment centers: A meta-analytic review. Pain 1992;49:221–230.

517. Hodges JM. Managing temporomandibular joint syndrome. Laryngoscope 1990;100:60–66.

518. Wright EF, Anderson GC, Schulte JK. A randomized clinical trial of intraoral soft splints and palliative treatment of masticatory muscle pain. J Orofac Pain 1995;9:192–199.

519. Danzig WN, VanDyke AR. Physical therapy as an adjunct to temporomandibular joint therapy. J Prosthet Dent 1983;49:96–99.

520. Michelotti A, de Wijer A, Steenks MH, Farella M. Home-exercise regimes for the management of nonspecific temporomandibular disorders. J Oral Rehabil 2005;32:779–785.

521. Poindexter RH, Wright EF, Murchison DF. Comparison of moist and dry heat penetration through orofacial tissues. Cranio 2002;20(1):28–33.

522. Rugh JD. Behavioral therapy. In: Mohl ND, Zarb GA, Carlsson GE, et al (eds). A Textbook of Occlusion. Chicago: Quintessence, 1988:329–338.

523. Oakley ME, McCreary CP, Clark GT, Holston S, Glover D, Kashima K. A cognitive-behavioral approach to temporomandibular dysfunction treatment failures: A controlled comparison. J Orofac Pain 1994;8:397–401.

524. Mealiea WL, McGlynn D. Temporomandibular disorders and bruxism. In: Hatch JP, Fisher JG, Rugh JD (eds). Biofeedback Studies in Clinical Efficacy. New York: Plenum, 1987:123–151.

525. Rugh JD. Psychological components of pain. Dent Clin North Am 1987;31:579–594.

526. Turner JA, Keefe FJ. Cognitive-behavioral therapy for chronic pain. In: Max M (ed). Pain 1999—An Updated Review. Seattle: IASP Press, 1999:523–533.

527. Dworkin SF, Massoth EL, Wilson L, Huggins KH, Truelove E. Guide to Temporomandibular Disorders: A Self-Management Approach. 1. Patient's Manual. Seattle: Univ of Washington, 1997.

528. Skevington SM. Psychology of Pain. Chichester, New York: Wiley, 1995.

529. Cannistraci AJ, Fritz G. Dental applications of biofeedback. In: Basmajiam JV (ed). Biofeedback, Principles and Practice for Clinicians. Baltimore: Williams & Wilkins, 1989:297–310.

530. Erlandson PM, Poppen R. Electromyographic biofeedback and rest position training of masticatory muscles in myofascial pain-dysfunction patients. J Prosthet Dent 1989;62:335–338.

531. Flor H, Birbaumer N. Comparison of the efficacy of electromyographic biofeedback, cognitive-behavioral therapy, and conservative medical interventions in the treatment of chronic musculoskeletal pain. J Consult Clin Psychol 1993;61:653–658.

532. National Institutes of Health Technology Assessment Conference on Integration of Behavioral and Relaxation Approaches Into the Treatment of Chronic Pain and Insomnia. Bethesda, MD: National Institutes of Health, 1995.

533. Crider AB, Glaros AG. A meta-analysis of EMG biofeedback treatment of temporomandibular disorders. J Orofac Pain 1999;13:29–37.

534. Dahlstrom L, Carlsson SG. Treatment of mandibular dysfunction: The clinical usefulness of biofeedback in relation to splint therapy. J Oral Rehabil 1984;11:277–284.

535. Funch DP, Gale EN. Factors associated with nocturnal bruxism and its treatment. J Behav Med 1980; 3:385–397.

536. Pierce CJ, Gale EN. A comparison of different treatments for nocturnal bruxism. J Dent Res 1988;67: 597–601.

537. Clark GT. A critical evaluation of orthopedic interocclusal appliance therapy: Design, theory and overall effectiveness. J Am Dent Assoc 1984;108:359–364.

538. Turk DC, Zaki HS, Rudy TE. Effects of intraoral appliance and biofeedback/stress management alone and in combination in treating pain and depression in patients with temporomandibular disorders. J Prosthet Dent 1993;70:158–164.

539. Caudill-Slosberg MA, Schwartz LM, Woloshin S. Office visits and analgesic prescriptions for musculoskeletal pain in US: 1980 vs. 2000. Pain 2004;109:514–519.

540. Kalso E, Edwards JE, Moore RA, McQuay HJ. Opioids in chronic non-cancer pain: Systematic review of efficacy and safety. Pain 2004;112:372–380.

541. Von Korff M, Deyo RA. Potent opioids for chronic musculoskeletal pain: Flying blind? Pain 2004;109:207–209.

542. Turk DC, Brody MC. Chronic opioid therapy for persistent noncancer pain: Panacea or oxymoron? Am Pain Soc Bull 1993;1:4–7.

543. Dionne RA. Pharmacologic Approaches. In: Laskin DM, Greene CS, Hylander WL (eds). TMDs. An Evidence-Based Approach to Diagnosis and Treatment. Chicago: Quintessence, 2006:347–357.

544. Tanaka TT. Differential diagnosis of arthritic disorders: Appendix, management of arthritic disorders with pharmaceuticals. Top Geriatr Rehabil 1990;5:47–49.

545. List T, Axelsson S, Leijon G. Pharmacological interventions in the treatment of temporomandibular disorders, atypical facial pain, and burning mouth syndrome. A qualitative systematic review. J Orofac Pain 2003:301–310.

546. Singer E, Dionne R. A controlled evaluation of ibuprofen and diazepam for chronic orofacial muscle pain. J Orofac Pain 1997;11:139–146.

547. Ta LE, Dionne RA. Treatment of painful temporomandibular joints with a cyclooxygenase-2 inhibitor: A randomized placebo-controlled comparison of celecoxib to naproxen. Pain 2004;111:13–21.

548. Mycek MJ, Harvey RA, Champe PC. Pharmacology, ed 2. Philadelphia: Lippincott-Raven, 1997.

549. Henry D, Drew A, Beuzeville S. Adverse drug reactions in the gastrointestinal system attributed to ibuprofen. In: Rainsford KD, Powanda MC (eds). Safety and Efficacy of Non-prescription (OTC) Analgesics and NSAIDs. London: Kluwer Academic, 1998:19–45.

550. Scheiman JM, Fendrick AM. Practical approaches to minimizing gastrointestinal and cardiovascular safety concerns with COX-2 inhibitors and NSAIDs. Arthritis Res Ther 2005;7(suppl 4):S23–S29.

551. Kopp S, Carlsson GE, Haraldson T, Wenneberg B. Long-term effect of intra-articular injections of sodium hyaluronate and corticosteroid on temporomandibular joint arthritis. J Oral Maxillofac Surg 1987;45:929–935.

552. Wenneberg B, Kopp S, Grondahl HG. Long-term effect of intra-articular injections of a glucocorticosteroid into the TMJ: A clinical and radiographic 8-year follow-up. J Craniomandib Disord Facial Oral Pain 1991;5:11–18.

553. Vallon D, Akerman S, Nilner M, Petersson A. Long-term follow-up of intra-articular injections into the temporomandibular joint in patients with rheumatoid arthritis. Swed Dent J 2002;26:149–158.

554. Wenneberg B, Kopp S. Short-term effects of intra-articular sodium hyaluronate, glucocorticoid, and saline injections on rheumatoid arthritis of the temporomandibular joint. J Craniomandib Disord Facial Oral Pain 1991;5:231–238.

555. Harkins SJ, Linford J, Cohen J, Kramer T, Cueva L. Administration of clonazepam in the treatment of TMD and associated myofascial pain: A double-blind pilot study. J Craniomandib Disord Facial Oral Pain 1991;5:179–186.

556. Russell IJ, Fletcher EM, Michalek JE, McBroom PC, Hester GG. Treatment of primary fibrositis/fibromyalgia syndrome with ibuprofen and alprazolam. A double-blind, placebo-controlled study. Arthritis Rheum 1991;34:552–560.

557. Montgomery MT, Nishioka GJ, Rugh JD, et al. Effect of diazepam on nocturnal masticatory muscle activity [abstract 96]. J Dent Res 1980;65(special issue):180.

558. Stanko JR. A review of oral skeletal muscle relaxants for the craniomandibular disorder (CMD) practitioner. Cranio 1990;9:234–243.

559. Saper JR, Lake AE III, Cantrell DT, Winner PK, White JR. Chronic daily headache prophylaxis with tizanidine: A double-blind, placebo-controlled, multicenter outcome study. Headache 2002;42:470–482.

560. Murros K, Kataja M, Hedman C, et al. Modified-release formulation of tizanidine in chronic tension-type headache. Headache 2000;40:633–637.

561. Borenstein DG, Korn S. Efficacy of a low-dose regimen of cyclobenzaprine hydrochloride in acute skeletal muscle spasm: Results of two placebo-controlled trials. Clin Ther 2003;25:1056–1073.

562. Turturro MA, Frater CR, D'Amico FJ. Cyclobenzaprine with ibuprofen versus ibuprofen alone in acute myofascial strain: A randomized, double-blind clinical trial. Ann Emerg Med 2003;41:818–826.

563. Tofferi JK, Jackson JL, O'Malley PG. Treatment of fibromyalgia with cyclobenzaprine: A meta-analysis. Arthritis Rheum 2005;15:9–13.

564. van Tulder MW, Touray T, Furlan AD, Solway S, Bouter LM. Muscle relaxants for nonspecific low back pain: A systematic review within the framework of the Cochrane collaboration. Spine 2003;28:1978–1992.

565. Herman CR, Schiffman EL, Look JO, Rindal DB. The effectiveness of adding pharmacologic treatment with clonazepam or cyclobenzaprine to patient education and self care for the treatment of jaw pain upon awakening: A randomized clinical trial. J Orofac Pain 2002;16:64–70.

566. Rizzatti-Barbosa CM, Martinelli DA, Ambrosano GM, de Albergaria-Barbosa JR. Therapeutic response of benzodiazepine, orphenadrine citrate and occlusal splint association in TMD pain. Cranio 2003;21:116–120.

567. Sharav Y, Singer E, Schmidt E, Dionne RA, Dubner R. The analgesic effect of amitriptyline on chronic facial pain. Pain 1987;31:199–209.

568. Brown BR, Bottomley WK. The utilization and mechanism of action of tricyclic antidepressant in the treatment of chronic facial pain: A review of the literature. Anesth Prog 1990;37:223–229.

569. Tura B, Tura SM. The analgesic effect of tricyclic antidepressants. Brain Res 1990;518:19–22.

570. Dionne RA. Antidepressants for chronic orofacial pain. Compend Contin Educ Dent 2000;21:822–824, 826, 828.

571. McQuay HJ, Tramer M, Nye BA, Carroll D, Wiffen PJ, Moore RA. A systematic review of antidepressants in neuropathic pain. Pain 1996;68(2-3):217–227.

572. Pettengill CA, Reisner-Keller L. The use of tricyclic antidepressants for the control of chronic orofacial pain. Cranio 1997;15:53–56.

573. Mohamed SE, Christensen LV, Penchas J. A randomized double-blind clinical trial of the effect of amitriptyline on nocturnal masseteric motor activity (sleep bruxism). Cranio 1997;15:326–332.

574. Raigrodski AJ, Christensen LV, Mohamed SE, Gardiner DM. The effect of four-week administration of amitriptyline on sleep bruxism. A double-blind crossover clinical study. Cranio 2001;19:21–25.

575. Raigrodski AJ, Mohamed SE, Gardiner DM. The effect of amitriptyline on pain intensity and perception of stress in bruxers. J Prosthodont 2001;10:73–77.

576. Brusie RW, Sullins KE, White NA, et al. Evaluation of sodium hyaluronate therapy in induced septic arthritis in the horse. Equine Vet J 1992;11(suppl):18–23.

577. Gaustad G, Larsen S. Comparison of polysulphated glycosaminoglycan and sodium hyaluronate with placebo in treatment of traumatic arthritis in horses. Equine Vet J 1995;27:356–362.

578. Xinmin Y, Jian H. Treatment of temporomandibular joint osteoarthritis with viscosupplementation and arthrocentesis on rabbit model. Oral Surg Oral Med Oral Pathol Oral Radiol Endod 2005;100(3):e35–e38.

579. Bertolami CN, Gay T, Clark GT, et al. Use of sodium hyaluronate in treating temporomandibular joint disorders: A randomized, double-blind, placebo-controlled clinical trial. J Oral Maxillofac Surg 1993;51:232–242.

580. Hirota W. Intra-articular injection of hyaluronic acid reduces total amounts of leukotriene C4, 6-keto-prostaglandin F1α, prostaglandin F2α and interleukin-1β in synovial fluid of patients with internal derangement in disorders of the temporomandibular joint. Br J Oral Maxillofac Surg 1998;36(1):35–38.

581. Alpaslan C, Bilgihan A, Alpaslan GH, Guner B, Ozgur YM, Erbas D. Effect of arthrocentesis and sodium hyaluronate injection on nitrite, nitrate, and thiobarbituric acid-reactive substance levels in the synovial fluid. Oral Surg Oral Med Oral Pathol Oral Radiol Endod 2000;89:686–690.

582. Sato S, Oguri S, Yamaguchi K, Kawamura H, Motegi K. Pumping injection of sodium hyaluronate for patients with non-reducing disc displacement of the temporomandibular joint: Two year follow-up. J Craniomaxillofac Surg 2001;29:89–93.

583. Sato S, Goto S, Kasahara T, Kawamura H, Motegi K. Effect of pumping with injection of sodium hyaluronate and the other factors related to outcome in patients with non-reducing disc displacement of the temporomandibular joint. Int J Oral Maxillofac Surg 2001;30:194–198.

584. Hepguler S, Akkoc YS, Pehlivan M, et al. The efficacy of intra-articular sodium, hyaluronate in patients with reducing displaced disc of the temporomandibular joint. J Oral Rehabil 2002;29:80–86.

585. Yeung RWK, Chow RLJ, Chiu K. Short-term therapeutic outcome of intra-articular high molecular weight hyaluronic acid injection for nonreducing disc displacement of the temporomandibular joint. Oral Surg Oral Med Oral Pathol Oral Radiol Endod 2006;102:453–461.

586. Kopp S, Akerman S, Nilner M. Short-term effects of intra-articular sodium hyaluronate, glucocorticoid, and saline injections on rheumatoid arthritis of the temporomandibular joint. J Craniomandib Disord Facial Oral Pain 1991;5:231–238.

587. Sato S, Ohta M, Ohki H, Kawamura H, Motegi K. Effect of lavage with injection of sodium hyaluronate for patients with nonreducing disc displacement of the temporomandibular joint. Oral Surg Oral Med Oral Pathol Oral Radiol Endod 1997;84:241–244.

588. Sato S, Sakamoto M, Kawamura H, Motegi K. Disc position and morphology in patients with nonreducing disc displacement treated by injection of sodium hyaluronate. Int J Oral Maxillofac Surg 1999;28:253–257.

589. Alpaslan GH, Alpaslan C. Efficacy of temporomandibular joint arthrocentesis with and without injection of sodium hyaluronate in treatment of internal derangements. J Oral Maxillofac Surg 2001;59:613–618.

590. Divine JG, Zazulak BT, Hewett TE. Viscosupplementation for knee osteoarthritis: A systematic review. Clin Orthop Relat Res 2007;455:113–122.

591. Shi Z, Guo C, Awad M. Hyaluronate for temporomandibular joint disorders. Cochrane Database Syst Rev 2004;(2):CD002970.

592. Kirk WS, Calabrese DK. Clinical evaluation of physical therapy in the management of internal derangement of the temporomandibular joint. J Oral Maxillofac Surg 1989;47:113–119.

593. Clark GT, Adachi NY, Dornan MR. Physical medicine procedures affect temporomandibular disorders: A review. J Am Dent Assoc 1990;121:151–161.

594. Carlsson J, Fahlcrantz A, Augustinsson LE. Muscle tenderness in tension headache treated with acupuncture or physiotherapy. Cephalalgia 1990;10:131–141.

595. Glass EG, McClynn FD, Glaros AG. A survey of treatments for myofascial pain dysfunction. Cranio 1991;9:165–168.

596. Feine JS, Lund JP. An assessment of the efficacy of physical therapy and physical modalities for the control of chronic musculoskeletal pain. Pain 1997;71:5–23.

597. Feine JS, Widmer CG, Lund JP. Physical therapy: A critique. Oral Surg Oral Med Oral Pathol Oral Radiol Endod 1997;83:123–127.

598. Wright EF. Using soft splints in your dental practice. Gen Dent 1999;47:506–510, 512.

599. Fricton JR. Clinical care for myofascial pain. Dent Clin North Am 1991;122:25–32.

600. Wright EF, Domenech MA, Fischer JR Jr. Usefulness of posture training for patients with temporomandibular disorders. J Am Dent Assoc 2000;131:202–210.

601. Olivo S, Bravo J, Magee D, Thie NM, Major PW, Flores-Mir C. The association between head and cervical posture and temporomandibular disorders: A systematic review. J Orofac Pain 2006;20:9–23.

602. Carlson CR, Okeson JP, Falace DA, Nitz AJ, Anderson D. Stretch-based relaxation and the reduction of EMG activity among masticatory muscle pain patients. J Craniomandib Disord Facial Oral Pain 1991;5:205–212.

603. Friedman MH, Weisberg J. Temporomandibular Joint Disorders: Diagnosis and Treatment. Chicago: Quintessence, 1985.

604. Au AR, Klineberg IJ. Isokinetic exercise management of temporomandibular joint clicking in young adults. J Prosthet Dent 1993;70:33–39.

605. Kraus SL. Physical therapy management of TMD. In: Kraus SL (ed). Temporomandibular Disorders, ed 2. New York: Churchill Livingstone, 1994:161–215.

606. VanDyke AR, Goldman SM. Manual reduction of displaced disc. Cranio 1990;8:350–352.

607. Minagi S, Nozaki S, Sato T, Tsuru H. A manipulation technique for treatment of anterior disc displacement without reduction. J Prosthet Dent 1991;65:686–691.

608. Segami N, Murakami K, Iizuka T. Arthrographic evaluation of disc position following mandibular manipulation technique for internal derangement with closed lock of the temporomandibular joint. J Craniomandib Disord Facial Oral Pain 1991;4:99–108.

609. Wolf SL. Electrotherapy: Clinics in Physical Therapy. New York: Churchill Livingstone, 1991.

610. Murphy GJ. Electrical physical therapy in treating TMJ patients. Cranio 1983;2:67–73.

611. Bettany JA, Fish DR, Mendel FC. Influence of high voltage pulsed direct current on edema formation following impact injury. Phys Ther 1988;4:219–224.

612. Reed BV. Effect of high voltage pulsed electrical stimulation on microvascular permeability to plasma proteins. Phys Ther 1988;4:491–495.

613. Moystad A, Krogstad BS, Larheim TA. Transcutaneous nerve stimulation in a group of patients with rheumatic disease involving the temporomandibular joint. J Prosthet Dent 1990;64:596–600.

614. Mohl ND, Ohrbach RK, Crow HC, Gross AJ. Devices for diagnosis and treatment of temporomandibular disorders. Part III. Thermography, ultrasound, electrical stimulation and EMG biofeedback. J Prosthet Dent 1990;63:472–477.

615. Ziskin MC, McDiarmid T, Michlovitz SL. Therapeutic ultrasound. In: Michlovitz SL (ed). Thermal Agents in Rehabilitation, ed 2. Philadelphia: Davis, 1990:134–169.

616. Hartley A. Ultrasound: A Monograph. Chattanooga, TN: Chattanooga Group, 1991.

617. Mannheimer JS. Therapeutic modalities. In: Kraus SL (ed). TMJ Disorders: Management of the Craniomandibular Complex. New York: Churchill Livingstone, 1988:311–337.

618. Cameron MH, Monroe LG. Relative transmission of ultrasound by media customarily used for phonophoresis. Phys Ther 1993;72:142–148.

619. van der Windt DA, van der Heijden GJ, van den Berg SG, ter Riet G, de Winter AF, Bouter LM. Ultrasound therapy for musculoskeletal disorders: A systematic review. Pain 1999;81:257–271.

620. Lark MR, Gangaros LP. Iontophoresis: An effective modality for the treatment of inflammatory disorders of the temporomandibular joint and myofascial pain. Cranio 1990;9:108–119.

621. Reid KI, Dionne RA, Sicard-Rosenbaum L, Lord D, Dubner RA. Evaluation of iontophoretically applied dexamethasone for painful pathologic temporo-mandibular joints. Oral Surg Oral Med Oral Pathol 1994;77:605–609.

622. Schiffman EL, Braun BL, Lindgren BR. Temporo-mandibular joint iontophoresis: A double-blind ran-domized clinical trial. J Orofac Pain 1996;10:157–165.

623. Jaeger B, Reeves JL. Quantification of changes in my-ofascial trigger point sensitivity with pressure al-gometer following passive stretch. Pain 1986;27:203–210.

624. Carlson CR, Okeson JP, Falace DA, Nitz AJ, Lin-droth JE. Reduction of pain and EMG activity in the masseter region by trapezius trigger point injection. Pain 1993;55:397–400.

625. Hong CZ. Lidocaine injection versus dry needling to myofascial trigger point. The importance of the local twitch response. Am J Phys Med Rehabil 1994;73:256–263.

626. Scicchitano J, Rounsefell B, Plilowsky I. Baseline cor-relates of the response to the treatment of chronic localized myofascial pain syndrome by injection of local anesthetic. J Psychosom Res 1996;40:75–85.

627. Hong CZ. Treatment of myofascial pain syndrome. Curr Pain Headache Rep 2006;10:345–349.

628. Zink W, Graf BM. Local anesthetic myotoxicity. Reg Anesth Pain Med 2004;29:333–340.

629. Raustia AM, Pohjola RT, Virtanen KK. Acupuncture compared with stomatognathic treatment for TMJ dysfunction. I. A randomized study. J Prosthet Dent 1985;54:581–585.

630. Raustia AM, Pohjola RT, Virtanen KK. Acupuncture compared with stomatognathic treatment for TMJ dysfunction. II. Components of the dysfunction index. J Prosthet Dent 1986;55:372–376.

631. Johansson A, Wenneberg B, Wagersten C, Harald-son T. Acupuncture in treatment of facial muscular pain. Acta Odontol Scand 1991;49:153–158.

632. List T, Helkimo M, Andersson S, Carlsson GE. Acu-puncture and occlusal splint therapy in the treat-ment of craniomandibular disorders. I. A compara-tive study. Swed Dent J 1992;16:125–141.

633. List T, Helkimo M, Karlsson R. Pressure pain thresholds in patients with craniomandibular dis-orders before and after treatment with acupuncture and occlusal splint therapy: A controlled clinical study. J Orofac Pain 1993;7:275–282.

634. Goddard G, Karibe H, McNeill C, Villafuerte E. Acupuncture and sham acupuncture reduce muscle pain in myofascial pain patients. J Orofac Pain 2002;16:71–76.

635. Mackler LS, Collender SL. Therapeutic uses of light in rehabilitation. In: Michlovitz SL (ed). Thermal Agents in Rehabilitation. Philadelphia: Davis, 1996:255–277.

636. Beckerman H, de Bie RA, Bouter LM, De Cuyper HJ, Oostendorp RA. The efficacy of laser therapy for musculoskeletal and skin disorders: A criteria-based meta-analysis of randomized clinical trials. Phys Ther 1992;72:483–491.

637. Gam AN, Thorsen H, Lonnberg F. The effect of low-level laser therapy on musculoskeletal pain: A meta-analysis. Pain 1993;52:63–66.

638. Bertolucci LE, Grey T. Clinical analysis of mid-laser versus placebo treatment of arthralgic TMJ degen-erative joints. Cranio 1995;13:26–29.

639. Gray RJM, Quayle AA, Hall CA, Schofield MA. Phys-iotherapy in the treatment of temporomandibular joint disorders: A comparative study of four treat-ment methods. Br Dent J 1994;176:257–261.

640. Bertolucci LE, Grey T. Clinical comparative study of microcurrent electrical stimulation to mid-laser and placebo treatment in degenerative joint disease of the temporomandibular joint. Cranio 1995;13:116–120.

641. Pinheiro AL, Cavalcanti ET, Pinheiro TI, et al. Low-level laser therapy is an important tool to treat dis-orders of the maxillofacial region. J Clin Laser Med Surg 1998;16:223–226.

642. Pinheiro AL, Cavalcanti ET, Pinheiro TI, Alves MJ, Manzi CT. Low-level laser therapy in the manage-ment of disorders of the maxillofacial region. J Clin Laser Med Surg 1997;15:181–183.

643. Conti PC. Low level laser therapy in the treatment of temporomandibular disorders (TMD): A double-blind pilot study. Cranio 1997;15:144–149.

644. Hansson TL. Infrared laser in the treatment of cran-iomandibular disorders, arthrogenous pain. J Pros-thet Dent 1989;61:614–617.

645. Kulekcioglu S, Sivrioglu K, Ozcan O, Parlak M. Ef-fectiveness of low-level laser therapy in temporo-mandibular disorder. Scand J Rheumatol 2003;32:114–118.

646. Cetiner S, Kahraman SA, Yucetas S. Evaluation of low-level laser therapy in the treatment of temporo-mandibular disorders. Photomed Laser Surg 2006;24:637–6741.

647. Ramfjord SP, Ash MM. Occlusion. Philadelphia: Saunders, 1983.

648. Posselt U. Treatment of bruxism by bite guards and bite planes. J Can Dent Assoc 1963;29:773–778.

649. Pavone B. Bruxism and its effect on natural teeth. J Prosthet Dent 1985;53:692–696.

650. Solberg WK, Clark GT, Rugh JD. Nocturnal elec-tromyographic evaluation of bruxism patients un-dergoing short term splint therapy. J Oral Rehabil 1975;2:215–223.

651. Clark GT, Beemsterboer PL, Rugh JD. Nocturnal masseter muscle activity and the symptoms of mas-ticatory dysfunction. J Oral Rehabil 1981;8:279–286.

652. Okeson JP, Kemper JT, Moody PM. A study of the use of occlusion splints in the treatment of acute and chronic patients with craniomandibular disorders. J Prosthet Dent 1982;48:708–712.

653. Laskin DM, Block L. Diagnosis and treatment of myofascial pain dysfunction syndrome. J Prosthet Dent 1986;56:76–84.

654. Kurita H, Ikeda K, Kurashina K. Evaluation of the effect of a stabilization splint on occlusal force in patients with masticatory muscle disorders. J Oral Rehabil 2000;27:79–82.

655. Carraro JJ, Caffesse RG. Effect of occlusal splints in TMJ symptomology. J Prosthet Dent 1978;40:563–566.

656. Goharian RK, Neff PA. Effect of occlusal retainers on temporomandibular joint and facial pain. J Prosthet Dent 1980;44:206–208.

657. Pruim GJ, de Jongh HJ, ten Bosch JJ. Forces acting on the mandible during bilateral static bite at different bite force levels. J Biomech 1980;13:755–763.

658. Spear FM. Fundamental occlusal therapy considerations. In: McNeill C (ed). Science and Practice of Occlusion. Chicago: Quintessence, 1997:421–434.

659. Conti PC, dos Santos CN, Kogawa EM, Conti AC, de Araujo C. The treatment of painful temporomandibular joint clicking with oral splints: A randomized clinical trial. J Am Dent Assoc 2006;137:1108–1114.

660. Farrar WB. Differentiation of temporomandibular joint dysfunction to simplify treatment. J Prosthet Dent 1972;28:629–636.

661. Farrar WB. Craniomandibular practice: The state of the art; definition and diagnosis. Cranio 1982;1:5–12.

662. Clark GT. Treatment of jaw clicking with temporomandibular repositioning: Analysis of 25 cases. Cranio 1984;2:263–270.

663. Lundh H, Westesson PL, Kopp S, Tillstrom B. Anterior repositioning splint in the treatment of temporomandibular joints with reciprocal clicking: Comparison with a flat occlusal splint and an untreated control group. Oral Surg Oral Med Oral Pathol 1985;60:131–36.

664. Pertes RA, Gross SC. Clinical management of temporomandibular disorders and orofacial pain. Chicago: Quintessence, 1995.

665. Kemper JT. Effect of occlusal retainers on temporomandibular joint and facial pain. J Prosthet Dent 1983;49:702–705.

666. Tsuga K, Akagawa Y, Sakaguchi R, et al. A short-term evaluation of the effectiveness of stabilization-type occlusal splint therapy for specific symptoms of temporomandibular joint dysfunction syndrome. J Prosthet Dent 1989;61:610–613.

667. Marbach JJ, Raphael KG. Future directions in the treatment of chronic musculoskeletal facial pain: The role of evidence based care. Oral Surg Oral Med Oral Pathol Oral Radiol Endod 1997;83:170–176.

668. Dao T, Lavigne GJ. Oral splints: The crutches for temporomandibular disorders and bruxism? Crit Rev Oral Biol Med 1998;9:345–361.

669. Kreiner M, Betancor E, Clark GT. Occlusal stabilization appliances. Evidence of their efficacy. J Am Dent Assoc 2001;132:770–777.

670. Turp JC, Komine F, Hugger A. Efficacy of stabilization splints for the management of patients with masticatory muscle pain: A qualitative systematic review. Clin Oral Investig 2004;179–195.

671. Forssell H, Kalso E, Koskela P, Vehmanen R, Puukka P, Alanen P. Occlusal treatments in temporomandibular disorders: A qualitative systematic review of randomized controlled trials. Pain 1999;83:549–560.

672. Forssell H, Kalso E. Application of principles of evidence based medicine to occlusal treatment for temporomandibular disorders: Are there lessions to be learned? J Orofac Pain 2004;18:9–22.

673. Al-Ani Z, Gray RJ, Davies SJ, Sloan P, Glenny AM. Stabilization splint therapy for the treatment of temporomandibular myofascial pain: A systematic review. J Dent Educ 2005;69:1242–1250.

674. Abbott DM, Bush FM. Occlusions altered by removable appliances. J Am Dent Assoc 1991;122:79–81.

675. Brown DT, Gaudet EL, Phillips C. Changes in vertical tooth position and face height related to long term anterior repositioning splint therapy. Cranio 1994;12:19–22.

676. Ekberg E, Vallon D, Nilner M. Treatment outcome of headache after occlusal appliance therapy in a randomized controlled trial among patients with temporomandibular disorders of mainly arthrogenous origin. Swed Dent J 2002;26:115–124.

677. Franco AA, Yamashita HK, Lederman HM, Cevidanes LH, Proffit WR, Vigorito JW. Frankel appliance therapy and the temporomandibular disc: A prospective magnetic resonance imaging study. Am J Orthod Dentofac Orthop 2002;121:447–457.

678. Linde C, Isacsson G, Jonsson BG. Outcome of 6-week treatment with transcutaneous electric nerve stimulation compared with splint on symptomatic temporomandibular joint disk displacement without reduction. Acta Odontol Scand 1995;53:92–98.

679. Bush FM. Tinnitus and otalgia in temporomandibular disorders. J Prosthet Dent 1987;58:495–498.

680. Major PW, Nebbe B. Use and effectiveness of splint appliance therapy: Review of literature. Cranio 1997;15:159–166.

681. Capp NJ. Occlusion and splint therapy. Br Dent J 1999;186:217–222.

682. Henrikson T, Nilner M. Temporomandibular disorders and the need for stomatognathic treatment in orthodontically treated and untreated girls. Eur J Orthod 2000;22:283–292.

683. Biondi DM. Headaches and their relationship to sleep. Dent Clin North Am 2001;45:685–700.

684. Andreasen JO, Andreasen FM, Mejare I, Cvek M. Healing of 400 intra-alveolar root fractures. 1. Effect of pre-injury and injury factors such as sex, age, stage of root development, fracture type, location of fracture and severity of dislocation. Dent Traumatol 2004;20:192–202.

685. Ekberg EC, Nilner M. Treatment outcome of short- and long-term appliance therapy in patients with TMD of myogenous origin and tension-type headache. J Oral Rehabil 2006;33:713–721.

686. Okeson JP. The effects of hard and soft splints on nocturnal bruxism. J Am Dent Assoc 1987;114:788–791.

687. Shan SC, Yun WH. Influence of an occlusal splint on integrated electromyography of the masseter muscle. J Oral Rehabil 1991;18:253–256.

688. Chung SC, Kim UK, Kim HS. Prevalence and patterns of nocturnal bruxofacets on stabilization splints in temporomandibular disorder patients. Cranio 2000;18:92–97.

689. Ingerslev H. Functional disturbances of the masticatory system in school children. J Dent Child 1983;50:446–450.

690. Harkins S, Marteney JL, Cueva O, Cueva L. Application of soft occlusal splints in patients suffering from clicking temporomandibular joints. Cranio 1988;6:71–76.

691. Pettengill CA, Growney MR Jr, Schoff R, Kenworthy CR. A pilot study comparing the efficacy of hard and soft stabilizing appliances in treating patients with temporomandibular disorders. J Prosthet Dent 1998;79:165–168.

692. Truelove E, Huggins KH, Manci L, Dworkin SF. The efficacy of traditional, low-cost and nonsplint therapies for temporomandibular disorder. A randomized controlled trial. J Am Dent Assoc 2006;137:1099–1107.

693. Singh BP, Berry DC. Occlusal changes following use of soft occlusal splints. J Prosthet Dent 1985;54:711–715.

694. Shankland WE. Nociceptive trigeminal inhibition—Tension supression system: A method of preventing migraine and tension headaches. Compend Contin Educ Dent 2002;23:105–108, 110, 112–113.

695. Shankland WE. Nociceptive trigeminal inhibition—Tension supression system: A method of preventing migraine and tension headaches. Compend Contin Educ Dent 2001;22:1075–1080, 1082 [erratum 2002:23:105–108, 112–113].

696. Jokstad A, Mo A, Krogstad BS. Clinical comparison between two different splint designs for temporomandibular disorder therapy. Acta Odontol Scand 2005;63:218–226.

697. Magnusson T, Adiels AM, Nilsson HL, Helkimo M. Treatment effect on signs and symptoms of temporomandibular disorders—Comparison between stabilization splint and a new type of splint (NTI). A pilot study. Swed Dent J 2004;28:11–20.

698. Gelb ML, Gelb H. Gelb appliance: Mandibular orthopedic repositioning therapy. Cranio Clin Int 1991;1(2):81–98.

699. Anderson GC, Schulte JK, Goodkind RJ. Comparative study of two treatment methods for internal derangements of the TMJ. J Prosthet Dent 1985;53:392–397.

700. Clark GT. TMJ repositioning appliance: A technique for construction, insertion, and adjustment. Cranio 1986;4:37–46.

701. Lundh H, Westesson PL, Jisander S, et al. Disc repositioning onlays in the treatment of temporomandibular joint disc displacement: Comparison with a flat plane occlusal splint and no treatment. Oral Surg 1988;66:155–162.

702. Tallents RH, Katzberg RW, Macher DJ, Roberts CA. Use of protrusive splint therapy in anterior disc displacement of the temporomandibular joint: A 1- to 3-year follow-up. J Prosthet Dent 1990;63:336–341.

703. Tallents RH, Katzberg RW, Miller TL, et al. Arthrographically assisted splint therapy: Painful clicking with a nonreducing meniscus. Oral Surg 1986;61:2–4.

704. Eberhard D, Bantleon HP, Steger W. The efficacy of anterior repositioning splint therapy studied by magnetic resonance imaging. Eur J Orthod 2002;24:343–352.

705. Simmons HC, Gibbs SJ. Anterior repositioning appliance therapy for TMJ disorders: Specific symptoms relieved and relationship to disk status on MRI. Cranio 2005;23:89–99.

706. Farrar WB. Diagnosis and treatment of painful temporomandibular joints. J Prosthet Dent 1968;20:345–351.

707. Orenstein ES. Anterior repositioning appliances when used for anterior disc displacement with reduction—A critical review. Cranio 1993;11:141–145.

708. Moloney F, Howard JA. Internal derangements of the temporomandibular joint. III. Anterior repositioning splint therapy. Aust Dent J 1986;31:30–39.

709. Okeson JP. Long-term treatment of disk-interference disorders of the temporomandibular joint with anterior repositioning occlusal splints. J Prosthet Dent 1988;60:611–616.

710. Summer JD, Westesson PL. Mandibular repositioning can be effective in treatment of reducing TMJ disc displacement. A long term clinical and MR imaging follow-up. Cranio 1997;15:107–120.

711. Widmalm SE. Use and abuse of bite splints. Compend Contin Educ Dent 1999;20:249–254.

712. Kirk WS. Magnetic resonance imaging and tomographic evaluation of occlusal appliance treatment for advanced internal derangement of the temporomandibular joint. J Oral Maxillofac Surg 1991;49:9–12.

713. Chung SC, Kim HS. The effect of stabilization splint on the TMJ closed lock. Cranio 1993;11:95–101.

714. Tecco S, Festa F, Salini V, Epifania E, D'Attilio M. Treatment of joint pain and joint noises associated with a recent TMJ internal derangement: A comparison of an anterior repositioning splint, a full-arch maxillary stabilization splint, and an untreated control group. Cranio 2004;22:209–219.

715. McNeill C. Temporomandibular disorders: Guidelines for diagnosis and management. J Calif Dent Assoc 1991;19:15–26.

716. Allanen PJ, Kirveskari PK. Disorders in TMJ research. J Craniomandib Disord Facial Oral Pain 1990;4:223–227.

717. De Boever JA, Carlsson GE, Klineberg IJ. Need for occlusal therapy and prosthodontic treatment in the management of temporomandibular disorders. Part II. Tooth loss and prosthodontic treatment. J Oral Rehabil 2000;27:647–659.

718. Just JK, Perry HT, Greene CS. Treating TM disorders: A survey on diagnosis, etiology and management. J Am Dent Assoc 1991;122:56–60.

719. Carlsson GE, Droukas BC. Dental occlusion and the health of the masticatory system. Cranio 1984;2:142–147.

720. Graham GS, Rugh JD. Maxillary splint occlusal guidance patterns and electromyographic activity of jaw closing muscles. J Prosthet Dent 1988;59:73–77.

721. Rugh JD, Graham GS, Smith JC, Ohrbach RK. Effects of canine versus molar occlusal splint guidance on nocturnal bruxism and craniomandibular symptomatology. J Craniomandib Disord Facial Oral Pain 1989;3:203–210.

722. Minagi S, Watanabe H, Sato T, Tsuru H. The relationship between balancing-side occlusal contact patterns and temporomandibular joint sounds in humans: Proposition of the concept of balancing-side protection. J Craniomandib Disord Facial Oral Pain 1990;4:251–256.

723. Denbo JA. Malocclusion. Dent Clin North Am 1990;34:103–109.

724. Michelotti A, Farella M, Gallo LM, Veltri A, Palla S, Martina R. Effect of occlusal interference on habitual activity of human masseter. J Dent Res 2005;84:644–648.

725. Koh H, Robinson PG. Occlusal adjustment for treating and preventing temporomandibular joint disorders. Cochrane Database Syst Rev 2003;(1):CD003812.

726. Fricton J. Current evidence providing clarity in management of temporomandibular disorders: Summary of a systematic review of randomized clinical trials for intra-oral appliances and occlusal therapies. J Evid Based Dent Pract 2006;6(1):48–52.

727. Hannam AG. Optimum occlusal relationships are essential for craniomandibular harmony [position paper]. In: Klineberg I, Sessle BJ (eds). Oro-facial Pain and Neuromuscular Dysfunction: Mechanisms and Clinical Correlates. Oxford: Pergamon Press, 1984.

728. Hylander WL. Mandibular function and temporomandibular joint loading. In: Carlson DS, McNamara JA Jr, Ribbens KA (eds). Developmental Aspects of Temporomandibular Joint Disorders. Craniofacial Growth Series, No. 16. Ann Arbor: Univ of Michigan, 1985.

729. Faulkner MG, Hatcher DC, Hay A. A three-dimensional investigation of temporomandibular joint loading. J Biomech 1987;20:997–1002.

730. Gausch K. Occlusal therapy of neuromuscular problems in the orofacial region. Int Dent J 1981;31:267–272.

731. Perry HT. Occlusal therapy: Repositioning. In: Laskin DM, Greenfield W, Gale E (eds). The President's Conference on the Examination, Diagnosis and Management of Temporomandibular Disorders. Chicago: American Dental Association, 1983:155–160.

732. Bradley GR. The Effect of Splint Therapy and Orthodontic Extrusion on TMJ Symptoms [thesis]. St Louis: St Louis University, 1989.

733. Greene CS. Orthodontics and the temporomandibular joint. Angle Orthod 1982;52:66–172.

734. Panchez H. The Herbst appliance—Its biologic effect and clinical use. Am J Orthod 1985;87:1–20.

735. Nielsen L, Melsen B, Terp S. TMJ function and the effects on the masticatory system on 14-16 year old Danish children in relation to orthodontic treatment. Eur J Orthod 1990;12:254–267.

736. Sadowsky C, BeGole EA. Long term status of temporomandibular joint function and functional occlusion after orthodontic treatment. Am J Orthod 1980;78:201–212.

737. Gold P. The Role of Orthodontic Treatment and Malocclusion in the Etiology of Mandibular Dysfunction [thesis]. Winnipeg, MB: Univ of Manitoba, 1980.

738. Janson M, Hasund A. Functional problems in orthodontic patients out of retention. Eur J Orthod 1981;3:172–179.

739. Sadowsky C, Polson AM. Temporomandibular disorders and functional occlusion after orthodontic treatments: Results of two long-term studies. Am J Orthod 1984;86:386–390.

740. Gross AJ, Gale E. Mandibular dysfunction and orthodontic treatment [abstract 1565]. J Dent Res 1984;63(special issue):354.

741. Eriksson I, Dahlberg G, Westesson PL, et al. Changes in TMJ disc position associated with orthognathic surgery. Oral Maxillofac Surg Clin North Am 1990; 2:691–698.

742. Reynder RM. Orthodontics and temporomandibular disorders: A review of the literature (1966–1988). Am J Orthod Dentofac Orthop 1990;97:463–471.

743. Dibbets JMH, van der Weele LT. Extraction, orthodontic treatment, and craniomandibular dysfunction. Am J Orthod Dentofac Orthop 1991;99:210–219.

744. Sadowsky C, Theisen TA, Sakol EI. Orthodontic treatment and temporomandibular joint sounds—A longitudinal study. Am J Orthod Dentofac Orthop 1991;99:441–447.

745. Kremenak CR, Kinser DD, Melcher TJ, et al. Orthodontics as a risk factor for temporomandibular disorders (TMD). II. Am J Orthod Dentofac Orthop 1992;101:21–27.

746. Hirata RH, Heft MW, Hernandez B, et al. Longitudinal study of signs of temporomandibular disorders (TMD) in orthodontically treated and untreated groups. Am J Orthod Dentofac Orthop 1992;101:35–40.

747. Rendell JK, Northon LA, Gay T. Orthodontic treatment and temporomandibular joint disorders. Am J Orthod Dentofac Orthop 1992;101:84–87.

748. Henrikson T. Temporomandibular disorders and mandibular function in relation to Class I malocclusion and orthodontic treatment. A controlled, prospective and longitudinal study. Swed Dent J Suppl 1999;134:1–144.

749. Egermark I, Magnusson T, Carlsson GE. A 20 year follow-up of signs and symptoms of temporomandibular disorders and malocclusions in subjects with and without orthodontic treatment in childhood. Angle Orthod 2003;73:109–115.

750. Mohlin BO, Derweduwen K, Pilley R, Kingdon A, Shaw WC, Kenealy P. Malocclusion and temporomandibular disorder: A comparison of adolescents with moderate to severe dysfunction with those without signs and symptoms of temporomandibular disorder and their further development to 30 years of age. Angle Orthod 2004;74:319–327.

751. Egermark I, Carlsson GE, Magnusson T. A prospective long-term study of signs and symptoms of temporomandibular disorders in patients who received orthodontic treatment in childhood. Angle Orthod 2005;75:645–650.

752. Spahl TJ, Witzig JW. The Clinical Management of Basic Maxillofacial Orthopedic Appliances, Vol I: Mechanics. Littleton, CO: PSG, 1987.

753. Palla S. Untersuchungen zur okklusionsbedingten Distraktion der Kiefergelenke nach orthodontish indizierter Pramolaren-Extraktion [thesis]. Zurich: Univ of Zurich, 1987.

754. Kundinger KK, Austin BP, Christensen LV, Donegan SJ, Ferguson DJ. An evaluation of temporomandibular joints and jaw muscles after orthodontic treatment involving premolar extractions. Am J Orthod Dentofac Orthop 1991;100:100–115.

755. Gianelly AA, Hughes HM, Wohlgemuth P, Gildea G. Condylar position and extract treatment. Am J Orthod Dentofac Orthop 1988;93:201–205.

756. Leucke PE, Johnston LE. The effect of maxillary first premolar extraction and incisor retraction on mandibular position: Testing the central dogma of "functional orthodontics." Am J Orthod Dentofac Orthop 1992;101:4–12.

757. Johnston LE Jr. EICO. Gnathologic assessment of centric slides in post-retention orthodontic patients. J Prosthet Dent 1988;60:712–715.

758. Leucke PE. The Effect of Maxillary Bicuspid Extraction Treatment of Class II, Division I Malocclusion on Mandibular Position [thesis]. St Louis: St Louis Univ, 1990.

759. Larsson E, Ronnerman A. Mandibular dysfunction symptoms in orthodontically treated patients ten years after completion of treatment. Eur J Orthod 1981;3:89–94.

760. Beattle JR, Paquewtte DE, Johnston LE. The functional impact of extraction and non-extraction treatments: A long-term comparison in patients with "borderline," equally susceptible Class II malocclusions. Am J Orthod Dentofac Orthop 1994;105:444–449.

761. Carlton KL, Nanda RS. Prospective study of posttreatment changes in the temporomandibular joint. Am J Orthod Dentofac Orthop 2002;122:486–490.

762. Egermark I, Thilander B. Craniomandibular disorders with special reference to orthodontic treatment: An evaluation from childhood to adulthood. Am J Orthod Dentofac Orthop 1992;101:28–34.

763. Luther F. TMD and occlusion. Part I. Damned if we do? Occlusion: The interface of dentistry and orthodontics. Br Dent J 2007;202(1):E2; discussion 38–39.

764. Solberg W, Seligman DA. Temporomandibular orthopedics: A new vista in orthodontics? In: Johnson LA (ed). New Vistas in Orthodontics. Philadelphia: Lea & Febiger, 1985.

765. Athanasiou AE, Melsen B, Eriksen J. Concerns, motivation and experiences of orthognathic surgery patients: A retrospective study of 152 patients. Int J Adult Orthod Orthognath Surg 1989;2:47–55.

766. Ochs M, La Banc JP, Dolwick MF. The diagnosis and management of concomitant dentofacial deformity and temporomandibular disorder. Oral Maxillofac Surg Clin North Am 1990;2:669–690.

767. Magnusson T, Ahbort G, Svartz K. Function of the masticatory system in 20 patients with mandibular hypo- or hyperplasia after correction by sagittal split osteotomy. Int J Oral Maxillofac Surg 1990;19:289–293.

768. Leshem D, Tompson B, Britto JA, Forrest CR, Phillips JH. Orthognathic surgery in juvenile rheumatoid arthritis patients. Plast Reconstr Surg 2006;117:1941–1946.

769. Aghabeigi B, Hiranaka D, Keith DA, Kelly JP, Crean SJ. Effect of orthognathic surgery on the temporomandibular joint in patients with anterior open bite. Int J Adult Orthod Orthognath Surg 2001;16:153–160.

770. Feinerman DM, Piecuch JF. Long-term effects of orthognathic surgery on the temporomandibular joint: Comparison of rigid and nonrigid fixation methods. Int J Oral Maxillofac Surg 1995;24:268–272.

771. American Society of Temporomandibular Joint Surgeons. Guidelines for diagnosis and treatment of disorders of the temporomandibular joint and related musculoskeletal disorders. Dallas, 1990.

772. Parameters of care for oral and maxillofacial surgery. A guide for practice, monitoring and evaluation (AAOMS Parameters of Care-92). American Association of Oral and Maxillofacial Surgeons. J Oral Maxillofac Surg 1992;50(7 suppl 2):i–xvi, 1–174.

773. Nitzan DW, Dolwick MF, Martinez GA. Temporomandibular joint arthrocentesis: A simplified treatment for severe, limited mouth opening. J Oral Maxillofac Surg 1991;49:1163–1167.

774. Dimitroulis G, Dolwick MF, Martinez GA. Temporomandibular joint arthrocentesis and lavage for the treatment of closed lock: A follow-up study. Br J Oral Maxillofac Surg 1995;33:23–27.

775. Nitzan DW, Price A. The use of arthrocentesis for the treatment of osteoarthritis of the temporomandibular joints. J Oral Maxillofac Surg 2001;59:1154–1159; discussion 1160.

776. Trieger N, Hoffman CH, Rodriguez E. The effect of arthrocentesis of the temporomandibular joint in patients with rheumatoid arthritis. J Oral Maxillofac Surg 1999;57:537–540.

777. Al-Belasy FA, Dolwick MF. Arthrocentesis for the treatment of temporomandibular joint closed lock: A review article. Int J Oral Maxillofac Surg 2007.

778. Heffez LB. Arthroscopy. In: Kaplan AS, Assael LA (eds). Temporomandibular Disorders. Philadelphia: Saunders, 1992:656.

779. Buckley MJ, Merrill RG, Braun TW. Surgical management of internal derangement of the temporomandibular joint. J Oral Maxillofac Surg 1993;51 (suppl 1):20–27.

780. Blaustein D, Heffez L. Diagnostic arthroscopy to the temporomandibular joint. Part II. Arthroscopic findings of arthographically diagnosed disc displacement. Oral Surg Oral Med Oral Pathol 1988;65:135–141.

781. Nitzan DW, Dolwick MF. An alternative explanation for the genesis of closed-lock symptoms in the internal derangement process. J Oral Maxillofac Surg 1991;49:810–815.

782. Montgomery MT, van Sickels JE, Harms SE. Success of temporomandibular joint arthroscopy in disc displacement with and without reduction. Oral Surg Oral Med Oral Pathol 1991;71:651–659.

783. Moses JJ, Sartoris D, Glass R, Tanaka T, Poker I. The effect of arthroscopic surgical lysis and lavage of the superior joint space on TMJ disc position and mobility. J Oral Maxillofac Surg 1989;47:674–678.

784. Gabler MJ, Greene CS, Palacios E, Perry HT. Effect of arthroscopic temporomandibular joint surgery on articular disc position. J Craniomandib Disord Facial Oral Pain 1989:191–202.

785. Nitzan DW, Dolwick MF, Heft MW. Arthroscopic lavage and lysis of the temporomandibular joint: A change of perspective. J Oral Maxillofac Surg 1990;48:798–801.

786. Perrott DH, Alborzi A, Kaban LB, et al. A prospective evaluation of the effectiveness of temporomandibular joint arthroscopy. J Oral Maxillofac Surg 1990;48:1029–1032.

787. Moses JJ, Topper C. A functional approach to the treatment of temporomandibular joint internal derangement. J Craniomandib Disord Facial Oral Pain 1991;5:19–27.

788. Ohnuki T, Fukuda M, Nakata A, et al. Evaluation of the position, mobility, and morphology of the disc by MRI before and after four different treatments for temporomandibular joint disorders. Dentomaxillofac Radiol 2006;35:103–109.

789. Kuwahara T, Bessette RW, Murayama T. A retrospective study on the clinical results of temporomandibular joint surgery. Cranio 1994;12:179–183.

790. Holmlund AB, Axelsson S, Gynther GW. A comparison of discectomy and arthroscopic lysis and lavage for the treatment of chronic closed lock of the temporomandibular joint: A randomized outcome study. J Oral Maxillofac Surg 2001;59:972–977; discussion 977–978.

791. Hall HD, Indresano AT, Kirk WS, Dietrich MS. Prospective multicenter comparison of 4 temporomandibular joint operations. J Oral Maxillofac Surg 2005;63:1174–1179.

792. Undt G, Murakami K, Rasse M, Ewers R. Open versus arthroscopic surgery for internal derangement of the temporomandibular joint: A retrospective study comparing two centres' results using the Jaw Pain and Function Questionnaire. J Craniomaxillofac Surg 2006;34:234–241.

793. Politi M, Sembronio S, Robiony M, Costa F, Toro C, Undt G. High condylectomy and disc repositioning compared to arthroscopic lysis, lavage, and capsular stretch for the treatment of chronic closed lock of the temporomandibular joint. Oral Surg Oral Med Oral Pathol Oral Radiol Endod 2007;103(1): 27–33.

794. Schiffman EL, Look JO, Hodges JS, et al. Randomized effectiveness study of four therapeutic strategies for TMJ closed lock. J Dent Res 2007;86:58–63.

795. Reston JT, Turkelson CM. Meta-analysis of surgical treatments for temporomandibular articular disorders. J Oral Maxillofac Surg 2003;61(1):3–10; discussion 10–12.

796. Anderson DM, Sinclair PM, McBride KM. A clinical evaluation of temporomandibular joint disk plication surgery. Am J Orthod Dentofac Orthop 1991; 100:156–162.

797. Hall HD, Nickerson JW Jr, McKenna SJ. Modified condylotomy for treatment of the painful temporomandibular joint with a reducing point. J Oral Maxillofac Surg 1993;51:133–142.

798. Trumpy IG, Lyberg T. Surgical treatment of internal derangement of the temporomandibular joint: Long-term evaluation of three techniques. J Oral Maxillofac Surg 1995;53:740-746; discussion 746–747.

799. Krug J, Jirousek Z, Suchmova H, Cermakova E. Influence of discoplasty and discectomy of the temporomandibular joint on elimination of pain and restricted mouth opening. Acta Medica (Hradec Kralove) 2004;47(1):47–53.

800. Silver CM. Long-term results of meniscectomy of the temporomandibular joint. Cranio 1984;3:46–57.

801. Eriksson L, Westesson PL. Long-term evaluation of meniscectomy of the temporomandibular joint. J Oral Maxillofac Surg 1985;43:263–267.

802. Hall HD. The role of discectomy for treating internal derangements of the temporomandibular joint. Oral Maxillofac Surg Clin North Am 1994;6:287–294.

803. Takaku S, Sano T, Yoshida M. Long-term magnetic resonance imaging after temporomandibular joint discectomy without replacement. J Oral Maxillofac Surg 2000;58:739–745.

804. Dimitroulis G. The use of dermis grafts after discectomy for internal derangement of the temporomandibular joint. J Oral Maxillofac Surg 2005;63: 173–178.

805. Nickerson JW Jr, Veaco NS. Condylotomy in surgery of the temporomandibular joint. Oral Maxillofac Surg Clin North Am 1989;1:303–327.

806. Nickerson JW Jr. The role of condylotomy in the management of temporomandibular joint disorders. In: Worthington P, Evans J Jr (eds). Controversies in Oral and Maxillofacial Surgery, ed 4. Philadelphia: Saunders, 1993.

807. Hall HD. A technique to improve predictability of condylar position with modified condylotomy. Oral Surg Oral Med Oral Pathol Oral Radiol Endod 1999;88:127–128.

808. Hall HD, Navarro EZ, Gibbs SJ. Prospective study of modified condylotomy for treatment of nonreducing disk displacement. Oral Surg Oral Med Oral Pathol Oral Radiol Endod 2000;89:147–158.

809. Hall HD, Navarro EZ, Gibbs SJ. One- and three-year prospective outcome study of modified condylotomy for treatment of reducing disc displacement. J Oral Maxillofac Surg 2000;58(1):7–17; discussion 18.

810. Friedman LM, Furberg CD, DeMets DL. Fundamentals of Clinical Trials, ed 2. St Louis: Mosby, 1985.

811. Silverman WA. Human Experimentation: A Guided Step into the Unknown. Oxford: Oxford Univ Press, 1985.

812. Feinstein AR. Clinical Judgment. Melbourne, FL: Krieger, 1967.

813. Feinstein AR. Clinical Epidemiology: The Architecture of Clinical Research. Philadelphia: Saunders, 1985.

# Cervicogenic Mechanisms of Orofacial Pain and Headaches

Neuromusculoskeletal structures within the cervical spine can contribute to orofacial pain dysfunction syndromes, separate from or in addition to temporomandibular disorders (TMDs). The clinician should be able to understand the mechanisms of referred cervicogenic pain, perform a screening evaluation so that an accurate diagnosis can be established, and initiate appropriate referral for further evaluation and comprehensive management.

*Cervical spine disorders* (CSDs) is a term that embraces a number of disorders involving the muscles, facet joints, discs, and nerves of the cervical spine. Symptoms vary with physical activity and/or static positioning but may develop spontaneously or follow trauma. Subclassification of CSDs includes an extensive list of traditional diag-

nostic terms, such as *cervical sprain/strain*, *discogenic disease*, *facet syndrome*, *myositis*, *fibrositis*, *fibromyositis*, and *articular hypo-* and *hypermobility*.[1] Patients may have two or three diagnoses by different physicians, depending on whether these physicians focused on pathophysiology, radiology, clinical symptoms, physical symptoms, duration of episode, or a combination of these factors.[1] In the absence of disease and fracture, determining the cause of cervical pain is difficult. To facilitate communication among health care professionals, a CSD subclassification scheme is proposed in Box 9-1. The proposal is adapted from guidelines used for low back pain and focuses on signs and symptoms that provide a better description of inclusion and exclusion criteria in a common language.[2,3]

1. *Convergence and central excitation of cervical sensory and motor neurons stimulates trigeminal motor neurons, causing an increase in masticatory activity.*

Stimulation of tissues innervated by the upper cervical segments has been demonstrated to influence motor activity of the trigeminal-innervated muscles of mastication.[39–42] Electrical stimulation applied to the central end of the ablated first cervical nerve has demonstrated EMG activity in masticatory muscles.[43] Experimental work has demonstrated that patients with an upper trapezius trigger point and ipsilateral masseter pain show decreased discomfort and a reduction in masseteric EMG activity after a single trigger-point injection in the upper trapezius.[40,43] Studies suggest that experimental trapezius pain can spread over a wide area to include the temporomandibular region, with elevation of masticatory activity and reduction of mouth opening.[44] Pain originating from the cervical spine also can cause changes in trigeminal-innervated musculature. It is speculated that a similar convergence and central excitation as seen with trigeminal and cervical sensory neurons may also exist for trigeminal motor neurons.[45,46]

2. *Masticatory muscles (antagonists) are activated in response to contraction of cervical spine muscles (agonists) by the process of cocontraction.*

Coordinated head, neck, and mandibular movements suggest a neurophysiologic and biomechanical interplay involving agonist/antagonist actions between the cervical and masticatory musculature.[47–50] The cervical and masticatory muscles can be viewed as agonistic and antagonistic to one another, and reciprocal innervation may play a role in modifying excitatory and inhibitory levels of appropriate neurons.[49–52] Daily events may cause the muscles of mastication to disproportionately contract in response to cervical muscles contracting. Isometric, isotonic, or eccentric contractions of cervical spine muscles occur during lifting, carrying, pushing, pulling, and reaching activities. When cervical spine muscles perform repetitive activity under load and over long duration, it is more likely that the muscles of mastication will disproportionately contract.[53]

# Screening Evaluation of the Cervical Spine

In the last two decades, classification criteria for TMDs and CSDs were proposed, which allow for standardization and replication of the physical examination used to recognize these disorders.[14,54,55] As these criteria evolve, validation of the taxonomic systems remains in process. Moreover, even though both disorders concern musculoskeletal structures, there is no universal diagnostic system that can be applied to both TMDs and CSDs.

Similar to the diagnostic process for TMDs, a chronologic history of treatments, sleep and work positions, functional limitations, and successful pain modifiers is critical to the diagnosis of a CSD. It is beyond the scope of this chapter to describe a thorough examination of the cervical spine.[56–58] The screening clinical examination may include assessment of the active range of motion and recording of responses to palpation of the cervical spine and associated muscles.

The active range of motion of the head and cervical spine may be observed and pain responses noted during extension, flexion, rotation, and side-bending head movements. Passive range of motion of the cervical spine should not be evaluated unless the clinician has had specific training in these techniques. For palpation evaluation, the same procedure used for the muscles of mastication may be used for assessing the cervical muscles. A neurologic examination consisting of muscle, reflex, and sensory testing will complete the cervical spine examination.

Important cervical muscles or muscle groups to evaluate are the sternocleidomastoid (SCM), suboccipital, paravertebral (scalenes), posterior deep cervical, and upper trapezius muscles. If further evaluation of the cervical region is indicated, referral to an appropriately trained clinician is recommended. Suboccipital pain syndromes are usually evaluated by physical therapists or spine specialists, who perform postural assessment as well as palpation for the presence of myalgic bands, trigger points, or tender facet joint pillars.[56,59-64] Craniofacial pain may either be triggered, reduced, or enhanced by manual segmental movement (compression/distraction), static and dynamic pain tests, or postural provocation testing techniques such as foraminal encroachment (Spurling test) and maximization of the forward head posture.[56,64,65]

Radiographs provide an ideal means by which mobility of the cervical spine is evaluated. Conventional radiography forms the basis of examination of the patient with acute cervical spine pathology, and a minimum of two views, preferably obtained in perpendicular planes, is essential. Typically, films are obtained with natural head position in neutral lateral, flexed, extended (retroflexion), oblique, and anteroposterior directions.[66-69]

If findings indicate nerve root involvement, further study with magnetic resonance imaging (MRI) or computerized tomography (CT) is recommended. Both MRI and CT techniques require the subject to be in a supine position, however, which eliminates the weight-bearing compression forces that are more pronounced by everyday postural situations and thus MRI and CT results may not be truly indicative of the effects of those functional and compressive forces. Obtaining, reading, or even requesting such imaging generally falls beyond the scope of the orofacial pain specialist. Patients not responding to physical therapy may need to have their source of pain verified and evaluated by the use of short-acting local anesthetic blocks to the suspected region or structure.[70-73]

## Craniofacial Pain Syndromes of Cervical Origin

Pain disorders of the cervical spine can involve a variety of structures, such as fascia, muscles, ligaments, joints, bones, and vascular and neural tissues. Symptoms such as dizziness, gastrointestinal complaints, and visual, memory, and cognition problems may accompany some of these disorders, and the presence of these symptoms may contribute to misdiagnosis.[74,75]

Knowledge of the anatomy and innervation of the various structures that make up the suboccipital spine is required to understand the myriad pain syndromes that originate from this region and often mimic forms of headache and orofacial pain. Also, understanding the referral patterns and characteristics of pain and dysfunction can provide the dental practitioner and physical therapist with the means by which to delineate the structure that is causing the pain.

## Innervation of the cervical spine

The cervical spine comprises the suboccipital and mid-lower cervical sections. The suboccipital spine is considered the switching station for all afferent and efferent transmission to the cranium and orofacial region. The first three cervical nerves (C1-C3) mediate pain at the suboccipital spine and may refer pain to the craniofacial region. These nerves innervate the ligaments and joints of the suboccipital spine, the anterior, posterior, and lateral suboccipital muscles, as well as the SCM and upper trapezius. They also innervate the posterior dura mater, tentorium and falx cerebelli, vertebral arteries, and the lateral walls of the posterior cranial fossa.

At the base of the occiput, the foramen magnum contains the meningeal branches of C1-C3, the vertebral and spinal arteries, and the spinal components of the spinal accessory nerve. The posterior cranial fossa contains the confluence of sinuses, the roots of the fifth to twelfth cranial nerves, the first two cervical nerves via the hypoglossal canal, the branches of C2-C3 through the foramen magnum, and the ascending branches of C1-C3, thus comprising several potential pathways for cervicogenic referral to the craniofacial region.[76-79] The greater occipital nerve branches off from the C2 dorsal root ganglia and thus may represent a source for occipital pain with or without retroorbital referral. Suboccipital spinal neurons have been shown to be excited by ipsilateral vagal input and correspond to dermatomal receptive fields of the upper cervical segments. They may represent another referral mechanism to the neck and jaw.[80,81]

The spinal accessory nerve, which arises from the C2-C4 levels, innervates the SCM and upper trapezius, both of which commonly refer pain to the craniofacial region. Spinal accessory fibers also cross the midline, providing implications for contralateral or bilateral frontal headache.[82-85]

Another source of cranial pain is transmitted via the C1-C3 sinuvertebral nerves, which innervate the cranial membranes, dura mater of the posterior cranial fossa, and epidural vasculature.[76,77] From the C3 level and below, the sinuvertebral nerves also provide innervation to the outer third of the intervertebral annular fibers as well as the cruciate, posterior longitudinal, and atlantoaxial ligaments.[76,78,79,86] The occipito-atlantal and atlantoaxial levels are devoid of intervertebral discs; however, sinuvertebral nerves are present at these two levels.

The SCM and upper trapezius are involved in positional control of the head in space along with the ligaments, facet joints, and capsules of the atlas and axis. Proper head position, balance, and equilibrium depend on a composite of visual and vestibular signals in addition to mechanical input from the suboccipital spine. Abnormal suboccipital afferent input can therefore contribute to torticollis, dizziness, nystagmus, vertigo, and disequilibrium in conjunction with craniofacial pain.[82,85,87,88]

## Common CSDs

While it is important for the dental practitioner to be aware of the cervical etiologic factors in orofacial pain, cervical disorders are not primarily managed in the dental setting. Patients with cervical disorders should be referred to a knowledgeable physical therapist or cervical spine specialist for evaluation and treatment.

## Cervicalgia (ICD-9 723.1)

*Cervicalgia* is a broad term meaning pain in the neck and represents the most common neck pain complaint. Although the pain may originate from any cervical structure, discomfort is primarily felt in the suboccipital area, SCM, and upper trapezius, with possible referral to the frontal, temporoparietal, occipital, vertex, and orbital regions. In addition, auditory, gastrointestinal, vestibular, and visual symptoms can occur as a result of vertebral artery involvement or convergence at the suboccipital region via neural interaction at the trigeminocervical complex with the spinal accessory and vagus nerves. Suboccipital discomfort is frequently associated with headache, nausea, vomiting, diplopia, dysphagia, and respiratory distress, which may cause the inexperienced clinician to immediately consider a primary vascular component. Dizziness can result from altered proprioception due to increased nociceptive input to cervical facet mechanoreceptors or to hyperactivity of the SCM.[41,56,74,75,88] Gastrointestinal disturbances may be due to involvement of the vagus nerve. The presence of these red flags should prompt the clinician to seek additional evaluation and care for such patients, which may include referral to an experienced physical therapist (Box 9-2).

Delayed referral in the presence of red flags and associated cervical hypomobility and/or postural dysfunction may lead to adaptive soft tissue shortening and joint restriction. Complications may progress to intervertebral disc bulging/herniation (*ICD-9 722.0*) as well as spondylosis (*ICD-9 721.0/ 721.1*). Intervertebral disc bulging or herniation may also occur as a result of acute trauma, whereas spondylosis and/or disc involvement can also be the result of cumu-

| **Box 9-2** Symptoms requiring referral |
| --- |
| Gradual worsening of symptoms |
| Constant upper quadrant pain |
| Upper extremity paresthesias |
| Marked postural changes |
| Marked limitation of cervical mobility |
| Disorientation |
| Respiratory distress |
| Dizziness, vertigo, nystagmus |
| Nausea, vomiting, dysphagia, globus |
| Visual deficits |
| Unrelenting headache |

lative microtrauma due to longstanding postural dysfunction. The association between cervicalgia and headache is significant.[89,90]

## Cervical strain (ICD-9 847.0)

The most frequent traumatic spinal injury encountered in medical practice is a sprain or strain of the cervical spine following a motor vehicle accident.[91] Other terms used to describe this disorder are *flexion-extension injury*, *acceleration-deceleration injury*, and *whiplash*. The location and nature of the injuries that occur as a result of head and neck strain vary depending on the severity of the trauma and the structures involved.[91-96] The incidence of soft tissue injury to the cervical spine and resultant neck pain along with postural changes is significant.[91,93-96] Depending on the mechanism of injury, a cervical strain can affect the anterior, posterior, or lateral structures of the cervical spine, as well as the shoulder girdle in whole or in part. Therefore, the Quebec Task Force suggests use of the term *whiplash-associated disorder*.[94] Recent studies show that patients with whiplash-associated disorder have significantly more signs and symptoms of TMDs than controls.[97–99]

The upper cervical spine usually sustains the greatest injury in flexion-extension injuries, because it is a pivot point. Acute suboccipital flexion and concomitant extension of the lower cervical spine may also result in increased dural tension and increased tension of the C1-C3 roots.[92] Postural factors such as a head-rest that is placed too low or a posteriorly inclined seat back may result in hyperextension of the head past the limit of stretch of the soft tissues of the neck, which can lead to a compression fracture of the posterior arch of the atlas.[96] Lateral whiplash can result in tractional injuries to the brachial plexus that may even cause nerve root avulsion, leading to Erb palsy.[91,93,96] In patients with preexisting cervical spondylosis, flexion-extension injuries may cause acute intervertebral disc herniation, giving rise to upper extremity myelopathy and radiculopathy.[95]

The onset of neck pain following acute trauma may be immediate or delayed for 24 to 48 hours, or in some instances, for several days. The onset of pain may occur as an "ache" or "stiffness" in the neck that is localized to the cervical paraspinal muscles depending on the mechanics of injury. Beside the common muscle guarding, stiffness, and local tenderness, pain referral to sites distant from the original injury is common. Headache, dizziness, tinnitus, dysphagia, and visual disturbances may occur with involvement of the suboccipital muscles, the SCM, and the upper trapezius.[74,75,91,96] Following the initial injury, neck pain is generally accompanied by limitations in range of motion secondary to involvement of the paraspinal musculature from either direct damage to the muscles (rupture or tear) or

by reflex response (splinting). Such injuries usually cause damage to both muscles and ligaments, and healing is often aggravated or delayed by sensory hyperactivity and abnormal function of the cervical spine.[73,100,101]

Patients with cervical strain injuries often present with subjective symptoms that are much greater than the objective signs. They often report a history of poor response to conventional therapeutic interventions and may present with psychologic and behavioral aspects common to chronic pain disorders. Consequently, these patients are often misclassified as hysterics or malingerers. Nevertheless, clinical and experimental evidence leaves little doubt that most cervical strain injuries can be explained on firm physiologic grounds. Evidence suggests that most patients with whiplash injuries recover within 2 months, but some may suffer from chronic cervical pain indefinitely.[94]

A history of trauma to the cervical spine is not always indicative of cervical strain. Other disorders that need to be considered in the differential diagnosis are degenerative osteoarthritis (OA), joint and ligamentous laxity, inflammatory diseases of muscle, vascular insufficiency, and neural compression syndromes. In addition, pathologic processes in other areas, such as the head, shoulders, or diaphragm, can cause pain that is referred to the neck. Such referred pain may be difficult to distinguish from primary cervical pathology.

Most minor cervical strains and spasms can be managed with rest, immobilization, anti-inflammatory drugs, and muscle relaxants until the patient is pain free and has regained full mobility of the cervical spine. Functional restoration may require an individualized and comprehensive physical therapy program, which may include short-term immobilization via a cervical collar.[102,103] Although the cervical collar is the most frequently used orthotic, it is recommended that it be used only until the acute pain has subsided for fear of creating hypomobility. A recent study did not find any difference in pain and disability scores between patients who wore a soft cervical collar for 2 versus 10 days.[103] Tendons can be injured as well, and may slow down recovery and necessitate physical therapy with postural reeducation that includes unloading and gradual reloading.[101]

## Cervical osteoarthritis (ICD-9 721.0)

Direct or indirect cumulative microtrauma to the weight-bearing joints of the cervical spine may lead to progressive degenerative arthritic changes. These changes may occur when the normally well-hydrated intervertebral discs lose their ability to withstand loading forces or are affected by abnormal postural factors.[104,105] There also may be degenerative changes to the vertebral body, adjacent uncinate processes (joints of Luschka), and posterior facet areas.[104] The cervical spine supports 10 to 15 pounds of weight through daily motions of the head. The most common load-bearing sites are in the area of C5-C6 and C6-C7, which are common regions of intervertebral disc disease.[106] Degenerative changes include inflammation of the joint linings with osteophyte formation, along with bony and cartilaginous exostoses. OA of the synovial joints is more usual in the more mobile upper cervical segments.[104]

OA is common in individuals aged 50 years and older, and may be associated with genetic predisposition. By the seventh decade of life, 75% of individuals display signs and symptoms of OA, and it is generally considered that 100% will develop it during the course of a normal lifetime.[105] As the elasticity of tissues decreases with age, there is a concomitant loss of range of motion, the neck becomes less resilient, and muscle strength declines. Early subjective complaints of OA include occasional episodes of neck pain triggered by activity, exertion, minor trauma, or weather changes, but postural factors should also be considered. Often these episodes will resolve in several days or a week with little more than rest. More advanced symptoms include stiffness, limitation of movements, crepitation, local pain, tenderness, and myalgia.

Early cervical OA may present without radiographic changes, while advanced cases frequently reveal radiographic evidence, such as alteration in curvature of the spine, loss of lordosis, narrowing of the intervertebral disc spaces, and anterior or posterior osteophytes.[69,106] Lateral neck movements, rotation, and extension are generally more limited than flexion. Progressive degeneration may lead to narrowing of the intervertebral spaces, and disc displacements may result in radiculopathy. Both sensory and motor roots may be involved, but sensory symptoms are more common and include pain, paresthesia, hypoesthesia, and hyperesthesia. With involvement of the C1-C3 nerve roots, pain may be referred to the head, neck, and shoulder girdle, and may be accompanied by suboccipital or occipital headaches, blurred vision, tinnitus, and dysphagia.[56,67-69] Involvement of the C4-T2 roots can cause interscapular, arm, and finger symptoms, all of which can be associated with painless or painful crepitation on active range of motion.[104,105,107] In advanced cervical OA, osteophytes and exostosis of neural foramina can lead to stenosis and nerve root compression, with subsequent cervical spondylotic myelopathy.

Mild and moderate stages of cervical OA will normally respond to comprehensive physical therapy management with or without medication. However, once osteoarthritic changes have reached the point of neural compression and radiculitis or myelopathy ensues, remission of symptoms is more difficult. Management at this stage may be accomplished by compliance with postural corrective guidelines, home use of a suboccipital traction device, and transcutaneous electrical nerve stimulation with or without medication.[108] Traction is preferably performed intermittently and in the supine position to avoid compressive forces on the temporomandibular joint (TMJ).[109]

## Compression, irritation, or distortion of upper cervical roots by structural lesions (IHS 13.12)

Entrapment or impingement of cervical rootlets, roots, ganglia, and peripheral nerves can occur throughout the cervical spine. Entrapment of C1-C3 may cause ipsilateral or contralateral headaches, facial pain, and associated sensory deficits. Compression, irritation, or distortion of the C1 root may produce orbital, frontal, and vertex pain.[86,110] C1-mediated pain may arise from irritation of the atlantooccipital joint, which may result in occipitofrontal headache.[86] C1-mediated pain may also be caused by vertebral dissection of the C1 horizontal segment, entrapment from posterior fossa tumors, or compression of the vertebral artery.[110,111]

The C2 root exits between the atlas and axis, and its peripheral distribution forms the greater occipital nerve, supplying sensation to the scalp from the occiput to the vertex. Disorders that affect the C2 dorsal rootlets, root, ganglion, or the peripheral branch may cause neuralgic pain, numbness, and dysesthesia, accompanied by a sensory deficit. The ventral ramus of the C2 root has meningeal branches to the hypoglossal and vagus nerves, which may account for throat and gastrointestinal symptoms.[112,113] Dull pain, primarily in the suboccipital, occipital, and frontal regions, may be due to lesions in anatomic structures innervated by peripheral branches of C2.[86,114] C3 and its distribution may refer pain in the preauricular region, with associated sensory deficits. Irritation or compression of the root of C3 may cause referred pain to the pinna, the angle of the jaw, the TMJ, and the retroorbital area.[86,114] Structures innervated by C3, such as the zygoapophyseal joints of C2-C3, may cause pain in the occipital region.[80,114] Space-occupying processes such as a tumor, vascular lesions (eg, arteriovenous malformation or aneurysm), or bony changes causing lesions of C2-C3 can also produce cephalic pain.

Cervical entrapment disorders should be referred to the proper health care professional for evaluation and management. If space-occupying lesions or malignant processes have been ruled out as the source of the pain, comprehensive noninvasive treatment may include definitive manual physical therapy, with education and instructions in proper postural corrective techniques and therapeutic exercises.

## Cervicogenic headache (IHS 11.2.1; ICD-9 723.2 or ICD-9 784.0)

Cervicogenic headache is defined as "referred pain perceived in any part of the head caused by a primary nociceptive source in the musculoskeletal tissues innervated by cervical nerves."[115–117] While there may be no single entity called cervicogenic headache it is reasonable to refer to headaches that originate in the cervical region as *cervicogenic* or *cervically mediated*, or as a *cervical-cranial syndrome*.[118]

Cervicogenic headache is characterized by a moderately severe, dull, dragging, unilateral headache without side-shift. The pain is provoked or aggravated by neck movements. The headache may last from 1 to 3 days and may be accompanied by myriad symptoms, including lacrimation, conjunctival hyperemia, dizziness, nausea, vomiting, and sensitivity to light and noise.[117] The IHS diagnostic criteria state that clinical signs need to imply that the source of the pain is a cervical structure and that the headache is abolished by diagnostic blockade of the source or its innervation.[119]

There are numerous structures in the region of the cervical spine that are pain sensitive and refer pain to the head. Craniofacial pain is mediated by the first three cervical nerves, the C1-C3 sinuvertebral nerves, and cranial nerves V, VII, IX, X, XI, and XII. Additional innervation is provided by sympathetic afferents that course with the first two thoracic nerves, synapsing in the trigeminal nucleus, as well as parasympathetic afferents traveling with cranial nerves VII and IX.[20,78] Irritating forces on these nerves at sites of neural compression can mediate craniofacial referral. The density of the suboccipital musculature along with the SCM and upper trapezius are prime sources of cervicogenic headache of myofascial origin. The myriad neural pathways that course through, connect with, or originate from the C1-C3 levels provide fertile ground for the development of discomfort in the suboccipital fossa, with referral to the occiput and vertex of the head. Anastomosis of the occipital to the supraorbital nerve, which is a trigeminal branch, provides a distinct neural pathway for headache in this region.[78] In addition, the myofascial connection between the occipitalis and frontalis muscles represents another mechanism behind the common occipital-frontal headache.[85] A decrease in the suboccipital space by occipitoatlantal approximation due to a forward head posture, which may be compounded by posterior cranial rotation, presents a mechanical mechanism for compression or irritation of the musculature, vasculature, and neural innervating components that compose the entire trigeminocervical complex.

Pain referred from the cervical muscles can be similar to that of a vascular or tension-type headache.[89,90,120-122] Referral of pain to the eye is quite common in headache of cervicogenic origin.[70] Pain can also be perceived in more than one area of the head and face.[85] A prime example is referral to the occipital, temporoparietal, and lateral orbital regions caused by hyperactivity of the upper trapezius, which in addition refers pain to the angle of the mandible in the masseteric region.[85]

The comorbidity of cervical and craniofacial pain is commonly seen by physical therapists, and this relationship has been well documented.[6,9-12,48,123-125] A definitive physical therapy evaluation of the upper quarter and temporomandibular complex is required to delineate the origin of headache as stemming from the cervical as opposed to the craniofacial region.

## Occipital neuralgia (IHS 13.8)

*Occipital neuralgia* is characterized by paroxysms of jabbing pain in the distribution of the greater or lesser occipital nerves, with the occasional persistence of aching between attacks. There may be a reduction of sensation or dysesthesia in the area, and the affected nerve is tender on palpation.

The pathogenesis is not always clear but may be related to trauma of the nerve. The differential diagnosis includes occipital referral of pain from the atlantoaxial or upper zygapophyseal joints, tender trigger points in neck muscles, and neoplasia or other lesions affecting the spine or occiput.[126]

A decrease in the suboccipital space by occipital-atlantal approximation due to a forward head posture, which may be compounded by posterior cranial rotation, presents a mechanical mechanism for compression or irritation of the musclulature, vasculature, and neural innervating components that comprise the entire trigemino-cervial complex. Manual or intermittant mechanical suboccipital traction or injection of local anesthetics and corticosteroids may provide temporary and even longlasting relief.[126]

## Dural headache (ICD-9 784.0)

The pain quality of dural headache is achy and can exist bilaterally or on alternate sides.[127] Dural pain is commonly triggered by abnormal movements, postures, or positions. Dural tension testing, such as in the form of the slump or the long-sitting test may recreate or increase the pain. It is therefore imperative that patients be asked about their sitting, working, and sleep postures, which may create tension on the spinal dura that emanates to the cranial region.[56,109] Posterior disc bulging or herniation at the C2-C3 or C3-C4 levels can also cause the outer annular fibers to press against the posterior longitudinal ligament and thus put pressure on the anterior dura, giving rise to craniofacial pain.[127–129] The anatomic relationship between the rectus capitis posterior minor in the suboccipital fossa and its attachment to the dura mater may also represent a source of dural headache.[130–134]

Chemical stimulation of the intracranial dura has demonstrated that all dura-sensitive neurons have cutaneous receptive fields, including one or more trigeminal divisions, the most common being the ophthalmic branch.[130–134] This evidence has implications for the origin of dural as well as vascular headache and the related eye pain that often accompanies these entities.

## Eagle syndrome

*Eagle syndrome*, which consists of either elongation or calcification of the stylohyoid ligament, has a variable presentation that may include sore throat, dysphagia, otalgia, glossodynia, headache, or vague orofacial pain, predominantly along the neck.[135,136] The patient may report pain on swallowing, yawning, or turning of the head. The pain is usually unilateral and has a neuralgic quality that may mimic glossopharyngeal neuralgia. Examination should include palpation of the stylohyoid area and tonsillar fossa, and provocation tests such as turning the head in an ipsi- as well as contralateral direction. Carotidynia is often confused with Eagle syndrome because of the close approximation of the styloid process and carotid artery. Spasm of the carotid artery can occur as a result of a traumatic hyperextension injury or contact irritation from an elongated styloid process. The SCM also courses in the same vicinity, and carotidymia or styloid compression may therefore excite the SCM and create a secondary occipital, frontal, or orbital headache. Radiographic examination will reveal the elongated/calcified stylohyoid process.[137] Treatment may consist of pharmacologic management with analgesics or anti-inflammatory agents and/or surgical excision via either an intraoral or extraoral approach.[135,136,138]

## Torticollis (ICD-9 723.5)

*Torticollis*, also known as *wry* or *stiff neck*, can occur from congenital absence of one SCM; musculoskeletal trauma; metabolic, infectious, or neurologic factors; and emotional triggers.[87,88,139] The resultant muscular rigidity, adversely affecting ipsilateral sidebending and contralateral rotation of the head, is caused by hyperactivity of the SCM and/or the upper trapezius, both of which cause myotomal referral to the craniofacial region. Bilateral SCM involvement will cause posterior cranial rotation.[140] The pain distribution from SCM referral depends in part on involvement of one or both heads of this muscle and can include the occiput, ear, forehead, and orbital region. Referral to the eye involves the superior, lateral, and inferior orbit, which may mimic migraine.[85] Frontal pain can be unilateral on the side of the involved SCM, contralateral, or bilateral due to the contralateral referral pattern of the SCM. The levator scapulae may also be involved, further contributing to the ipsilateral sidebending. Since these muscles also control positioning of the head, dizziness and visual disturbances may become evident. Congenital absence of one SCM is rare, but acute torticollis after a throat or glandular infection is seen in childhood. A cumulative involvement can occur in the adolescent stage by a slowly increasing C2-C3 or C3-C4 posterolateral intervertebral nuclear migration.[69,122]

The idiopathic spasmodic variety accounts for only 5% to 10% of all cases and usually has a familial neurologic origin that may cause concomitant facial dystonia.[69] Postencephalitis produces a paroxysmal twisting movement of the head, while a spastic scenario presents a fixed position of ipsilateral sidebending and contralateral rotation of the head. A fixed forward head posture with posterior cranial rotation can also occur due to bilateral involvement of the SCMs, giving rise to antecollis with concomitant dysphagia and vocal disturbance.[87] It is important to understand that the addition of posterior cranial rotation causes increased approximation of the occiput on the atlas/axis, therefore maximizing suboccipital compression. Torticollis may also be caused by hypothyroidism, alcoholism, and emotional stress disorders. Physical therapy intervention in the form of manual soft tissue release techniques, postural correction, and EMG biofeedback have demonstrated effectiveness in the management of torticollis.[141,142] Botox injections can be beneficial for recalcitrant torticollis or headache associated with torticollis.[143]

## Neck-tongue syndrome (IHS 13.9)

*Neck-tongue syndrome* is a rare disorder characterized by infrequent attacks of unilateral pain in the upper neck that last from 15 seconds to several minutes. The pain radiates toward the ear, with simultaneous numbness, paresthesia, or the sensation of involuntary movement involving the ipsilateral half of the tongue. A sudden rotational movement of the head will elicit the attack contralateral to the side of rotation.[144] Additional findings have been described, including upper extremity tingling or pain (usually on the same side), sensory changes of the oropharynx with subsequent dysphagia, and a sensation of choking.[145]

The proposed mechanism is compromise of the C2 ventral ramus by subluxation of the lateral atlantoaxial joint, which produces occipital pain. Numbness of the tongue arises because afferent fibers from the tongue pass from the ansa hypoglossi into the C2 ventral ramus.[114] Most individuals with this syndrome have significant pathology of the atlantoaxial joint, and it has also occurred in patients with rheumatoid arthritis or congenital joint laxity. Hypomobility in the contralateral atlantoaxial joint may be a predisposing factor.[144]

In the absence of pathologic findings the disorder appears benign, and conservative management with cervical collars,[146] manipulation,[147] analgesics, antiepileptic drugs, antidepressants,[146] steroids, muscle relaxants, and injections of local anesthetics may be effective.

### Vertebral artery syndrome (ICD-9 435.1)

Vertebral artery involvement can also contribute to various cervicogenic headaches. Conditions with similar symptoms include vertebral artery compression syndrome (ICD-9 721.1), vertebral basilar syndrome (ICD-9 435.3), and benign positional vertigo (ICD-9 386.11). The major extracranial region of the vertebral artery is protected by the vertebral canal and the surrounding soft tissue structures, but the area from C2 to the foramen magnum is vulnerable. Vertebral artery injury in the suboccipital region can result from severe cervical spine trauma, such as a fracture of the atlas, whereas vertebral artery compression may be associated with Barré-Liéou syndrome.[148] Red flags, such as disorientation, nausea, vomiting, visual disturbances, dizziness, or vertigo that occur with change from a non–weight-bearing (supine) to a weight-bearing (sitting or standing) position, should immediately necessitate further testing to rule out vertebral artery involvement.[148–151] An experienced physician or physical therapist should perform the assessment, which may be cur-tailed in favor of neurologic and radiologic testing if any of the above red flags recur or intensify during the evaluation.

Active cervical spine range of motion and provocation testing in positions of rotation, sidebending, and extension can be used to stretch, narrow, or kink the ipsilateral and/or contralateral vertebral artery, but this testing must be performed with great caution, and the reliability is suspect unless performed by an experienced clinician.[148–151] The delineation between labyrinthine and vertebral artery involvement should also be considered. The trained clinician can auscultate the carotid and subclavian arteries for bruits with the patient in a seated position and the head in a neutral position, but further testing in positions of cervical rotation and extension to each side should be designated to others.[148]

### Barré-Liéou syndrome (ICD-9 723.2)

Irritation of the vertebral artery or posterior cervical sympathetic network via stretching or compression forces can give rise to Barré-Liéou syndrome, also known as *posterior cervical sympathetic syndrome*.[152] This rare syndrome, characterized by intracranial vasoconstriction, may cause widespread facial and cranial symptoms that can mimic migraine, tension-type headache, sinusitis, and craniofacial dysautonomia, due to involvement of the trigeminal spinal tract, upper cervical roots, posterior sympathetic fibers, and the vertebral artery. Head and neck pain that falls into the Barré-Liéou category is usually continuous but variable, with qualitative characteristics that consist of throbbing, burning, stinging, or pinching.[152–154] Tinnitus, decreased auditory perception, a feeling of dust in the eye, blurred vision, tearing, nasal irritation, and hoarseness may also be present. One or more of these symptoms in addition to pain may become evident or exacerbated by active range of motion and positional or manual suboccipital testing. It is imperative that any positive findings be further evaluated by a definitive neurologic examination. This syndrome is very controversial, as it may simply fall into the category of a vertebral artery syndrome associated with other compressive forces within the suboccipital fossa.[154]

## Arnold-Chiari syndrome (ICD-9 348.4)

Herniation of the cerebellar tonsils into the foramen magnum of 3 to 5 mm or distally to the C2 level represents a structural malformation of the brainstem and dura known as *Arnold-Chiari syndrome*.[155] This syndrome is commonly delineated by the type of abnormality and may include hydrocephalus, myelomeningocele, syringomyelia, spinal cord cavitations (syrinx), as well as the components of the posterior fossa. Headaches, hemifacial spasm, coughing with or without symptoms of sleep apnea, inability to speak, dysphagia, and nystagmus may be associated symptoms.[155-160] An Arnold-Chiari malformation causes traction or compression of one or more cranial nerves and is confirmed with a definitive neurologic assessment as well as MRI evaluation. Surgical decompression is often required.

## Summary

The composite of neural elements that converge at the trigeminocervical complex can cause, mimic, or contribute to TMDs, orofacial pain, or headaches as well as associated gastrointestinal, aural, laryngeal, pharyngeal, and equilibrium disturbances. Determination of the level and structures that give rise to the perceived nociception and associated symptoms requires a comprehensive upper-quarter physical therapy evaluation.[56] It is imperative for the clinician to understand that disorders of the suboccipital spine refer pain proximally and are often described as headache variants. Associated sensory deficits are common in these disorders and help establish the proper diagnosis.

Current evidence has shown that specific and individualized intervention consisting of early and comprehensive posture correction, ergonomic adaptation, therapeutic exercise, and manual therapy by experienced physical therapists can assist the clinician in effectively managing cervicogenic factors to reduce pain, restore function, and prevent recurrence.[100,109,161-173]

## References

1. Scientific approach to the assessment and management of activity-related spinal disorders. A monograph for clinicians. Report of the Quebec Task Force on Spinal Disorders. Spine 1987;12(7 suppl):S1–S59.
2. Spitzer WO, Skovron ML, Salmi LR, et al. Scientific monograph of the Quebec Task Force on Whiplash-Associated Disorders: Redefining "whiplash" and its management. Spine 1995;20(8 suppl):S1–S73.
3. Abenhaim L, Rossignol M, Valat JP, et al. The role of activity in the therapeutic management of back pain. Report of the International Paris Task Force on Back Pain. Spine 2000;25(4 suppl):1S–33S.
4. Linton SJ. A review of psychological risk factors in neck and back pain. Spine 2000;25:1148–1156.
5. Svensson P, Graven-Nielsen T. Craniofacial muscle pain: Review of mechanisms and clinical manifestations. J Orofac Pain 2001;15:117–145.
6. de Wijer A, de Leeuw JR, Steenks MH, Bosman F. Temporomandibular and cervical spine disorders. Self-reported signs and symptoms. Spine 1996;21:1638–1646.

7. Mannheimer JS, Rosenthal RM. Acute and chronic postural abnormalities as related to craniofacial pain and temporomandibular disorders. Dent Clin North Am 1991;35(1):185–208.

8. Kirveskari P, Alanen P, Karskela V, et al. Association of functional state of stomatognathic system with mobility of cervical spine and neck muscle tenderness. Acta Odontol Scand 1988;46:281–286.

9. De Wijer A. Temporomandibular and Cervical Spine Disorders [thesis]. The Netherlands: Utrecht Univ, 1995.

10. De Laat A, Meuleman H, Stevens A, Verbeke G. Correlation between cervical spine and temporomandibular disorders. Clin Oral Investig 1998;2:54–57.

11. Clark GT, Green EM, Dornan MR, Flack VF. Craniocervical dysfunction levels in a patient sample from a temporomandibular joint clinic. J Am Dent Assoc 1987;115:251–256.

12. Ciancaglini R, Testa M, Radaelli G. Association of neck pain with symptoms of temporomandibular dysfunction in the general adult population. Scand J Rehabil Med 1999;31(1):17–22.

13. Visscher CM, Lobbezoo F, de Boer W, van der Zaag J, Naeije M. Prevalence of cervical spinal pain in craniomandibular pain patients. Eur J Oral Sci 2001;109: 76–80.

14. Okeson J. Orofacial Pain. Guidelines for Assessment, Diagnosis, and Management. Chicago: Quintessence, 1996.

15. Balasubramaniam R, de Leeuw R, Zhu H, Nickerson RB, Okeson JP, Carlson CR. Prevalence of temporomandibular disorders in fibromyalgia and failed back syndrome patients: A blinded prospective comparison study. Oral Surg Oral Med Oral Pathol Oral Radiol Endod 2007;104:204–216.

16. Wright EF, Des Rosier KF, Clark MK, Bifano SL. Identifying undiagnosed rheumatic disorders among patients with TMD. J Am Dent Assoc 1997;128:738–744.

17. Aaron LA, Burke MM, Buchwald D. Overlapping conditions among patients with chronic fatigue syndrome, fibromyalgia, and temporomandibular disorder. Arch Intern Med 2000;160:221–227.

18. Aaron LA, Buchwald D. Chronic diffuse musculoskeletal pain, fibromyalgia and co-morbid unexplained clinical conditions. Best Pract Res Clin Rheumatol 2003;17:563–574.

19. Sollecito TP, Stoopler ET, DeRossi SS, Silverton S. Temporomandibular disorders and fibromyalgia: Comorbid conditions? Gen Dent 2003;51:184–187; quiz 88–89.

20. Brodie AG. Anatomy and physiology of head and neck musculature. Am J Orthod 1950;36(11):831–844.

21. Amiri M, Jull G, Bullock-Saxton J, Darnell R, Lander C. Cervical musculoskeletal impairment in frequent intermittent headaches. Part 2: Subjects with concurrent headaches. Cephalalgia 2007;27:891–898.

22. Kraus S. Clinics in Physical therapy, ed 2. New York: Churchill Livingstone, 1994.

23. Juhl J, Miller S, Roberts G. Roentgenographic variations in the normal cervical spine. Radiology 1962;78: 591–597.

24. Visscher CM, de Boer W, Naeije M. The relationship between posture and curvature of the cervical spine. J Manipulative Physiol Ther 1998;21:388–391.

25. Lawrence E, Razook S. Nonsurgical management of mandibular disorders. In: Kraus S (ed). Temporomandibular Disorders, ed 2. New York: Churchill Livingstone, 1994.

26. Yemm R. The mandibular rest position: The roles of tissue elasticity and muscle activity. J Dent Assoc S Afr 1975;30(1):203–208.

27. Darling DW, Kraus S, Glasheen-Wray MB. Relationship of head posture and the rest position of the mandible. J Prosthet Dent 1984;52(1):111–115.

28. Goldstein DF, Kraus SL, Williams WB, Glasheen-Wray M. Influence of cervical posture on mandibular movement. J Prosthet Dent 1984;52:421–426.

29. Forsberg CM, Hellsing E, Linder-Aronson S, Sheikholeslam A. EMG activity in neck and masticatory muscles in relation to extension and flexion of the head. Eur J Orthod 1985;7:177–184.

30. Boyd CH, Slagle WF, Boyd CM, Bryant RW, Wiygul JP. The effect of head position on electromyographic evaluations of representative mandibular positioning muscle groups. Cranio 1987;5(1):50–54.

31. Woda A, Pionchon P, Palla S. Regulation of mandibular postures: Mechanisms and clinical implications. Crit Rev Oral Biol Med 2001;12:166–178.

32. Hackney J, Bade D, Clawson A. Relationship between forward head posture and diagnosed internal derangement of the temporomandibular joint. J Orofac Pain 1993;7:386–390.

33. Lee WY, Okeson JP, Lindroth J. The relationship between forward head posture and temporomandibular disorders. J Orofac Pain 1995;9:161–167.

34. Visscher CM, De Boer W, Lobbezoo F, Habets LL, Naeije M. Is there a relationship between head posture and craniomandibular pain? J Oral Rehabil 2002;29:1030–1036.

35. Olivo SA, Bravo J, Magee DJ, Thie NM, Major PW, Flores-Mir C. The association between head and cervical posture and temporomandibular disorders: A systematic review. J Orofac Pain 2006;20(1):9–23.

36. Armijo Olivo S, Magee DJ, Parfitt M, Major P, Thie NM. The association between the cervical spine, the stomatognathic system, and craniofacial pain: A critical review. J Orofac Pain 2006;20:271–287.

37. Visscher CM, Huddleston Slater JJ, Lobbezoo F, Naeije M. Kinematics of the human mandible for different head postures. J Oral Rehabil 2000;27:299–305.

38. Eriksson PO, Zafar H, Nordh E. Concomitant mandibular and head-neck movements during jaw opening-closing in man. J Oral Rehabil 1998;25:859–870.

39. McCouch GP, Deering ID, Ling TH. Location of receptors for tonic neck reflexes. J Neurophysiol 1951; 14:191–195.

40. Wyke B. Neurology of the cervical spinal joints. Physiotherapy 1979;65:72–76.

41. Sumino R, Nozaki S, Katoh M. Trigemino-neck reflex. In: Kawamura Y, Dubner R (eds). Oral-Facial Sensory and Motor Functions. Tokyo: Quintessence, 1981:81.

42. Hu JW, Yu XM, Vernon H, Sessle BJ. Excitatory effects on neck and jaw muscle activity of inflammatory irritant applied to cervical paraspinal tissues. Pain 1993; 55:243–250.

43. Funakoshi M, Amano N. Effects of the tonic neck reflex on the jaw muscles of the rat. J Dent Res 1973;52: 668–673.

44. Svensson P, Wang K, Arendt-Nielsen L, Cairns BE, Sessle BJ. Pain effects of glutamate injections into human jaw or neck muscles. J Orofac Pain 2005;19: 109–118.

45. Sessle BJ, Hu JW, Amano N, Zhong G. Convergence of cutaneous, tooth pulp, visceral, neck and muscle afferents onto nociceptive and non-nociceptive neurones in trigeminal subnucleus caudalis (medullary dorsal horn) and its implications for referred pain. Pain 1986;27:219–235.

46. Carlson CR, Okeson JP, Falace DA, Nitz AJ, Lindroth JE. Reduction of pain and EMG activity in the masseter region by trapezius trigger point injection. Pain 1993;55:397–400.

47. Sumino R, Nozaki S. Trigemino-neck reflex: Its peripheral and central organization. In: Anderson DJ, Matthews B (eds). Pain in the Trigeminal Region. Amsterdam: Elsevier/North-Holland Biomedical Press, 1977:365–374.

48. Clark GT, Browne PA, Nakano M, Yang Q. Co-activation of sternocleidomastoid muscles during maximum clenching. J Dent Res 1993;72:1499–1502.

49. Ehrlich R, Garlick D, Ninio M. The effect of jaw clenching on the electromyographic activities of 2 neck and 2 trunk muscles. J Orofac Pain 1999;13: 115–120.

50. Eriksson PO, Haggman-Henrikson B, Nordh E, Zafar H. Co-ordinated mandibular and head-neck movements during rhythmic jaw activities in man. J Dent Res 2000;79:1378–1384.

51. Sherrington CS. The Integrative Action of the Nervous System. New Haven, CT: Yale Press, 1906.

52. Ralston HJ, Libet B. The question of tonus in skeletal muscle. Am J Phys Med 1953;32(2):85–92.

53. Kraus S. Head and orofacial pain: Cervical spine implications. In: Gremillion H (ed). Denl Clin North Am 2007;51:161–193.

54. Mersky H, Bogduk N. Classification of Chronic Pain, ed 2. Descriptions of Chronic Pain Syndromes and Definitions of Pain Terms. Task Force on Taxonomy of the International Association for the Study of Pain. Seattle: IASP Press, 1994.

55. Dworkin SF, LeResche L. Research Diagnostic Criteria for Temporomandibular Disorders: Review, criteria, examinations and specifications, critique. J Craniomandib Disord 1992;6:301–355.

56. Mannheimer JS, Dunn JJ. Cervical spine evaluation and relation to temporomandibular disorders. In: Kaplan A, Assael LA (eds). Textbook of Craniomandibular Disorders. Philadelphia: Saunders, 1991.

57. Braun B, Schiffman EL. The validity and predictive value of four assessment instruments for evaluation of the cervical and stomatognathic systems. J Craniomandib Disord 1991;5:239–244.

58. Dvorak J. Epidemiology, physical examination, and neurodiagnostics. Spine 1998;23:2663–2673.

59. Meloche JP, Bergeron Y, Bellavance A, Morand M, Huot J, Belzile G. Painful intervertebral dysfunction: Robert Maigne's original contribution to headache of cervical origin. The Quebec Headache Study Group. Headache 1993;33:328–334.

60. Farmer JC, Wisneski RJ. Cervical spine nerve root compression. An analysis of neuroforaminal pressures with varying head and arm positions. Spine 1994;19:1850–1855.

61. Simons DG. Review of enigmatic MTrPs as a common cause of enigmatic musculoskeletal pain and dysfunction. J Electromyogr Kinesiol 2004;14(1):95–107.

62. Hall T, Robinson K. The flexion-rotation test and active cervical mobility—A comparative measurement study in cervicogenic headache. Man Ther 2004;9: 197–202.

63. Yi X, Cook AJ, Hamill-Ruth RJ, Rowlingson JC. Cervicogenic headache in patients with presumed migraine: Missed diagnosis or misdiagnosis? J Pain 2005;6:700–703.

64. Zito G, Jull G, Story I. Clinical tests of musculoskeletal dysfunction in the diagnosis of cervicogenic headache. Man Ther 2006;11:118–129.

65. Visscher CM, Lobbezoo F, de Boer W, van der Zaag J, Verheij JG, Naeije M. Clinical tests in distinguishing between persons with or without craniomandibular or cervical spinal pain complaints. Eur J Oral Sci 2000;108:475–483.

66. Rocabado M. Biomechanical relationship of the cranial, cervical, and hyoid regions. Cranio 1983;1(3):61–66.

67. Wackenheim A. Cervico-Occipital Joint Radiography. Berlin: Springer-Verlag, 1985.

68. Harris JH, Edeiken-Monroe B. The Radiology of Acute Cervical Spine Trauma. Baltimore: Williams & Wilkins, 1987.

69. Henderson DJ, Staines M. Radiographic evaluation of the upper cervical spine. In: Vernon H (ed). Upper Cervical Syndrome: Chiropractic Diagnosis and Treatment. Baltimore: Williams & Wilkins, 1988:18–47.

70. Ellis B, Kosmorsky G. Referred occular pain relieved by suboccipital injection. Headache 1987:101–103.

71. Bovim G, Berg R, Dale LG. Cervicogenic headache: Anesthetic blockades of cervical nerves (C2-C5) and facet joint (C2/C3). Pain 1992;49:315–320.

72. Bovim G, Fredriksen TA, Stolt-Nielsen A, Sjaastad O. Neurolysis of the greater occipital nerve in cervicogenic headache. A follow up study. Headache 1992;32:175–179.

73. Vincent M. Greater occipital nerve blockades in cervicogenic headache. Funct Neurol 1998;13(1):78–79.

74. Treleaven J, Jull G, Sterling M. Dizziness and unsteadiness following whiplash injury: Characteristic features and relationship with cervical joint position error. J Rehabil Med 2003;35(1):36–43.

75. Malik H, Lovell M. Soft tissue neck symptoms following high-energy road traffic accidents. Spine 2004;29(15):E315–E317.

76. Bogduk N. The clinical anatomy of the cervical dorsal rami. Spine 1982;7:319–330.

77. Retzlaff E, Mitchell F. The Cranium and Its Sutures. New York: Springer-Verlag, 1987.

78. Berkowitz B, Moxham B. A Textbook of Head and Neck Anatomy. London: Wolfe, 1988.

79. Bogduk N. The anatomical basis for cervicogenic headache. J Manipulative Physiol Ther 1992;15(1):67–70.

80. Janda V. Some aspects of extracranial causes of facial pain. J Prosthet Dent 1986;56:484–487.

81. Razook JC, Chandler MJ, Foreman RD. Phrenic afferent input excites C1-C2 spinal neurons in rats. Pain 1995;63(1):117–125.

82. Jaeger B. Are "cervicogenic" headaches due to myofascial pain and cervical spine dysfunction? Cephalalgia 1989;9:157–164.

83. Smith MV, Hodge CJ Jr. Response properties of upper cervical spinothalamic neurons in cats. A possible explanation for the unusual sensory symptoms associated with upper cervical lesions in humans. Spine 1992;17(10 suppl):S375–S382.

84. Dunteman E, Turner MS, Swarm R. Pseudo-spinal headache. Reg Anesth 1996;21:358–360.

85. Simons DG, Travell JG, Simons LS. Myofascial Pain and Dysfunction. The Trigger Point Manual, ed 2. Baltimore: Williams & Wilkins, 1999.

86. Poletti CE. C2 and C3 radiculopathies. APS Journal 1992;1:272–275.

87. Duane DD. Spasmodic torticollis. Adv Neurol 1988;49:135–150.

88. Galm R, Rittmeister M, Schmitt E. Vertigo in patients with cervical spine dysfunction. Eur Spine J 1998;7(1):55–58.

89. Fishbain DA, Cutler R, Cole B, Rosomoff HL, Rosomoff RS. International Headache Society headache diagnostic patterns in pain facility patients. Clin J Pain 2001;17(1):78–93.

90. Sjaastad O, Wang H, Bakketeig LS. Neck pain and associated head pain: Persistent neck complaint with subsequent, transient, posterior headache. Acta Neurol Scand 2006;114:392–399.

91. Barnsley L, Lord S, Bogduk N. Whiplash injury. Pain 1994;58:283–307.

92. Cusick JF, Pintar FA, Yoganandan N. Whiplash syndrome: Kinematic factors influencing pain patterns. Spine 2001;26:1252–1258.

93. Croft S. Management of soft tissue injuries. In: Foreman S, Croft A (eds). Whiplash Injuries: The Cervical Acceleration/Deceleration Syndrome, ed 3. Baltimore: Lippincott Williams & Wilkins, 2002:541–560.

94. McClune T, Burton AK, Waddell G. Whiplash associated disorders: A review of the literature to guide patient information and advice. Emerg Med J 2002;19:499–506.

95. Rao SK, Wasyliw C, Nunez DB Jr. Spectrum of imaging findings in hyperextension injuries of the neck. Radiographics 2005;25:1239–1254.

96. Kumar S, Ferrari R, Narayan Y. Looking away from whiplash: Effect of head rotation in rear impacts. Spine 2005;30:760–768.

97. Klobas L, Tegelberg A, Axelsson S. Symptoms and signs of temporomandibular disorders in individuals with chronic whiplash-associated disorders. Swed Dent J 2004;28(1):29–36.

98. Eriksson PO, Haggman-Henrikson B, Zafar H. Jaw-neck dysfunction in whiplash-associated disorders. Arch Oral Biol 2007;52:404–408.

99. Carroll LJ, Ferrari R, Cassidy JD. Reduced or painful jaw movement after collision-related injuries: A population-based study. J Am Dent Assoc 2007;138(1):86–93.

100. Sterling M, Jull G, Vicenzino B, Kenardy J. Sensory hypersensitivity occurs soon after whiplash injury and is associated with poor recovery. Pain 2003;104:509–517.

101. Davenport TE, Kulig K, Matharu Y, Blanco CE. The EdUReP model for nonsurgical management of tendinopathy. Phys Ther 2005;85:1093–1103.

102. Soderlund A, Lindberg P. An integrated physiotherapy/cognitive-behavioural approach to the analysis and treatment of chronic whiplash associated disorders, WAD. Disabil Rehabil 2001;23:436–447.

103. Dehner C, Hartwig E, Strobel P, Scheich M, Schneider F, Elbel M, et al. Comparison of the relative benefits of 2 versus 10 days of soft collar cervical immobilization after acute whiplash injury. Arch Phys Med Rehabil 2006;87:1423–1427.

104. Bland J. Disorders of the Cervical Spine: Diagnosis and Medical Management. Philadelphia: Saunders, 1987.

105. Christian C. Medical management of cervical sprine diseases. In: Camins M, O'Leary P (eds). Disorders of the Cervical Spine. Baltimore: Williams & Wilkins, 1992:147–155.

106. Abdulkarim JA, Dhingsa R, L Finlay DB. Magnetic resonance imaging of the cervical spine: Frequency of degenerative changes in the intervertebral disc with relation to age. Clin Radiol 2003;58:980–984.

107. Tanaka Y, Kokubun S, Sato T, Ozawa H. Cervical roots as origin of pain in the neck or scapular regions. Spine 2006;31:E568–E573.

108. Mannheimer J, Lampe G. Clinical Transcutaneous Electrical Nerve Stimulation. Philadephia: Davis, 1984.

109. Mannheimer JS. Prevention and restoration of abnormal upper quater posture. In: Gelb H, Gelb M (eds). Postural Considerations in the Diagnosis and Treatment of Cranio-Cervical-Mandibular and Related Chronic Pain Disorders. London: Mosby-Wolfe, 1994:277–323.

110. Wilson PR. Cervicogenic headache. Am Pain Soc J 1992;1:259–264.

111. Kerr RW. A mechanism to account for frontal headache in cases of posterior-fossa tumors. J Neurosurg 1961;18:605–609.

112. Renehan WE, Zhang X, Beierwaltes WH, Fogel R. Neurons in the dorsal motor nucleus of the vagus may integrate vagal and spinal information from the GI tract. Am J Physiol 1995;268(5 pt 1):G780–G790.

113. Kobashi M, Koga T, Mizutani M, Matsuo R. Suppression of vagal motor activities evokes laryngeal afferent-mediated inhibition of gastric motility. Am J Physiol Regul Integr Comp Physiol 2002;282:R818–R827.

114. Bogduk N. An anatomical basis for the neck-tongue syndrome. J Neurol Neurosurg Psychiatry 1981;44:202–208.

115. Sjaastad O, Saunte C, Hovdahl H, Breivik H, Gronbaek E. "Cervicogenic" headache. An hypothesis. Cephalalgia 1983;3:249–256.

116. Pfaffenrath V, Dandekar R, Pollmann W. Cervicogenic headache—The clinical picture, radiological findings and hypotheses on its pathophysiology. Headache 1987;27:495–499.

117. Sjaastad O, Fredriksen TA, Pfaffenrath V. Cervicogenic headache: Diagnostic criteria. Headache 1990;30:725–726.

118. Edmeads J. The cervical spine and headache. Neurology 1988;38:1874–1878.

119. The International Classification of Headache Disorders, ed 2. Cephalalgia 2004;24(suppl 1):9–160.

120. Saadah HA, Taylor FB. Sustained headache syndrome associated with tender occipital nerve zones. Headache 1987;27:201–205.

121. Bansevicius D, Sjaastad O. Cervicogenic headache: The influence of mental load on pain level and EMG of shoulder-neck and facial muscles. Headache 1996;36:372–378.

122. Chen TY. The clinical presentation of uppermost cervical disc protrusion. Spine 2000;25:439–442.

123. De Leeuw JRJ. Psychosocial Aspects and Symptom Characteristics of Craniomandibular Dysfunction [thesis]. The Netherlands: Utrecht Univ, 1993.

124. Lobbezoo-Scholte AM, de Leeuw JR, Steenks MH, et al. Diagnostic subgroups of craniomandibular disorders. Part I. Self-report data and clinical findings. J Orofac Pain 1995;9:24–36.

125. Browne PA, Clark GT, Kuboki T, Adachi NY. Concurrent cervical and craniofacial pain. A review of empiric and basic science evidence. Oral Surg Oral Med Oral Pathol Oral Radiol Endod 1998;86:633–640.

126. Raskin NH. Facial pain. Headache, ed 2. New York: Churchill Livingstone, 1988:333–373.

127. Burstein R, Yamamura H, Malick A, Strassman AM. Chemical stimulation of the intracranial dura induces enhanced responses to facial stimulation in brain stem trigeminal neurons. J Neurophysiol 1998;79:964–82.

128. Strassman AM, Raymond SA, Burstein R. Sensitization of meningeal sensory neurons and the origin of headaches. Nature 1996;384(6609):560–564.

129. Schepelmann K, Ebersberger A, Pawlak M, Oppmann M, Messlinger K. Response properties of trigeminal brain stem neurons with input from dura mater encephali in the rat. Neuroscience 1999;90:543–554.

130. Kimmel DL. Innervation of spinal dura mater and dura mater of the posterior cranial fossa. Neurology 1961;11:800–809.

131. Alix ME, Bates DK. A proposed etiology of cervicogenic headache: The neurophysiologic basis and anatomic relationship between the dura mater and the rectus posterior capitis minor muscle. J Manipulative Physiol Ther 1999;22:534–539.

132. Bartsch T, Goadsby PJ. Stimulation of the greater occipital nerve induces increased central excitability of dural afferent input. Brain 2002;125(pt 7):1496–1509.

133. Hack GD, Hallgren RC. Chronic headache relief after section of suboccipital muscle dural connections: A case report. Headache 2004;44(1):84–89.

134. Nash L, Nicholson H, Lee AS, Johnson GM, Zhang M. Configuration of the connective tissue in the posterior atlanto-occipital interspace: A sheet plastination and confocal microscopy study. Spine 2005;30:1359–1366.

135. Beder E, Ozgursoy OB, Karatayli Ozgursoy S. Current diagnosis and transoral surgical treatment of Eagle's syndrome. J Oral Maxillofac Surg 2005;63:1742–1745.

136. Mendelsohn AH, Berke GS, Chhetri DK. Heterogeneity in the clinical presentation of Eagle's syndrome. Otolaryngol Head Neck Surg 2006;134:389–393.

137. Beder E, Ozgursoy OB, Karatayli Ozgursoy S, Anadolu Y. Three-dimensional computed tomography and surgical treatment for Eagle's syndrome. Ear Nose Throat J 2006;85:443–445.

138. Cheifetz I. Intraoral treatment of Eagle's syndrome. J Oral Maxillofac Surg 2006;64:749.

139. Kohno S, Yoshida K, Kobayashi H. Pain in the sternocleidomastoid muscle and occlusal interferences. J Oral Rehabil 1988;15:385–392.

140. Smith AM. The coactivation of antagonist muscles. Can J Physiol Pharmacol 1981;59:733–747.

141. Smania N, Corato E, Tinazzi M, Montagnana B, Fiaschi A, Aglioti SM. The effect of two different rehabilitation treatments in cervical dystonia: Preliminary results in four patients. Funct Neurol 2003; 18:219–225.

142. Konrad C, Vollmer-Haase J, Anneken K, Knecht S. Orthopedic and neurological complications of cervical dystonia—Review of the literature. Acta Neurol Scand 2004;109:369–373.

143. Ondo WG, Gollomp S, Galvez-Jimenez N. A pilot study of botulinum toxin A for headache in cervical dystonia. Headache 2005;45:1073–1077.

144. Bertoft ES, Westerberg CE. Further observations on the neck-tongue syndrome. Cephalalgia 1985;5(suppl 3):312–313.

145. Orrell RW, Garsden CD. The neck-tongue syndrome. J Neurol Neurosurg Psychiatry 1994;57:348–352.

146. Fortin CJ, Biller J. Neck tongue syndrome. Headache 1985;25:255–258.

147. Terrett AGJ. Neck tongue syndrome and spinal manipulative therapy. In: Vernon H (ed). Upper Cervical Syndrome: Chiropractic Diagnosis and Treatment. Baltimore: Williams & Wilkins, 1988:223–229.

148. Sakaguchi M, Kitagawa K, Hougaku H, et al. Mechanical compression of the extracranial vertebral artery during neck rotation. Neurology 2003;61: 845–847.

149. Zaina C, Grant R, Johnson C, Dansie B, Taylor J, Spyropolous P. The effect of cervical rotation on blood flow in the contralateral vertebral artery. Man Ther 2003;8:103–109.

150. Mitchell JA. Changes in vertebral artery blood flow following normal rotation of the cervical spine. J Manipulative Physiol Ther 2003;26:347–351.

151. Mitchell J, Keene D, Dyson C, Harvey L, Pruvey C, Phillips R. Is cervical spine rotation, as used in the standard vertebrobasilar insufficiency test, associated with a measureable change in intracranial vertebral artery blood flow? Man Ther 2004;9:220–227.

152. Gayral L, Neuwirth E. Oto-neuroophthalmologic manifestations of cervical origin; posterior cervical sympathetic syndrome of Barré-Liéou. N Y State J Med 1954;54:1920–1926.

153. Wight S, Osborne N, Breen AC. Incidence of ponticulus posterior of the atlas in migraine and cervicogenic headache. J Manipulative Physiol Ther 1999;22(1):15–20.

154. Foster CA, Jabbour P. Barré-Liéou syndrome and the problem of the obsolete eponym. J Laryngol Otol 2006:1–4.

155. Penarrocha M, Okeson JP, Penarrocha MS, Angeles Cervello M. Orofacial pain as the sole manifestation of syringobulbia-syringomyelia associated with Arnold-Chiari malformation. J Orofac Pain 2001; 15:170–173.

156. Taylor FR, Larkins MV. Headache and Chiari I malformation: Clinical presentation, diagnosis, and controversies in management. Curr Pain Headache Rep 2002;6:331–337.

157. Wynn R, Goldsmith AJ. Chiari Type I malformation and upper airway obstruction in adolescents. Int J Pediatr Otorhinolaryngol 2004;68:607–611.

158. Tubbs RS, Soleau S, Custis J, Wellons JC, Blount JP, Oakes WJ. Degree of tectal beaking correlates to the presence of nystagmus in children with Chiari II malformation. Childs Nerv Syst 2004;20:459–461.

159. Botelho RV, Bittencourt LR, Rotta JM, Tufik S. Adult Chiari malformation and sleep apnoea. Neurosurg Rev 2005;28:169–176.

160. Colpan ME, Sekerci Z. Chiari type I malformation presenting as hemifacial spasm: Case report. Neurosurgery 2005;57:E371; discussion E71.

161. Watson DH, Trott PH. Cervical headache: An investigation of natural head posture and upper cervical flexor muscle performance. Cephalalgia 1993;13: 272–284; discussion 232.

162. Vernon H, McDermaid CS, Hagino C. Systematic review of randomized clinical trials of complementary/alternative therapies in the treatment of tension-type and cervicogenic headache. Complement Ther Med 1999;7:142–155.

163. Whorton R, Kegerreis S. The use of manual therapy and exercise in the treatment of chronic cervicogenic headaches. J Man Manipulative Ther 2000;8:193–203.

164. Jull G, Trott P, Potter H, et al. A randomized controlled trial of exercise and manipulative therapy for cervicogenic headache. Spine 2002;27:1835–1843; discussion 1843.

165. Wang WT, Olson SL, Campbell AH, Hanten WP, Gleeson PB. Effectiveness of physical therapy for patients with neck pain: An individualized approach using a clinical decision-making algorithm. Am J Phys Med Rehabil 2003;82:203–218; quiz 219–221.

166. Biondi DM. Physical treatments for headache: A structured review. Headache 2005;45:738–746.

167. McLean L. The effect of postural correction on muscle activation amplitudes recorded from the cervicobrachial region. J Electromyogr Kinesiol 2005;15:527–535.

168. Sjogren T, Nissinen KJ, Jarvenpaa SK, Ojanen MT, Vanharanta H, Malkia EA. Effects of a workplace physical exercise intervention on the intensity of headache and neck and shoulder symptoms and upper extremity muscular strength of office workers: A cluster randomized controlled cross-over trial. Pain 2005;116(1-2):119–128.

169. Torelli P, Lambru G, Manzoni GC. Psychiatric comorbidity and headache: Clinical and therapeutical aspects. Neurol Sci 2006;27(suppl 2):S73–S76.

170. van Ettekoven H, Lucas C. Efficacy of physiotherapy including a craniocervical training programme for tension-type headache: A randomized clinical trial. Cephalalgia 2006;26:983–991.

171. Fernandez-de-las-Penas C, Alonso-Blanco C, San-Roman J, Miangolarra-Page JC. Methodological quality of randomized controlled trials of spinal manipulation and mobilization in tension-type headache, migraine, and cervicogenic headache. J Orthop Sports Phys Ther 2006;36:160–169.

172. Fernandez-de-Las-Penas C, Cuadrado ML, Pareja JA. Myofascial trigger points, neck mobility and forward head posture in episodic tension-type headache. Headache 2007;47:662–672.

173. Fernandez-de-Las-Penas C, Simons D, Cuadrado ML, Pareja JA. The role of myofascial trigger points in musculoskeletal pain syndromes of the head and neck. Curr Pain Headache Rep 2007;11:365–372.

# Extracranial and Systemic Causes of Head and Facial Pain

Although head or facial pain frequently arises from teeth or other masticatory structures, it can originate from *any* of the tissues or organs in the head and neck as well as from systemic disease. If orofacial pain or headache is associated with a serious or life-threatening illness, timely recognition and referral to a physician is crucial. In cases where the cause of head or facial pain is not readily apparent, nonmasticatory, extracranial, and systemic pain sources should be considered in the differential diagnosis. This chapter briefly summarizes these pain sources, based on the current classification methods of the International Headache Society (IHS),[1] and provides lists of associated disorders and symptoms for easy reference. For further information, the reader is referred to other chapters in the text or to standard medical references.

## Cranial Bones (IHS 11.1)

Most lesions that affect the bones of the skull are not painful.[2] Lesions of the skull most likely to produce pain are those that are rapidly expansile, aggressively osteoclas-

tic, or have an inflammatory component.[3] In this case, pain is received by nociceptors of the underlying periosteum. Included among this group of lesions are osteomyelitis, multiple myeloma, and Paget disease.

## Eyes (IHS 11.3.x)

Patients with eye pain often have obvious ocular signs accompanying the pain, making diagnosis relatively easy in such cases. Most ocular diseases are not painful, however.

Ocular pain may be either primary or referred (Box 10-1). Primary pain arises from the ophthalmic division of the trigeminal nerve, although the maxillary division supplies most of the lower eyelid through its infraorbital branch.[4] The retina and optic nerve are not capable of nociception; however, the cornea, conjunctiva, and iris have an abundant supply of nociceptors, as do the extraocular muscles, the dural sheath of the optic nerve, and the periorbita, which produce pain when stretched. Pain may be perceived as originating in the orbit when the optic nerve is stimulated at any point along its path from the face to the cortex.

**Box 10-1** Head and facial pain arising from the eyes (IHS 11.3.x)

| Primary pain | Referred pain |
|---|---|
| Glaucoma (IHS 11.3.1) | Saccular aneurysms (IHS 6.3.1) |
| Convergence disorders (IHS 11.3.3) | Cavernous sinus inflammation |
| (heterophoria or heterotropia) | Carotidocavernous fistula (IHS 6.3.3) |
| Ocular inflammation (IHS 11.3.4) | Carotid artery dissection (IHS 6.5.1) |
| Corneal diseases | Myofascial pain |
| Painful ophthalmoplegia | Orbital apex syndrome |
| Superior orbital fissure syndrome | Parasellar syndrome |
| Orbital tumors | |

**Box 10-2** Head and facial pain arising from the ears

| Primary pain | Referred pain |
|---|---|
| Infections of the auricle, external auditory canal, tympanic membrane, and middle ear (IHS 11.4) | Temporomandibular disorders |
| | Myofascial pain |
| Cholesteatoma (IHS 11.4) | Toothache |
| Mastoiditis | Auriculotemporal syndrome |
| Ramsay Hunt syndrome | Carotid artery dissection (IHS 6.5.1) |
| Herpes simplex virus | Red ear syndrome |
| Herpes zoster virus | Hypopharynx pain |
| Tumors | Larynx pain |
| | Nasopharynx pain |
| | Oromucosal pain |
| | Sinus pain |
| | Tongue pain |

Possible stimuli include intracranial tumors, tumors of the orbit or paranasal sinuses, cavernous sinus inflammation, and carotid aneurysms.[5] Facial, cervical, and pericranial muscles are common sources of pain referred to the orbit or periorbital areas.[6]

Pain quality and associated symptoms can often provide clues as to the nature or origin of the pain. For example, deep, aching ocular pain originates from the uveal tract, especially the iris, and this pain can be referred to the ipsilateral teeth.[5] Ocular pain associated with inflammation is often accompanied by photophobia and conjunctival hyperemia. Pain with eye movement can be due to optic neuritis or anterior sinusitis.[5] Asthenopic symptoms such as strained, burning, or sore eyes are common complaints experienced by computer users.[7] Refractive errors are unlikely to cause eye pain or headaches. Although headache is often accompanied by ocular or periorbital pain, in the absence of ocular or periocular findings, it should be assumed that the pain is not due to a primary ocular disorder, and further testing should be done.[5]

# Ears (IHS 11.4)

About 50% of earaches are due to structural lesions of the external or middle ear.[8] The remainder are cases of referred pain, arising from disorders such as toothache, temporomandibular disorders, pharyngeal or laryngeal disorders, and cervical disorders.[9,10]

Sensory innervation of the ear is supplied by numerous nerves, including branches of the second and third cervical nerves and fifth, seventh, ninth, and tenth cranial nerves. Thus, pain originating in the regions that supply these numerous nerve branches may be perceived as pain in or around the ears. Otalgia from primary disorders of the ear can originate in the auricle, external ear canal, tympanic membrane, or middle ear (Box 10-2) and may be accompanied by symptoms such as vertigo, deafness, or tinnitus.[11]

# Nasal-Paranasal Sinus Complex

The nasal cavity is surrounded by the paranasal sinuses, which include the maxillary, ethmoid, frontal, and sphenoid sinuses. The sinuses are lined by ciliated respiratory epithelia and drain through openings, or *ostia*, into the nasal cavity via an osteomeatal complex. If the ostia become blocked due to inflammation or obstruction, fluid and bacteria accumulate, leading to signs and symptoms of sinusitis. Obstruction of the

ostia can also be due to anatomic variations and tumors.

Acute rhinosinusitis is typically sudden in onset, lasts up to 4 weeks, and resolves with antibiotic treatment. Chronic rhinosinusitis lasts longer than 12 weeks.[12] The bacteria most commonly isolated in acute sinusitis are *Streptococcus pneumoniae, Haemophilus influenzae,* and *Moraxella catarrhalis,* while anaerobes and *Staphylococcus aureus* are most commonly found in chronic sinusitis.[13]

The symptoms of rhinosinusitis commonly include nasal obstruction, nasal congestion, nasal discharge, nasal purulence, postnasal drip, facial pressure and pain, alteration in the sense of smell, cough, fever, halitosis, fatigue, dental pain, pharyngitis, otalgia, and headache.[12] Sensory innervation of the nasal-paranasal sinus complex is supplied by the first and second division of the trigeminal nerve.[8] Early studies demonstrated that the mucosal lining of the sinuses and the nasal septum is relatively insensitive to pain; however, the sinus ostia and nasal turbinates are highly sensitive.[14,15] It is noteworthy that in a study of the symptoms of acute sinusitis,[16] maxillary toothache was highly specific (93%), but only 11% of patients with sinusitis had this symptom. Headache had a sensitivity of 68% and a specificity of only 30%. The so-called sinus headache is a common complaint; however, the exact nature and cause of this association is not clear.[17]

It may be that the maxillary sinuses alone are involved in acute rhinosinusitis. Isolated disease of the ethmoid, frontal, or sphenoid sinuses is uncommon. The location of pain experienced may often provide clues as to which of the sinuses is primarily involved. For example, maxillary sinusitis may cause infraorbital or cheek discomfort, ethmoidal sinusitis may cause tenderness over the

**Box 10-3** Head and facial pain arising from the nasal-paranasal sinus complex

| Primary pain | Referred pain |
|---|---|
| Rhinosinusitis (IHS 11.5) | Toothache |
| Acute or chronic sinusitis (IHS 11.5) | Temporomandibular disorders |
| Vestibulitis | Myofascial pain |
| Septal deviation | |
| Hypertrophic turbinates | |
| Nasal polyposis | |
| Septal abscess/hematoma | |
| Sarcoidosis | |
| Wegener granulomatosis | |
| Tumors | |
| Infections | |

lacrimal region, frontal sinusitis characteristically causes headache in the forehead over the orbits, and pain due to sphenoidal sinusitis radiates to the occiput and vertex areas.[18] Box 10-3 lists painful disorders of the nasal-paranasal sinus complex.

## Throat

The throat, or *pharynx*, is divided into the nasopharynx, which is located posterior to the nasal cavities and superior to the soft palate; the oropharynx, which extends from the junction of the hard and soft palate to the vallecula; and the hypopharynx, which is posterior to the larynx and trachea and includes the pyriform fossae.[19] Surrounding the pharynx are three circumferential muscles: the superior, middle, and inferior constrictor muscles.[20] Also in this region are the adenoids, palatine tonsils, and accessory lymphoid tissues, which surround the upper airway as the *Waldeyer tonsillar ring*.

Pharyngeal tissues are innervated by the branches of the glossopharyngeal and vagus nerves.[20] Because of the significant overlap of innervation of these structures, throat pain is often poorly localized, and pain referral to the ear is common.[11] In addition to inflammation, other painful disorders of the throat can be developmental, neuropathic, or neoplastic (Box 10-4).

## Lymphatic System

The lymphatic system is composed of an extensive network of lymphatic capillaries, larger lymphatic vessels, and lymph nodes. The lymphatic system functions as a supplementary drainage system that collects interstitial fluid, protein, and cells and returns them to the circulation. Once fluid enters the lymphatic capillaries, it is called *lymph* and is propelled through the system by intermittent skeletal muscle contraction, contraction of the lymphatic vessels, and an ex-

---

**Box 10-4** Head and facial pain arising from the throat

| Primary pain | Referred pain |
|---|---|
| Pharyngitis | Temporomandibular disorders |
| Tonsillitis | Myofascial pain |
| Tracheitis | |
| Tonsillar abscess | |
| Stylohyoid syndrome (Eagle syndrome) | |
| Sarcoidosis | |
| Wegener granulomatosis | |
| Cricoarytenoid arthritis | |
| Glossopharyngeal neuralgia | |
| Tumors | |

---

tensive system of one-way valves.[21] If the volume of the interstitial fluid exceeds the drainage capacity of the vessels, fluid collects in the interstitial tissues and gives rise to edema.

In the head and neck, lymph nodes are grouped into chains, located both subcutaneously and in the deeper muscle tissues and fascial planes. The lymph chains include the occipital, preauricular, postauricular, parotid, buccal, mandibular, submandibular, submental, superficial cervical, internal jugular, spinal accessory, and supraclavicular lymph nodes.

In health, lymph nodes generally are not palpable. Enlarged, palpable nodes, called *lymphadenopathy*, may indicate pathology, possibly due to inflammation, infection, or neoplasia.[22] Inflammatory/infective causes may be local or systemic and include bacterial and viral disease. Inflammatory lymphadenopathy may also indicate a noninfective disorder such as sarcoidosis or connective tissue disease. Neoplastic enlargement can

be due to primary lymph node disease or to metastatic disease.

In the head and neck, the most common node to become enlarged is the jugulodigastric node, which is inflamed secondary to a viral upper respiratory tract infection.[22] This node is located just inferior and anterior to the angle of the mandible. Solitary enlarged nodes generally are due to a local or regional problem, while multiple enlarged nodes suggest systemic disease. The character of an enlarged node can often give clues as to its nature or cause. Enlarged nodes that are soft, freely movable, and tender are likely inflammatory. Nodes that are firm or rubbery, fixed to underlying tissue, or matted together and nontender are likely neoplastic. The differential diagnosis of nonpainful lymphadenopathies should include Hodgkin and non-Hodgkin lymphoma, leukemia, and plasmacytoma. Most painful disorders associated with the lymphatic system will occur secondary to a regional acute inflammatory/infectious process (Box 10-5).

---

**Box 10-5**  Head and facial pain arising from the lymphatic system[22]

**Primary pain**

Local or systemic bacterial infections

Local or systemic viral infections

Systemic protozoal infections

Toxoplasmosis

Leishmaniasis

Kawasaki disease

Sarcoidosis

Crohn disease

Connective tissue disease

Leukemia

Lymphoma

Metastatic disease

Drug-induced pain

---

**Box 10-6**  Head and facial pain arising from blood vessels

**Primary pain**

Subarachnoid hemorrhage (IHS 6.2.2)

Unruptured vascular malformation (IHS 6.3)

Saccular aneurysm (IHS 6.3.1)

Arteriovenous malformation (IHS 6.3.2)

Giant cell arteritis (IHS 6.4.1)

Primary intracranial angiitis (IHS 6.4.2)

Systemic lupus erythematosus (IHS 6.4.3)

Carotid or vertebral artery dissection (IHS 6.5.1)

Postcarotid endarterectomy (IHS 6.5.2)

Cerebral venous thrombosis (IHS 6.6)

Arterial hypertension (IHS 10.3)

---

## Blood Vessels

Vascular disease may be a source of head and facial pain (Box 10-6). Orofacial pain is a common presenting symptom of *giant cell arteritis*, a condition caused by granulomatous inflammation of the temporal artery or other branches of the aortic arch. Giant cell arteritis is found predominantly in elderly, white patients and is characterized by headache, jaw claudication, visual loss, hip and shoulder girdle pain, and constitutional symptoms.[23] Other features of the disease include a swollen, tender superficial temporal artery and a markedly elevated erythrocyte sedimentation rate. Blindness can occur due to inflammation of the posterior ciliary arteries with anterior ischemic optic neuropathy.[23] Thus, prompt, accurate diagnosis and treatment with steroids is necessary.

*Carotidynia* is a term that has been used to describe a disorder characterized by unilateral neck pain with projection of pain to the ipsilateral side of the head and tenderness over the carotid artery. In recent years, this diagnosis has fallen into disfavor due to a lack of specificity, and a critical review of the literature revealed that it is not a valid entity.[24]

## Salivary Glands

There are three pairs of major salivary glands: the parotid, submandibular, and sublingual glands. The parotid is the largest of the three glands and is located inferior and anterior to the ear, superficial to the masseter muscle. The parotid duct, or the *Stensen duct*, arises from the superior, anterior aspect of the gland and courses beneath the zygomatic arch to enter the oral cavity at about the level of the second maxillary molar. Sensory fibers are supplied by the auriculotemporal branch of the trigeminal nerve, while the secretory fibers are supplied by the glossopharyngeal nerve but transported via the auriculotemporal nerve.[25] The submandibular gland is located in the posterior floor of the mouth, inferior and posterior to the mylohyoid muscle. The submandibular duct arises from the deep aspect of the gland and courses forward, superior to the mylohyoid muscle, and enters the oral cavity at the base of the lingual frenum. The sublingual gland, the smallest of the three glands, lies in the anterior floor of the mouth superior to the mylohyoid muscle just beneath the mucosa and is tucked under the apices of the mandibular canines and premolars. The gland empties via several small ducts directly into the oral cavity or into the submandibular duct. Both the submandibular and sublingual glands derive their sensory nerve supply from the lingual nerve, while the secretory fibers are from the chorda tympani.[25]

Pain originating in the salivary glands is typically of inflammatory, infectious, traumatic, or neoplastic origin. Common salivary gland disorders that are accompanied by pain include sialoadenitis, sialolithiasis, epidemic parotitis, and tumors. Usually, diagnosis of salivary gland pain is not difficult, due to the accompanying signs or symptoms, such as pain occurring on eating, or swelling, firmness, or tenderness of the affected gland.

## Systemic Causes

There are a multitude of systemic diseases and disorders that are accompanied by

> **Box 10-7** Head and facial pain arising from systemic disease
>
> Anemia
>
> Adrenal insufficiency
>
> Arthritides
>    Rheumatoid arthritis
>    Osteoarthritis
>    Psoriatic arthritis
>    Systemic lupus erythematosus
>
> Chronic pulmonary failure with hypercapnia
>
> Diabetes mellitus
>
> Fibromyalgia
>
> Hashimoto thyroiditis
>
> Herpes zoster virus
>
> HIV/AIDS
>
> Hypertension/pheochromocytoma
>
> Infectious mononucleosis
>
> Ischemic heart disease
>
> Lyme disease
>
> Menopause
>
> Menstruation
>
> Metastatic malignancies
>
> Multiple sclerosis
>
> Primary malignancies
>
> Renal failure (uremia)/dialysis

headache and facial pain. Included among these are metabolic and endocrine disorders, infectious disease, autoimmune disease, cardiovascular disease, renal disease, and pulmonary disease. Box 10-7 lists some of the more common of these systemic diseases, but it is beyond the scope of this chapter to discuss them. However, the practitioner should include systemic disease in the differential diagnosis when facial pain is accompanied by systemic signs or symptoms, such as fever, malaise, generalized aches and pains, unintentional weight loss or gain, chronic fatigue, tachycardia or palpitations, chest pain, shortness of breath, extreme hunger or thirst, and skin lesions. In these instances, the practitioner must guard against the trap of attempting to treat facial pain when a much more serious underlying problem is present. In addition to these disorders, the reader is referred to chapter 4 for a discussion of other worrisome constitutional symptoms.

# References

1. The International Classification of Headache Disorders, ed 2. Cephalalgia 2004;24(suppl 1):9–160.
2. Weiss HD, Stern BJ, Goldberg J. Post-traumatic migraine: Chronic migraine precipitated by minor head or neck trauma. Headache 1991;31:451–456.
3. Göbel H, Edmeads JG. Disorders of the skull and cervical spine. In: Olesen J, Goadsby PJ, Ramadan NM, Tfelt-Hansen P, Welch KM (eds). The Headaches. Philadelphia: Lippincott Williams & Wilkins, 2006: 1003–1011.
4. Beck RW, Smith CH. Trigeminal nerve. In: Duane TD, Jaeger EA (eds). Biomedical Foundations in Ophthalmology. Philadelphia: Harper & Row, 1983:1–16.
5. Orcutt JC. Ocular and periocular pain. In: Loeser JD (ed). Bonica's Management of Pain. Philadelphia: Lippincott Williams & Wilkins, 2001:925–935.
6. Jaeger B. Head and neck pain: Overview of head and neck region. In: Simons DG, Travell JG, Simons LS (eds). Travell & Simons' Myofascial Pain and Dysfunction: The Trigger Point Manual. Baltimore: Lippincott Williams & Wilkins, 1999:237–277.
7. Blehm C, Vishnu S, Khattak A, Mitra S, Yee RW. Computer vision syndrome: A review. Surv Ophthalmol 2005;50:253–262.
8. Göbel H, Baloh RW. Disorders of ear, nose, and sinus. In: Olesen J, Goadsby PJ, Ramadan NM, Tfelt-Hansen P, Welch KM (eds). The Headaches. Philadelphia: Lippincott Williams & Wilkins, 2006:1019–1027.
9. Simons DG, Travell JG, Simons LS. Travell & Simons' Myofascial Pain and Dysfunction: The Trigger Point Manual. Baltimore: Lippincott Williams & Wilkins, 1999.
10. Wright EF. Referred craniofacial pain patterns in patients with temporomandibular disorder. J Am Dent Assoc 2000;131:1307–1315.
11. Dray TG, Weymuller EA. Pain in the ear, midface, and aerodigestive tract. In: Loeser JD (ed). Bonica's Management of Pain. Philadelphia: Lippincott Williams & Wilkins, 2001:936–947.
12. Lanza DC, Kennedy DW. Adult sinusitis defined. Otolaryngol Head Neck Surg 1997;117:S1–S7.
13. Brook I. The role of bacteria in chronic rhinosinusitis. Otolaryngol Clin North Am 2005;38:1171–1192.
14. Wolff HG. Wolff's Headache and Other Head Pain. New York: Oxford Univ Press, 1948.
15. McAuliffe GW, Goodell H, Wolff HG. Experimental studies on headache: Pain from the nasal and paranasal structures. Res Publ Assoc Res Nerv Ment Dis 1943;23:185–206.
16. Williams JW, Simel DL, Roberts L, et al. Clinical evaluation of sinusitis. Ann Intern Med 1992;117:705–710.
17. Silberstein SD, Willcox TO. Nasal disease and sinus headache. In: Silberstein SD, Lipton RB, Dalessio DJ (eds). Wolff's Headache and Other Head Pain. New York: Oxford Univ Press, 2001:494–508.
18. Hadley JA, Schafer SD. Clinical evaluation of rhinosinusitis: History and physical examination. Otolaryngol Head Neck Surg 1997;117:S8–S11.
19. Viani L, Donnelly M. Non-malignant diseases of the pharynx. In: Jones ES, Phillips DE, Hilgers FJ (eds). Diseases of the Head and Neck, Nose and Throat. London: Arnold, 1998:574–585.
20. Sharp J, Watkinson JC. Surgical anatomy of the head and neck. In: Jones AS, Phillips DE, Hilgers FJ (eds). Diseases of the Head and Neck, Nose and Throat. London: Arnold, 1998:11–23.
21. Berne RM, Levy M N. Physiology. St Louis: Mosby, 1998.
22. Scully C, Porter S. Orofacial disease: Update for the dental clinical team. II. Cervical lymphadenopathy. Dent Update 2000;27:44–47.
23. Wall M, Corbett JJ. Arteritis. In: Olesen J, Goadsby PJ, Ramadan NM, Tfelt-Hansen P, Welch KMA (eds). The Headaches. Philadelphia: Lippincott Williams & Wilkins, 2006:901–910.
24. Biousse V, Bousser M. The myth of carotidynia. Neurology 1994;44:993–995.
25. Bradley PJ. Tumors of the salivary gland. In: Jones AS, Phillips DE, Hilgers FJ (eds). Diseases of the Head and Neck, Nose and Throat. London: Arnold, 1998:329–346.

# Axis II: Biobehavioral Considerations

## Foundation of the Biobehavioral Model

Scientific advances in understanding modulatory control of ascending and descending neural circuits involved in pain processing have highlighted the important roles that nonbiologic variables, such as emotions, attention, and expectations, play in pain transmission. The fact that emotions and cognitions can facilitate or inhibit orofacial pain[1] requires the adoption of a biobehavioral model of disease. Behavioral factors encompass a broad spectrum of behavioral science theory (eg, principles of learning, interpersonal processes, family systems, and social learning) and techniques for change (eg, relaxation training, interpersonal psychotherapy, biofeedback, cognitive therapy, and breathing entrainment). When behavioral factors are discussed in the context of how they contribute to the functioning of biologic systems, it is appropriate to use the term *biobehavioral*. For reviews of the role of biobehavioral factors in the development and management of orofacial pain disorders, the reader is referred to other texts.[2,3]

As discussed in chapter 1, Engel[4] noted that the biomedical model, with its focus on pathobiology, does not fully explain the development of disease states. Therefore, he introduced the term *biopsychosocial* to describe the complex interactions among biology, psychologic states, and social conditions that bring about and/or maintain (dys)function. Using the term *biobehavioral* parallels the use of the word *biomedical*, and both concepts are subsumed in Engel's biopsychosocial model. Using the word *biobehavioral* calls attention to behavioral factors as they contribute to the functioning of biologic systems.

Adopting the biobehavioral model of orofacial pain requires that a linear, unidirectional model of treatment be replaced by a bidirectional approach to treatment. Whether the practitioner provides dental or psychologic treatment, a mechanistic (eg, identify the one cause, treat the one cause, observe recovery), linear model for understanding orofacial pain conditions is an incomplete model that will yield incomplete clinical care. Unless behavioral, psychologic, and social dimensions of a patient's presenting complaints and current adaptive strategies are addressed in the treatment plan, effective management of the pain condition will not likely be achieved. This multidisciplinary philosophy of treatment does not necessarily require a multispecialty clinic with dental practitioners, psychologists, physical therapists, and physicians. More so, it requires a worldview by the practitioners themselves that embraces the biobehavioral perspective.

Pain is a complex phenomenon influenced by both biologic and psychologic factors. Nociception that reaches thalamocortical–basal ganglia circuitry in the brain evokes the sensation of pain. However, since pain is a perceptual experience, it can be modified by factors other than the intensity of the nociceptive stimuli themselves. For example, excitatory factors that could amplify the pain experience would include fear, anxiety, attention, and expectations of pain. Conversely, self-confidence, positive emotional state, relaxation, and beliefs that the pain is manageable can reduce reports of pain.[5]

The biobehavioral approach to pain disorders involves assessing the underlying behavioral, psychologic, and physiologic disturbances that may be associated with the pain condition and helping the patient learn new skills for dealing with these disturbances, which may involve referral to a mental health professional. Effective biobehavioral symptom management, of both physical and psychologic aspects of symptoms, may be elusive for many patients, especially for those whose pain has become chronic (eg, lasting longer than than 3 to 6 months). These patients may have adopted coping patterns to enable them to maintain some level of functioning. However, sometimes these efforts at coping contribute to the development of maladaptive patterns that extend beyond the pain condition and into the aspects of

daily life. For example, a patient who stops engaging in pleasurable daily activities because of pain may be prone to developing depression. When maladaptive patterns emerge, it is important that the orofacial pain clinician be prepared to recognize and manage them appropriately, as failure to do so will likely prolong suffering (an individual's negative emotional reaction to pain) and prevent effective symptom management. It is also possible that maladaptive coping patterns were in practice before the pain condition's onset and may have contributed to or intensified the problem. There are also conditions under which an acute pain experience, if unresolved for an extended period of time, becomes chronic and results in the development and maintenance of behavioral, emotional, and cognitive patterns that significantly disrupt the patient's personal, interpersonal, and vocational life. The severity of the disruptions may even take the form of one of a variety of psychopathologic conditions that are discussed in later sections of this chapter.

The biobehavioral perspective introduces a model whereby the assessment process includes an interview component that focuses on the patient's psychosocial processes thus providing a broader perspective from which to understand and to conceptualize treatment for a patient's presenting pain symptoms. It is rare that pain reports are based entirely on psychologic or psychogenic factors. It is equally rare, however, to find that pain, especially chronic pain of 3 to 6 months' duration, is not influenced by psychologic factors to some degree. Psychologic factors may also account for the individual differences in response to similar levels of pain. For example, a person may report a pain intensity of "7" on a scale of 0 to 10, where 0 represents "no pain" and 10 represents "the most extreme pain," and yet be completely disabled by that level of pain. Another person who reports a pain intensity of "7" may be adaptively coping with the pain and continue with most routine activities. Because there can be substantial individual variability in response to painful conditions, the perceived intensity of pain may not necessarily be linked to an individual's expressed reaction to the pain.

It is often difficult to predict outcomes for the treatment of many chronic pain conditions without knowing the full psychosocial history. Often patients can be helped considerably by learning to manage their orofacial pain conditions for extended periods of time, but ongoing biobehavioral issues may either promote or prevent the use of such skills for symptom management. The reality is, however, that it is not a matter of "curing" pain, but learning to manage pain with the physical and psychologic tools developed and refined through the practice of science.

## Developing a Biobehavioral Framework

Orofacial pain clinicians need to develop a strategy by which they can evaluate the role of biobehavioral issues during the initial interview. Of course, the task is not to establish a biobehavioral diagnosis. Rather, the dental practitioner's role is to judge the level of complexity of the patient's clinical presentation through screening and to decide whether additional resources outside the scope of dental practice should be included in the treatment plan. This screening can include questionnaires that have demonstrated validity and reliability for use in identifying potential mental dysfunction. Objec-

tive questionnaires provide the clinician with an actuarial approach to decision-making rather than relying on clinical judgments formed in the initial interview alone. There is, for example, evidence that dental practitioners have difficulty in making accurate judgments of the psychologic status of pain patients.[6] More specifically, Oakley et al[6] reported that dentists tend to overreport psychopathology. These results suggest that the use of screening instruments may help improve the accuracy of clinical decision-making.

One screening method involves evaluating the patient's current pain intensity, the extent of the pain's interference in normal daily activity, the ability to control the pain, the impact of pain on work, and the presence of indicators (eg, level of depression or anxiety) of a need for more extensive psychologic or psychiatric consultation. Current pain intensity is most easily assessed using the 0 to10 pain scale. There are data suggesting that rating "current pain level," "average pain level," and "worst pain level" and then averaging the three items will provide a good overall index of pain intensity.[7] Likewise, the extent of interference in daily activities, the ability to control pain, and the impact of work on pain can be assessed using similar approaches. High self-rated levels of pain, interference, and impact, along with low ability to control pain, suggest the need for further biobehavioral evaluation.[7,8]

Screening instruments that have proven validity and reliability may be useful in certain cases. The Symptom Checklist-90-Revised (SCL-90-R),[9] for example, provides the clinician with an objective and validated screening instrument for symptoms of significant psychologic dysfunction. Its use requires training in administration, scoring, and interpretation that is beyond the scope of this chapter but can be readily obtained through continuing education or other formalized training programs. Other standardized screening questionnaires exist for specific categories, such as depression and anxiety.[10-12]

# Implementation of Dual-Axis Coding

To reflect the recognition of a psychologic component in the etiology of orofacial pain, a multiaxial nosology for these disorders has been created and implemented. Similar to the development of axial coding systems for psychiatric disorders by the American Psychiatric Association[13] and pain disorders by the International Association for the Study of Pain, the Research Diagnostic Criteria for Temporomandibular Disorders (RDC/TMD) were developed by a group of scientists and clinicians in 1992.[14] The Axis I domain focuses on the physical nature of the disease and includes the variety of orofacial pain conditions discussed in earlier chapters. The Axis II domain focuses on the patient's adaptation to the pain experience and pain-related disability that may result from the pain itself and assesses the extent to which the orofacial pain condition is associated with psychologic distress, disability, or impairment of functioning (significant disruption in normal activities), based on the use of standardized and validated assessment methods. The RDC/TMD Axis II was an attempt to codify the emotional sequelae and functional limitations that accompany chronic orofacial pain conditions and to determine whether there is need for referral of patients to appropriate providers (eg, psychiatrists, clinical psychologists) for formal diagnosis and treatment of psychiatric disorders.

There is a distinction between the RDC/TMD Axis II in its original form and the Axis II that was first presented in the American Academy of Orofacial Pain (AAOP) 1996 guidelines.[15] Intitially, the goal of the AAOP Axis II was merely to provide an introduction to the common psychiatric conditions observed among patients with orofacial pain conditions. The RDC/TMD Axis II was created to examine the psychologic and behavioral components of orofacial pain and the role they play in the onset and maintenance of chronic orofacial pain conditions. For more detailed information regarding the use of the Axis II RDC/TMD, the reader is referred elsewhere for a comprehensive introduction to these measures.[8,14]

# Definitions and General Features of Common Disorders

Stressful life events, such as conflicts in home or work relationships, financial problems, and cultural readjustment may contribute to illness and chronic pain.[16,17] Environmental stressors may heighten tensions, insecurities, and dysphoric effects that may lead in turn to increased adverse loading (clenching or bruxing) of the masticatory system as stress is converted to muscle tension and increased parafunctional behaviors.[18] While it is not necessarily the case that all stressors will lead to increases in muscle tension and that increases in muscle tension will always create pain, it is a distinct possibility to consider when evaluating an individual's clinical presentation. Although many mental conditions can be influenced by, or result from, orofacial pain disorders, only a select group is addressed in this chapter. For a more complete description of other mental conditions, the reader is encouraged to review the current *Diagnostic and Statistical Manual for Mental Disorders, Fourth Edition (DSM IV)*.[13] Gatchel and colleagues[19] have reported that the most frequently occurring mental disorders are major depression, anxiety disorders, and personality disorders. The other disorders presented in this chapter have a much lower frequency of occurrence, but the orofacial pain clinician should be aware of them to assist in making a successful referral for definitive diagnosis and treatment.

## Major depressive disorder (ICD-9 296.2x)13

Major depression has been identified as one of the most common mental disorders in patients with orofacial pain.[19] Recent clinical data suggest that almost one of every three patients presenting for treatment of orofacial pain may be experiencing symptoms consistent with a diagnosis of depression.[20] The diagnosis of major depression requires at least five of the following symptoms over a 2-week period, with at least one of the symptoms being depressed mood or loss of interest/pleasure: (1) depressed mood most of the day, (2) decreased interest or pleasure in all or most daily activities, (3) weight loss or appetite change, (4) insomnia or hypersomnia, (5) daily psychomotor agitation or retardation, (6) fatigue or loss of energy, (7) feelings of worthlessness or guilt, (8) reduced ability to think or concentrate, and (9) thoughts of death or suicide. When these symptoms cause distress and impair functioning, and are not due to a medical condition or substance use, the diagnosis of major depression is likely.

Depression can have a significant impact on pain perception and perceived control.[21] Depression can also diminish an individual's capacity to engage in self-care, including complying with pain treatment regimens. Major depression is a serious, potentially life-threatening condition, and referral to appropriate health care providers for effective treatment is essential along with care for the pain disorder.

## Anxiety disorders

### Generalized anxiety disorder (ICD-9 300.02)[13]

*Generalized anxiety disorder* (GAD) is diagnosed when an individual has persistent and excessive anxiety or worry for a period of 6 months or longer. The patient with GAD is not able to control these feelings, and at least three of the following symptoms are present: restlessness, fatigue, difficulty concentrating, irritability, muscle tension, and sleep disturbance. In addition, the anxiety and worry are not associated with another mental disorder, substance use, or medical condition, and the symptoms cause significant impairment of interpersonal functioning or work performance. It is estimated that between 10% and 30% of the orofacial pain population may be experiencing GAD. Referral for treatment of GAD may be delayed to determine first whether treatment of the orofacial pain condition itself may begin to alter symptoms.

### Panic disorder (ICD-9 300.01)[13]

Although much less common than GAD, *panic disorder* involves a sudden, intense onset of fear and terror that is often accompanied by thoughts of impending disaster. It is not uncommon for the individual to feel as though he or she is dying because of the associated chest pain, palpitations, and shortness of breath. Individuals having a panic attack report sensations of choking/smothering and are afraid of losing control of their thoughts. Panic disorder is diagnosed when a panic attack has occurred, and at least one of the following criteria has been present for at least 1 month: persistent concern about having another attack, worry about the implications or consequences of the attack, and a notable change in behavior related to the attacks or fear thereof. In addition, the panic attacks must not be due to a medical condition or substance use. Even though panic disorder is not common, it is a condition that, if present, requires immediate attention and coping skills.

## Posttraumatic stress disorder (*ICD-9* 309.81)[13]

Considerable professional interest and burgeoning public concern has focused on the sequelae of traumatic experiences. It is now well recognized that physical and sexual abuse are implicated in the etiology of a broad spectrum of physical and emotional symptoms. The essential feature of posttraumatic stress disorder (PTSD) is the onset of characteristic symptoms following exposure to a traumatic event involving direct personal experience or witnessing of an event that involves actual or threatened death or serious injury, or the threat to one's physical and psychologic integrity. Typical symptoms include persistent reexperiencing of the traumatic event; persistent avoidance of stimuli associated with the trauma and numbing of general responsiveness; and persistent symptoms of increased arousal. The full symptom picture must be present for more than 1 month, and the disturbance must cause clinically significant distress or impairment in daily functioning. For children, sexually traumatic events may include developmentally inappropriate sexual experiences without threatened or actual violence or injury. The disorder may be especially severe or longlasting when the traumatic experience has been created by deliberate human intent (eg, torture or rape) as contrasted with naturally occurring disasters. The likelihood of this disorder developing may increase as the intensity of and physical proximity to the event increases.

Psychologic reexperiencing of the traumatic event may occur as recurrent and intrusive recollections, distressing dreams, and, in rare instances, brief dissociative states or flashbacks during which components of the event are relived and the person behaves as though experiencing the event at that moment. Intense psychologic distress or physiologic reactions often occur when the person is exposed to triggering events that resemble or symbolize an aspect of the traumatic event (for example, entering an elevator for a person who may have been assaulted or raped in an elevator; or any intraoral pain or manipulation for individuals who may have been sexually violated or traumatized in their mouth).

Typically, people with this condition make deliberate efforts to avoid thoughts, feelings, or conversations about the traumatic event and in some instances may develop amnesia for important aspects of it. Diminished psychologic responsiveness, referred to as *psychic numbing* or *emotional anesthesia* may be accompanied by markedly diminished interest in previously enjoyed activities and marked reduced capacity of emotional responsiveness (especially in intimate, tender, and sexual situations). The individual has persistent symptoms of anxiety and increased arousal that were not present before the trauma, along with sleep disturbance, nightmares, hypervigilence, and an exaggerated startle response. This increased arousal is frequently accompanied by activation of the autonomic nervous system, measurable by electrocardiography, electromyography, and sweat gland activity.

In younger children, distressing dreams of the event may change into generalized nightmares. Rather than having a sense of reliving the past as a memory, young children often recreate versions of the trauma through repetitive play. For example, a child involved in a motor vehicle accident may reenact scenes of toy cars crashing, and sexually traumatized children may depict genital contact occurring between toy animals.

Not all psychopathology in individuals exposed to trauma should be attributed to PTSD, however. Symptoms of avoidance, numbing and increased arousal that are present *before* exposure to the stressor do not meet criteria for the diagnosis of PTSD and require further consideration for a diagnosis such as a mood or anxiety disorder. Acute stress disorder is distinguished from PTSD because the symptoms appear and subsequently resolve within 4 weeks of the trauma. Adjustment disorder is diagnosed when the response to an extreme stressor does not meet the criteria for PTSD or when the stressor itself is not that extreme.

Recent evidence indicates that a significant proportion of orofacial pain patients are likely to meet lifetime criteria for having experienced PTSD.[22,23] This relatively high rate of occurrence is consistent with other data suggesting that exposure to traumatic life events is common among patients with orofacial pain[24] and other pain conditions as well.[25] Given these data, it is necessary that clinicians have an awareness of the signs and symptoms of PTSD and be able to make appropriate referrals for treatment. The autonomic activation, perceptual distortion, and denial of one's own needs that are characteristic of this disorder may prevent significant therapeutic gains unless the underlying disorder is addressed.

Some of the symptoms of PTSD may share aspects with other disorders and therefore need to be carefully differentiated. In obsessive-compulsive disorder, for example, recurrent intrusive thoughts are experienced as inappropriate and are not related to an experienced traumatic event. Flashbacks in PTSD must be distinguished from illusions, hallucinations, and other perceptual disturbances that occur in schizophrenia and other psychotic conditions. Finally, malingering must be ruled out in those situations in which financial gain or forensic determinations play a role, as has recently been witnessed in some of the widely publicized cases of "false memory syndrome."

## Substance use disorders[13]

It is not uncommon for patients with orofacial pain to have ongoing or previous substance use disorders. These disorders include dependence, abuse, intoxication, and withdrawal. *Substance dependence* is defined as a pattern of substance use that leads to clinically significant impairment or distress. *Substance abuse* refers to a pattern of substance use that has significant negative consequences such as failure to meet obligations of work, school, or home; behaviors that are physically hazardous, like driving a car when impaired; legal problems; or interpersonal problems related to the continued substance use. *Substance intoxication* refers to the reversible signs and symptoms associated with the intake of a substance that can produce physical, behavioral, or psychologic changes. *Withdrawal* refers to substance-specific physical, behavioral, or psychologic changes that occur with the reduction or stoppage of a substance that has been used over a period of time.

The orofacial pain clinician should also be familiar with the terms, *addiction* and *pseudoaddiction*. *Addiction* involves one or more of the following characteristics: impaired control over drug use, compulsive use of drug(s), continued use despite harm, and craving. A person with an addiction often does not take medications according to prescription or schedule, has multiple visits to multiple practitioners, and likely reports on a frequent basis that his or her prescriptions have been lost or stolen. It is important to distinguish addiction from pseudoaddiction in patients with chronic pain.[26,27] *Pseudoaddiction* looks like addiction, in that the same behaviors are typically present, but the patient has identifiable nociception (eg, cancer pain, neuropathic pain, or postsurgical pain) that is undermedicated, so the individual is in constant search of effective treatment. When such a person is given adequate medication, the addiction-like behaviors cease. Clearly, separating a person with pseudoaddiction related to undermedication of active nociception from the person seeking opioids for a stated complaint of pain requires good knowledge of the patient by the clinician. In the case of pseudoaddiction in particular, progress notes should clearly document the contingent nature of the medication seeking along with the appropriateness of the medication to the identified nociception.

These disorders can occur within 11 broad classes of substances that include alcohol, amphetamines or similar compounds, caffeine, cannabis, cocaine, hallucinogens, inhalants, nicotine, opioids, phencyclidine or similar compounds, and sedatives/hypnotics/anxiolytics. The pain practitioner must be alert to potential abuse disorders. Unless the practitioner has specialty training in the management of addiction disorders, referral to a health care provider who does is the appropriate standard of care. It is important to develop a rapport with patients who have problems with substance abuse to foster successful referral.

## Sleep disorders[13]

There are two major sleep disorders, *primary insomnia* (ICD-9 307.42) and *breathing-related sleep disorder* (eg, sleep apnea, ICD-9 780.59), that the pain practitioner is likely to encounter. Other sleep disorders such as narcolepsy or night terrors are not as common in the chronic pain environment. *Primary insomnia* involves difficulty in starting or maintaining sleep for a period of at least 1 month. This condition can adversely affect a patient's life in a number of ways, including relationships and employment. For a diagnosis of primary insomnia to be made, it must be clear that depression, anxiety, or medication/substance use is not contributing to the disruptions in sleep.

*Breathing-related sleep disorder* is disordered breathing that disrupts sleep, often causing daytime sleepiness. The breathing problem is usually the result of either obstructive or central sleep apnea, but it can be the result of central alveolar hypoventilation syndrome. These latter conditions represent medical disorders that merit a referral to physicians trained in sleep medicine. Sleep disorders in patients with chronic pain are common, and appropriate management of the sleep disorder itself is an important component of a biobehavioral approach to patient management.

## Psychologic factors affecting physical condition (ICD-9 316)[13]

When the primary presenting complaint is a medical (physical) condition and there are one or more psychologic or behavioral issues influencing that condition, the diagnosis of psychologic factors affecting physical condition can be made. Typically, the diagnosis will link the psychologically related issues with the physical condition as in the example, "stress and anger toward significant other affecting masticatory muscle pain." The issues identified must be contributing to the disorder by (1) having a close temporal connection between the beginning of the physical condition and the onset of the psychologic/behavioral factors, (2) interfering with the treatment of the condition, (3) increasing health risk, or (4) increasing physiologic activation that brings on or intensifies the physical condition.

This diagnostic category provides the practitioner with the means to codify a comorbid psychologic condition that may be contributing to the patient's ability to manage a medical problem. Since chronic pain complaints represent a complex interaction between psychologic and physiologic factors, the use of this diagnostic category is common. In addition, this label may also be more acceptable to some patients than other labels of psychiatric conditions.

## Personality disorders[13]

Recent data suggest that a significant number of orofacial pain patients have a personality disorder.[19] Generally speaking, a personality disorder is a long-term pattern of thinking and acting that is significantly different from the general population and results in significant adverse consequences to the individual and those around the individual. These abnormal patterns may be manifested as exaggerations or dysfunction of certain dimensions of personality. Personality disorders represent a serious challenge to the pain practitioner.

There are three basic groups of personality disorders that share common clinical presentations. *Cluster A* includes odd or eccentric disorders (paranoid, schizoid, and schizotypal); *Cluster B* includes emotional, dramatic, or unpredictable disorders (antisocial, borderline, histrionic, and narcissistic); and *Cluster C* includes anxious and fearful disorders[13] (avoidant, dependent, and obsessive-compulsive).

Within Cluster A, *paranoid personality disorder (ICD-9 301.0)* describes an individual who does not trust others and is very suspicious. These patients may overinterpret what the clinician is saying, or they may be unforgiving of others for perceived injury or insult. Patients with *schizoid personality disorder (ICD-9 301.2)* are detached from others and have very limited emotional expression. A person with this disorder has few, if any, close friends or family and usually does things alone. The *schizotypal personality disorder (ICD-9 301.22)* shares the features of detachment and limited emotional expression but is also characterized by substantial distortions of thought and very unusual behavior. Thought distortions include magical thinking, belief in telepathy, and weird fantasies. Unusual behaviors might involve acting out the use of "special powers" or listening to "voices for direction."

Within Cluster B, the *antisocial personality disorder* (ICD-9 301.7) is characterized by little or no regard for the rights of others. This personality disorder requires at least three of the following characteristics to be present: *(1)* doing things that could lead to arrest, *(2)* lying, *(3)* not planning ahead, *(4)* being irritable and aggressive to the point of getting into fights, *(5)* disregarding safety of self and others, *(6)* being irresponsible, and *(7)* not expressing remorse or sorrow for behavior that hurts others. *Borderline personality disorder* (ICD-9 301.83) represents a repeated pattern of instability of relationships and impulsivity in action. The instability takes the form of leaving and entering relationships in a recurrent pattern, as well as frequent changes in the nature of the relationship. The patient with borderline personality disorder often does not want to be abandoned. These patients exhibit impulsive self-destructive behavior, such as substance abuse, unsafe sex, binge eating, and reckless driving, and engage in repeated threats and gestures of self-harm, including suicide. There is also marked emotional instability and intense, inappropriate anger and extremes in thinking (eg, at one point the clinician is "the best doctor ever"; several weeks later the clinician is "an incompetent toad"). Finally, the borderline personality can manifest paranoid thoughts or dissociative symptoms.

*Histrionic personality disorder* (ICD-9 301.5) is characterized by pronounced emotional expression and attention seeking. These patients can be provocative and sexually seductive; they are easily suggestible; and they may perceive relationships as more intimate than they really are, possibly blurring boundaries normally maintained by patients. The patient with *narcissistic personality disorder* (ICD-9 301.81) acts in a grandiose manner and has an intense need for the admiration of others, while displaying little empathy. This patient will expect the clinician to respond to his or her needs at all hours, including during the weekends.

Cluster C disorders involve persons who are overly anxious or afraid as a predominant feature of their everyday experience. *Avoidant personality disorder* (ICD-9 301.82) is associated with feeling socially inhibited, inadequate, and being overly sensitive to any criticism. The patient with *dependent personality disorder* (ICD-9 301.6) has a pervasive need to be taken care of, so that there is excessive clinging and fear of being abandoned. These individuals will continue to seek care for their condition despite lack of improvement over time, or even harm done. With *obsessive-compulsive personality disorder* (ICD-9 301.4),[28,29] a drive for perfection, orderliness, and being in control rules a person's day-to-day life. There is limited openness to new ideas, and rules, details, and lists are very important. Patients with obsessive-compulsive personality disorder do not like to work with others, keep everything they have owned, even if it is worthless, and hoard their resources in case something should happen in the future.

## Somatoform disorders[13]

In this group of mental conditions, the patient reports somatic complaints, yet no physical evidence of organic disease is present. Somatoform disorders are subdivided into the following categories: somatization disorders, undifferentiated somatoform disorders, conversion disorders, somatoform pain disorders, hypochondriasis, body dysmorphic disorders (BDD), and somatoform disorders not otherwise specified.

## Somatization disorder (*ICD-9* 300.81)

This disorder features recurrent and multiple somatic complaints of several years' duration for which treatment has been sought but for which no organic cause has been ascertained. In addition, there is significant disarray or distress in the person's life for which no treatment is sought. Clinical characteristics include preoccupation with somatic complaints, denial of difficulty in life, high level of treatment-seeking for somatic complaints but poor adherence and compliance to treatment, and amplification of symptoms. The disorder begins before the age of 30 years and has a chronic but fluctuating course. Historically, this condition was referred to as *hysteria* or *Briquet syndrome*. Complaints are often presented in a dramatic, vague, or exaggerated manner, or are part of a complicated dental and/or medical history in which many physical diagnoses have been considered. These individuals frequently receive dental care from a number of practitioners, sometimes simultaneously. Complaints often extend to multiple organ systems.

For the diagnosis of somatization disorder, there must be a history of pain related to at least four different sites (eg, head, abdomen, back joints, extremities, chest, rectum) or functions (eg, mastication, menstruation, sexual intercourse, and urination). There also must be a history of at least two gastrointestinal symptoms other than pain. Most individuals with this disorder complain of abdominal bloating and nausea; vomiting, diarrhea, and food intolerance are less frequent symptoms. Also, there must be a history of at least one sexual or reproductive symptom plus one pseudoneurologic symptom other than pain. It should be emphasized that the unexplained symptoms in somatization disorder are not intentionally feigned or produced.

Somatization disorder is relatively rare, but somatization as a style or as a major characteristic is fairly common in the orofacial pain population.[30] It has also been demonstrated that there is a significant relationship between number of tender muscles on an RDC/TMD examination and somatization scores on the SCL-90-R.[31] These clinical data highlight somatization as a style of coping among patients with orofacial pain.

Anxiety and depressed mood are extremely common, and suicide threats/attempts, antisocial behavior, and occupational, interpersonal, and marital difficulties frequently accompany the syndrome. The clinical course is typically chronic but fluctuating in nature and rarely remits spontaneously. Through seeking numerous evaluations, diagnostic tests, multiple trials on medication, and frequently submitting unwittingly to unnecessary surgery, these patients often experience iatrogenic complications both in and out of the hospital.

The differential diagnosis necessitates ruling out physical disorders that present with vague, multiple, and confusing somatic symptoms. In addition, schizophrenia with multiple somatic delusions, dysthymic disorder, generalized anxiety disorder, panic disorder, and conversion disorder need to be excluded from this specific diagnostic classification.

245

## Undifferentiated somatoform disorder (*ICD-9* 300.81)

When one or more physical complaints persist for 6 months or longer, and these symptoms cannot be fully explained either by any known dental or general medical condition, or incident or substance (eg, the effects of injury, substance use, or medication side effects), undifferentiated somatoform disorder is likely. Alternatively, the physical complaints or resultant impairments are grossly in excess of what would be expected from the history, physical examination, or laboratory findings. The symptoms must cause clinically significant distress or impairment in social, occupational, or other areas of adaptive functioning. This is a residual category for those persistent somatoform presentations that do not meet the full criteria for somatization disorder or another somatoform disorder.

It should be noted that unexplained medical and/or dental symptoms and worry about physical illness do not always indicate psychopathology. The highest frequency of unexplained physical complaints occurs in young women of low socioeconomic status, but such symptoms are not limited to any age, sex, or sociocultural group. *Neurasthenia*, a syndrome characterized by fatigue and weakness, is classified as an undifferentiated somatoform disorder if symptoms have persisted for longer than 6 months and are not attributable to any other organic illness or mental disorder.

## Conversion disorder (*ICD-9* 300.11)

Patients with conversion disorder present a loss of or alteration in physical functioning that suggests a physical disorder but instead is an expression of psychologic conflict or need. The disturbance is not under voluntary control and cannot be explained by any physical disorder or known pathophysiologic mechanism. Conversion disorder is not likely when conversion symptoms are limited to pain (see somatoform pain disorder) or to a circumscribed disturbance in sexual functioning.

Two mechanisms have been suggested to explain the psychologic advantages accomplished by the development of conversion symptoms. In one mechanism, the individual achieves "primary gain" by keeping an internal conflict or need out of conscious awareness. In these instances, there is often a temporal relationship between an environmental stimulus that heightens a psychologic conflict or need and the initiation or exacerbation of the symptom. In such cases, the symptom has symbolic value as a representation of and partial solution for the underlying psychologic conflict.

In the other mechanism, the patient achieves "secondary gain" by avoiding a particular activity that is noxious to him or her or by obtaining support from the environment that otherwise would not be forthcoming. A conversion symptom is likely to involve a single symptom during a given episode, but may vary in site and nature if there are subsequent episodes.

Usually the symptom develops in a setting of extreme psychologic stress and appears suddenly. Hysterical personality traits are common but not invariably present. *La belle indifference*, an attitude toward the symptom that suggests a relative lack of concern, out of keeping with the severe nature of the impairment, is sometimes present. This feature has little diagnostic value, however, since it is also found in some seriously ill medical patients who are stoic about their situation.

The usual age of onset is late childhood or early adulthood, and rarely before age 10 or after age 35 years. When an apparent conversion disorder first develops in middle or old age, the probability of an occult neurologic or other general medical condition is high.

Some physical disorders that present with vague, multiple, somatic symptoms (eg, multiple sclerosis or systemic lupus erythematosus) may be misdiagnosed early in their course as conversion symptoms. A diagnosis of conversion disorder is suggested if the symptoms are inconsistent with the actual known physical disorder, or if complaints are obviously inconsistent with the anatomic distribution of the nervous system. Permanent remission of symptoms through suggestion, hypnosis, or narcoanalysis also suggests the diagnosis of conversion disorder (although transient improvement in response to suggestion is also encountered in some patients with organic disease).

Somatization disorder and, more infrequently, schizophrenia may have conversion symptoms. However, the diagnosis of conversion disorder should not be made when such symptoms are due to either of these pervasive disorders. Some psychogenic pain can be conceptualized as a conversion symptom, but because of the different course and treatment implications, all such cases should be coded as somatoform pain disorder. On the other hand, some parafunctions and atypical jaw movement disorders in the absence of pain may fit appropriately in the diagnostic category of conversion disorder.

In hypochondriasis, preoccupation with physical symptoms is typical, but there is usually no actual loss or distortion of bodily function. In factitious disorder with physical symptoms, the symptoms are, by definition, under voluntary control, and the simulated illness rarely takes the form of neurologic symptoms that would be confused with conversion symptoms. In malingering, the symptom production is under the patient's voluntary control and is in pursuit of a goal that is obviously recognizable, given the individual's environmental circumstances. Such goals frequently involve the prospect of material benefit or the avoidance of unpleasant work or responsibility.

## Somatoform pain disorder (*ICD-9 308.8x*)

This disorder presents a clinical picture in which complaints of pain are prominent, in the absence of adequate physical findings, and in association with evidence of psychologic factors that have a role in the onset, severity, exacerbation, and maintenance of the pain.

Somatoform pain disorder is not diagnosed if the pain is better accounted for by a mood, anxiety, or psychotic disorder. However, the pain may be an associated or exacerbating factor contributing to other emotional conditions.

*Somatoform pain disorder associated with psychologic factors (ICD-9 307.80)* is diagnosed when psychologic factors are judged to have a major role, and when general medical or dental conditions have either minimal or no role in the onset and maintenance of pain. This subtype is not diagnosed if criteria are met for somatization disorder.

*Somatoform pain disorder associated with both psychologic factors and general medical condition (ICD-9 307.89)* is diagnosed when psychologic factors and a medical condition (eg, TMDs) coexist with the onset and maintenance of pain.

Both of these subtypes may be further specified as *acute* (if the pain is of less than 6 months' duration) or *chronic* (if the pain has been present for 6 months or longer). For somatoform pain disorder associated with dental or medical conditions, the diagnostic code for the pain is selected based on the associated physical diagnosis if one has been established or the anatomic location of the pain if the physical diagnosis remains uncertain.

In somatoform pain disorder, the pain symptom either is inconsistent with the anatomic distribution of the nervous system or, if it mimics a known disease, cannot be adequately accounted for by organic pathology. Similarly, no pathophysiologic mechanism accounts for the pain (in contrast, for example, with tension-type headaches associated with pericranial muscle tenderness). A psychologic origin of pain may be inferred when a temporal relationship exists between an environmental stimulus that is apparently related to a psychologic conflict or need and the initiation or exacerbation of the pain. Alternatively, the pain may permit an individual to avoid some activity that is noxious to him or her or to get support from the environment that would otherwise not be forthcoming.

Somatoform pain disorder may be accompanied by other localized sensory or motor changes, such as paresthesias and muscle spasm. There often are frequent visits to health care practitioners in search for relief despite medical reassurance; excessive use of analgesics without relief of pain; requests for surgery; and the assumption of an "invalid role" (eg, chronic pain syndrome). The patient usually refuses to consider the role of psychologic factors in the pain. In some cases the pain may have symbolic significance, such as pain mimicking "being slapped in the face" for a patient whose spouse is unfaithful. A history of conversion symptoms is common. However, histrionic personality traits are seldom present, nor is la belle indifference, though concern about the pain symptom is usually less intense than its stated severity. Dysphoric moods are common.

This disorder can occur at any stage of life, from childhood to old age, but seems to begin most frequently in adolescence or early adulthood. The pain usually appears suddenly and increases in severity over a few days or weeks. The symptom may subside with appropriate intervention or termination of a precipitating event, or it may persist for months or years if reinforced. The degree of impaired functioning varies with the intensity and duration of pain and may range from a slight disturbance of social or occupational performance to total incapacity and need for hospitalization. The most serious complications are iatrogenic, including dependence on minor tranquilizers and narcotic analgesics and repeated, unnecessary diagnostic procedures and treatment interventions.

Severe psychosocial stress is known to predispose to somatoform pain disorder. There is no information available on its general prevalence, but the disorder is most frequently diagnosed in women. Relatives of individuals with this disorder have had more painful injuries and illnesses than occur in the general population.

The dramatic presentation of pain complaints is *not* sufficient grounds for diagnosing somatoform pain disorder; certain patients with histrionic personality traits or cultural styles of communication may be prone to being overly dramatic (but psychiatrically normal) when expressing organic discomfort.

Patients with somatization disorder, depressive disorders, or schizophrenia may complain of various aches and pains, but the pain rarely dominates the clinical picture. Somatoform pain disorder should not be the primary diagnosis if pain is associated with other mental conditions. In such cases, an additional diagnosis of somatoform pain disorder should be considered only if the pain is an independent focus of clinical attention, leads to clinically significant distress or impairment, and is in excess of that usually associated with the other mental disorder. The pain associated with muscle contraction headaches, bruxism, or parafunctional movements and posturing would not be diagnosed as somatoform pain disorder because there is a pathophysiologic mechanism that accounts for the pain (a subset of such patients meeting diagnostic criteria for conversion disorder).

The Task Force on Taxonomy of The International Association for the Study of Pain[32] proposed a five-axis system for categorizing chronic pain: *(I)* regions; *(II)* systems; *(III)* temporal characteristics of pain and pattern of occurrence; *(IV)* patient's statements of intensity and time since the onset; and *(V)* etiology.

This five-axis system focuses primarily on the physical manifestations of pain and provides for comments on psychologic factors on both the second axis (where the involvement of a mental disorder can be coded) and the fifth axis (where possible causes include psychophysiologic and psychologic).

## Hypochondriasis (*ICD-9* 300.70)

The predominant feature of this disorder is an unrealistic interpretation of physical signs and sensations as abnormal, leading to preoccupation with the fear of or belief in having a serious disease. These unrealistic fears and beliefs persist despite medical and dental reassurance and cause impairment in social and occupational functioning. The preoccupation may be with bodily functions or with minor physical abnormalities that the patient interprets as symptoms or signs of serious disease. More than one organ system may be involved simultaneously.

Such patients frequently present their medical/dental history in great detail and at length; have a history of "doctor shopping," with frequent deterioration in the doctor-patient relationship (with frustration and anger on both sides); and are frequently convinced that they are being deprived of appropriate care. Physical complaints may be used secondarily to exert control over relationships with family and friends. Anxiety, depressed mood, and compulsive personality traits are common. The distinction between *hypochondriasis* and *somatization* is the unrealistic nature of the interpretation of symptoms and the strong fear of the unknown disease.

The most common age at onset is in early adulthood, although frequently the disorder begins in the fourth decade for men and the fifth decade for women. The overall course is usually chronic, with waxing and waning of symptoms. It appears that acute onset, general medical comorbidity, the absence of a personality disorder, and the absence of secondary gain are favorable prognostic indicators. This disorder may stem from either learning history associated with developmental issues or iatrogenically due to interactions with the medical system.

Social and occupational functioning are usually impaired, and relationships are often strained because the individual is preoccupied with disease. The impairment is severe when the individual adopts an invalid lifestyle and becomes bedridden. Hypochon-driac concerns can range from simple (but excessive) worry to experiencing psycho-physiologic responses, the latter resulting in the patient feeling justified.

Complications are secondary to efforts to obtain medical and dental care. Because multiple physical symptoms without or-ganic basis become the focus, organic path-ology may be overlooked. In addition, doc-tor shopping carries the added danger of repeated diagnostic procedures and the ia-trogenicity sometimes associated with un-necessary pharmacologic, biomechanical, and surgical interventions. A past experience with organic disease in one's self or a fam-ily member and generalized psychosocial stress apparently predispose to the devel-opment of this disorder. Because these pa-tients are often offended at the suggestion that their fears or beliefs may be unrealistic, they frequently refuse referral for mental health care. The most important differential diagnostic considerations are general med-ical diseases. However, the presence of or-ganic pathology does not rule out the pos-sibility of coexisting hypochondriasis.

In some psychotic disorders, such as schizophrenia and major depression with psychotic features, there may be somatic delusions of having a disease. In hypochon-driasis, the belief of having a disease gener-ally does not have the fixed quality of a true somatic delusion, in that the individual af-fected with hypochondriasis can usually en-tertain the possibility that the feared disease is not present. A specifier is provided to allow the clinician to designate whether the condition is of the "with poor insight" type. If symptoms of hypochondriacal preoccu-pation are present in psychotic disorders, the added diagnosis of hypochondriasis should not be made.

In dysthymic disorder, panic disorder, GAD, obsessive-compulsive disorder, and somatization disorder, the symptom of hypo-chondriac preoccupation may appear, but generally is not the predominant distur-bance. In somatization disorder, there tends to be preoccupation with symptoms rather than fear of having a specific disease. When the criteria for any of these other syndromes are met and the hypochondriac preoccupa-tion is due to one of these disorders, the ad-ditional diagnosis of hypochondriasis is not made.

## Body dysmorphic disorder (ICD-9 300.7)

The essential feature of BDD is either a pre-occupation with a defect in appearance that is imagined or, if a slight physical anomaly is present, concern that is markedly excessive. The preoccupation must cause significant distress or impairment and must not be bet-ter explained by the presence of another mental disorder (eg, dissatisfaction with body shape and size in anorexia nervosa).

Common preoccupations include the shape, size, or some other aspect of the nose, eyes, eyelids, eyebrows, ears, mouth, lips, teeth, jaw, chin, cheeks, or head. How-ever, any other body part may be the focus of concern. Because of embarrassment over their concerns, some individuals with BDD avoid describing their "defects" in detail and may instead refer only to their general "ugliness." Most of these patients experi-ence marked distress over their supposed deformity, often describing their preoccu-pations as "intensely painful," "tormenting," or "devastating." Thoughts about their "de-fect" frequently dominate their lives, lend-ing to social avoidance and significant im-pairment in general functioning.

Associated features of BDD include frequent mirror checking of the "defect" and excessive preoccupation with grooming. Attempts at reassurance about the defect result in temporary, if any, relief. Ideas of people making references that are related to the imagined defect are also common. The distress and dysfunction associated with this disorder, although highly variable, can lead to repeated hospitalization, suicide attempts, and completed suicide.

Individuals with BDD often pursue and receive general medical, dental, or surgical treatments to rectify their imagined defects. Such treatments may cause the disorder to worsen, leading to new or intensified preoccupations, chronic dissatisfaction, anger, and litigation toward the health care professional involved. Preliminary evidence suggests that BDD is diagnosed with approximately equal frequency in women and men.

The onset usually occurs during adolescence and may be either gradual or abrupt. The course tends to be fairly continuous, with few symptom-free intervals, although the intensity of preoccupation and impairment in social adjustment may wax and wane over time. The part of the body on which concern is focused may change or remain the same.

BDD should not be diagnosed if the excessive preoccupation is limited to the usual concerns of patients with anorexia nervosa or gender identity disorder or the mood-congruent rumination during a major depressive episode. Individuals with avoidant personality disorder or social phobia may worry about embarrassment by real defects in appearance, but this concern is usually not prominent, persistent, distressing, time consuming, and impairing. A separate diagnosis of obsessive-compulsive disorder is given to individuals with BDD only when obsessions and compulsions are not restricted to concerns about appearance. Patients with BDD can receive an additional diagnosis of delusional disorder, somatic type, if their preoccupations with an imagined defect are held with delusional intensity. An example of BDD in the orofacial pain setting might be that individual who presents with excessive demands for surgery for an otherwise unproblematic temporomandibular joint click in the hopes that the surgery will correct the deformity. This patient is not amenable to reassurances that the click may be normal.

## Somatoform disorder, not otherwise specified (ICD-9 300.81)

This category includes those conditions with somatoform symptoms that do not meet the criteria of any specific somatoform disorder. Examples include pseudocyesis; nonpsychotic hypochondriac symptoms of less than 6 months' duration; and any disorder involving unexplained physical complaints (eg, fatigue, orofacial pain, or body weakness) of less than 6 months' duration that are not due to another mental disorder or general medical or dental condition.

## Factitious disorders[13]

Factitious means not real, genuine, or natural. Factitious disorders are therefore characterized by physical and/or psychologic symptoms that are produced by the individual and are under voluntary control. The judgment that the patient is willfully creating his or her symptoms is based, in part, on the patient's ability to simulate illness in such a way as to avoid detection. However, such acts also have a compulsive quality, because the individual is unable to refrain from a particular behavior, even if its dangers are known. These conditions should therefore be considered *voluntary* only in the sense that they are deliberate and purposeful, but not in the sense that the patient adopts or sustains the pathologic behavior intentionally. The presence of factitious psychologic or physical symptoms does not preclude the coexistence of true psychologic or physical illness.

Factitious disorders are distinguished from acts of malingering. In malingering, the individual is also in voluntary control of the symptoms, but is in pursuit of obvious and recognizable benefits through willful falsification. In contrast, in a factitious disorder, there is no apparent goal other than to assume the patient role. Whereas an act of malingering may be considered adaptive under certain circumstances, by definition, a diagnosis of a factitious disorder always implies psychopathology (most often a severe personality disturbance). In the past, some of the disorders classified here would have been subsumed under the category of *hysteria*.

Factitious disorders may present with psychologic or physical symptoms and are coded according to the subtype that characterizes the predominant symptoms. These subtypes include: *(1)* factitious disorder with predominantly psychological signs and symptoms (*ICD-9* 300.16); *(2)* factitious disorder with predominantly physical signs and symptoms (*ICD-9* 300.19); *(3)* factitious disorder with combined psychological and physical signs and symptoms (*ICD-9* 300.19); and *(4)* factitious disorder not otherwise specified (*ICD-9* 300.19).

Factitious disorder with predominantly physical signs and symptoms, for example, is the patient's plausible presentation of factitious physical symptoms of such a degree that he or she is able to obtain and sustain multiple hospitalizations. This person's entire life may consist of trying either to be admitted or to remain in hospitals. All organ systems are potential targets, and the symptoms presented are limited only by the individual's medical and dental knowledge, sophistication, and imagination. This disorder has also been called *Munchausen syndrome*.

These patients usually present their history with great dramatic flair, but are extremely vague and inconsistent when questioned in more detail. There may be uncontrollable, pathologic lying (*pseudologia fantastica*), and, after an extensive workup of their initial chief complaints proves negative, they will often complain of other physical problems and produce more factitious symptoms. Complaints of pain and requests for analgesics are very common. Individuals with this disorder often eagerly undergo multiple invasive diagnostic procedures and surgical interventions. When confronted with evidence of their factitious symptoms, they either deny the allegations or rapidly discharge themselves against medical advice.

Substance abuse, particularly of prescribed analgesics and sedatives, is frequently present. The onset is usually in early adult life, often with an initial hospitalization for physical illness. Rapidly thereafter, a pattern of successive hospitalizations begins and becomes a lifelong pattern. This disorder is extremely incapacitating. Multiple hospitalizations frequently lead to iatrogenically induced physical problems.

Factitious disorders may be predisposed by past physical illness with extensive medical/dental treatment and hospitalization; a grudge against the dental or medical profession, sometimes due to previous mismanagement; employment in the dental field as a nurse, technician, or other paraprofessional; underlying dependent, exploitative, or masochistic personality traits; identification with a dentist or physician in the past (for example, identifying with a family member who is a health professional); or a traumatic experience with a health care professional, such as being sexually abused by a physician or dentist.

The major differential diagnostic consideration is obviously to rule out a general medical condition. A high index of suspicion for factitious disorder should be aroused if any combination of the following is noted: *(1)* pseudologica fantastica, with emphasis on the dramatic presentation; *(2)* disruptive behavior, including noncompliance with rules, regulations, and arguing excessively with health care providers; *(3)* extensive knowledge of dental/medical terminology and hospital routine; *(4)* continued use of analgesics for "pain"; and *(5)* a fluctuating clinical course with a rapid production of "complications" or new "pathology" once the initial workup results are negative.

In somatoform disorders also, there are physical complaints not due to bonafide organic disease. However, the symptom production is not under voluntary control, and admissions to hospitals are rarely as common as in factitious disorder. Patients with malingering may seek hospitalization by producing symptoms in attempts to obtain obvious benefits or compensation. However, the goal is usually apparent, and they can "stop" the symptom when it is no longer useful to them. Antisocial personality disorder is often incorrectly diagnosed on the basis of the pseudologica fantastica, the lack of close relationships with others, and the occasionally associated drug and criminal histories that these patients present. However, antisocial personality disorder differs from this disorder by its earlier onset

and its rare association with chronic hospitalization as a way of life. Schizophrenia is often incorrectly diagnosed because of the bizarre lifestyle that these patients present. However, the characteristic psychotic symptoms of schizophrenia are not present in patients with factitious disorder.

## Malingering (ICD-9 V65.2)[13]

The essential feature of *malingering* is the voluntary production and presentation of false or grossly exaggerated physical or psychologic symptoms. The symptoms are produced in a conscious and voluntary pursuit of a goal, having obvious benefit to the individual (for example, to avoid work or military conscription, obtain financial compensation, evade criminal prosecution, or obtain drugs).

A high index of suspicion for malingering should be aroused when any combination of the following is noted: *(1)* medicolegal context of presentation (for example, when the person has been referred by an attorney to the dentist/physician); *(2)* marked discrepancy between the person's claim of distress or disability and the objective findings; *(3)* lack of cooperation with diagnostic evaluations and prescribed treatment regimens; and *(4)* the presence of antisocial personality disorder. In contrast, persons with factitious disorder evidence an intrapsychic need to maintain the sick role independent of practical costs vs benefits. Thus, the diagnosis of factitious disorder excludes the diagnosis of malingering.

Malingering is differentiated from conversion disorder and the other somatoform disorders by the voluntary production of symptoms and by the obvious, recognizable goal. The malingering individual is much less likely to present his or her symptoms in the context of emotional conflict, and the symptoms presented are less likely to be symbolic of an underlying emotional conflict. Symptom relief in malingering is not often obtained by suggestions, hypnosis, or intravenous barbiturates, as it frequently is in conversion disorder.

## Summary

There are a broad range of factors that may influence the development and course of orofacial pain conditions. The astute clinician will recognize the contributions of psychosocial factors. The biobehavioral frame of reference enables the clinician to explore the complexities of chronic orofacial pain in the initial interview and to mobilize resources to address the multifactorial nature of pain conditions. When the presence of mental disorders is suspected, the astute clinician will make an effective referral to competent clinicians with the skills to diagnose and treat mental disorders in persons with orofacial pain. Appropriate care of orofacial pain disorders includes management of the cognitive, emotional, and behavioral features that present with these conditions.

## References

1. Fields HL. Pain modulation: Expectation, opioid analgesia and virtual pain. Prog Brain Res 2000;122:245–253.
2. Dworkin SF. Perspectives on the interaction of biological, psychological and social factors in TMD. J Am Dent Assoc 1994;125:856–863.
3. Turk DC. Psychosocial and behavioral assessment of patients with temporomandibular disorders: Diagnostic and treatment implications. Oral Surg Oral Med Oral Pathol Oral Radiol Endod 1997;83:65–71.
4. Engel GL. The need for a new medical model: A challenge for biomedicine. Science 1977;196:129–136.
5. Carlson CR. Psychological factors associated with orofacial pain. Dent Clin North Am 2007;51:145–160.
6. Oakley ME, McCreary CP, Flack VF, Clark GT, Solberg WK, Pullinger AG. Dentists' ability to detect psychological problems in patients with temporomandibular disorders and chronic pain. J Am Dent Assoc 1989;118:727–730.
7. Von Korff M, Ormel J, Keefe FJ, Dworkin SF. Grading the severity of chronic pain. Pain 1992;50:133–149.
8. Dworkin SF. Psychosocial issues. In: Lund GLJP, Dubner R, Sessle B (eds). Orofacial Pain: From Basic Science to Clinical Management. Chicago: Quintessence, 2001:115–127.
9. Derogatis LR. The SCL 90R: Administration, Scoring and Procedure Manual. Baltimore: Clinical Psychology Research, 1977.
10. Beck AT. Beck Depression Inventory. San Antonio, TX: The Pyschological Corporation, 1978.
11. Spielberger CD. State-Trait Anxiety Inventory. Palo Alto, CA: Consulting Psychologists Press, 1983.
12. Beck AT. Beck Anxiety Inventory. San Antonio, TX: The Psychological Corporation, 1993.
13. Diagnostic and Statistical Manual of Mental Disorders, ed 4. Washington, DC: American Psychiatric Association, 1994.
14. Dworkin SF, LeResche L. Research Diagnostic Criteria for Temporomandibular Disorders: Review, criteria, examinations and specifications, critique. J Craniomandib Disord 1992;6:301–355.
15. Okeson JP. Orofacial Pain: Guidelines for Classification, Assessment, and Management. Chicago: Quintessence, 1996.
16. Dworkin SF, Burgess JA. Orofacial pain of psychogenic origin: Current concepts and classification. J Am Dent Assoc 1987;115:565–571.
17. Rugh JD, Davis SE. Temporomandibular disorders: Psychological and behavioral aspects. In: Sarnat BG, Laskin DM (eds). The Temporomandibular Joint: A Biological Basis for Clinical Practice. Philadelphia: Saunders, 1992:329–345.
18. Bertrand PM. The management of facial pain. American Association of Oral and Maxillofacial Surgery Knowledge Update Series. Rosemont, IL: AAOMS, 2001;3:79–109.
19. Gatchel RJ, Garofalo JP, Ellis E, Holt C. Major psychological disorders in acute and chronic TMD: An initial examination. J Am Dent Assoc 1996;127:1365–1370, 1372, 1374.
20. Korszun A, Hinderstein B, Wong M. Comorbidity of depression with chronic facial pain and temporomandibular disorders. Oral Surg Oral Med Oral Pathol Oral Radiol Endod 1996;82:496–500.
21. Turk DC, Okifuji A. Pain management. In: Nezu AM, Nezu CM, Geller PA (eds). Handbook of Psychology. New York: Wiley, 2003:299–300.

22. Sherman JJ, Carlson CR, Wilson JF, Okeson JP, Mc-Cubbin JA. Post-traumatic stress disorder among patients with orofacial pain. J Orofac Pain 2005;19:309–317.

23. De Leeuw R, Bertoli E, Schmidt JE, Carlson CR. Prevalence of post-traumatic stress disorder symptoms in orofacial pain patients. Oral Surg Oral Med Oral Pathol Oral Radiol Endod 2005;99:558–568.

24. Curran SL, Sherman JJ, Cunningham LL, Okeson JP, Reid KI, Carlson CR. Physical and sexual abuse among orofacial pain patients: Linkages with pain and psychologic distress. J Orofac Pain 1995;9:340–346.

25. Wurtele SK, Kaplan GM, Keairnes M. Childhood sexual abuse among chronic pain patients. Clin J Pain 1990;6:110–113.

26. Heit HA. The truth about pain management: The difference between a pain patient and an addicted patient. Eur J Pain 2001;(5 suppl A):27–29.

27. Weissman DE. Understanding pseudoaddiction. J Pain Symptom Manage 1994;9:74.

28. Kinney RK, Gatchel RJ, Ellis E, Holt C. Major psychological disorders in chronic TMD patients: Implications for successful management. J Am Dent Assoc 1992;123:49–54.

29. Kight M, Gatchel RJ, Wesley L. Temporomandibular disorders: Evidence for significant overlap with psychopathology. Health Psychol 1999;18:177–182.

30. Dworkin SF. Somatization, distress and chronic pain. Qual Life Res 1994;3(suppl 1):S77–S83.

31. Wilson L, Dworkin SF, Whitney C, LeResche L. Somatization and pain dispersion in chronic temporomandibular disorder pain. Pain 1994;57:55–61.

32. International Association for the Study of Pain, Task Force on Taxonomy. Scheme for coding chronic pain diagnoses. In: Merskey H, Bogduk N (eds). Classification of Chronic Pain. Descriptions of Chronic Pain Syndromes and Definitions of Pain Terms, ed 2. Seattle: IASP Press, 1994:3–4.

# Glossary

## A

**abducens nerve** motor cranial nerve (CN VI) supplying the lateral rectus muscle of the eye

**abduction** turning outward or laterally—*ant: adduction*

**ablation** removal or detachment of a body part, usually by surgery

**abrasion, tooth** wearing away of the tooth structure by tooth-to-tooth contact; in contrast with chemical erosion or *attrition*

**abscess** localized collection of pus within preformed cavities formed by tissue disintegration

**acceleration-deceleration injury** —**see** *flexion-extension injury*

**accommodation** adjustment of the focus of the eye for various distances; *also* the rise in threshold of a nerve during constant, direct stimulation

**acoustic meatus** external cartilaginous and internal bony auditory canal that leads to the tympanic membrane—*syn: external auditory meatus*

**acoustic myography** electronic recording of muscle sounds, reflecting the mechanical component of muscle contraction

**acoustic nerve** sensory cranial nerve (CN VIII) with cochlear (hearing) and vestibular (equilibrium) fibers

**acoustic neuroma** benign tumor within the auditory canal arising from the acoustic nerve (CN VIII); frequently causes headache, hearing loss, tinnitus, facial pain, or numbness

**acquired disorder** postnatal aberration, change, or disturbance of normal development or condition that is not congenital but incurred after birth

**acromegaly** chronic metabolic condition caused by overproduction of growth hormone in the anterior pituitary gland and characterized by a gradual and marked elongation and enlargement of bones and soft tissues of the distal portion of the face, maxilla and mandible, and extremities

**activation, muscle** energy release in muscle tissue resulting in muscle contraction

**activation, nerve** depolarization of a neuron

**active mandibular opening** mandibular motion due to voluntary dominant contraction of the agonist (jaw-opening) muscles relative to the antagonist (jaw-closing) muscles

**active resistive stretch** motion voluntarily forced against resistance of muscle, tendons, capsule, or intra-articular structures

**active trigger point** —**see** *myofascial trigger point: active*

**acupuncture** traditional Chinese practice of inserting needles into specific points along the "meridians" of the body to induce anesthesia, to alleviate pain, or for therapeutic purposes; experimental evidence shows that acupuncture produces an analgesic effect by triggering the release of enkephalin, a naturally occurring endorphin that has opiate-like effects—*see endorphin, enkephalin*

**acute** having recent onset, severe symptoms, or short course—*ant: chronic*

**acute malocclusion** sudden alteration in the occlusal condition secondary to a disorder that is either perceived by the patient or clinically apparent

**acute onset** development that is sudden and recent—*ant: insidious onset*

**acute pain** unpleasant sensation with a duration limited to the normal healing time or the time necessary for neutralization of the initiating or causal factors

**adamantinoma** —*see* ameloblastoma

**adaptation** the progressive adjustive changes in sensitivity that regularly accompany continuous sensory stimulation or lack of stimulation; the process by which an organism responds to stress in its environment

**adaptive capacity** relative ability to adjust to any type of change—*syn: adaptive potential, adaptive response*

**adaptive potential** —*see* adaptive capacity

**adaptive response** —*see* adaptive capacity

**addiction, substance** a state characterized by an overwhelming compulsion to continue use of a substance and to obtain it by any means, with a tendency to increase the dosage, a psychologic and usually a physical dependence on its effects, and a detrimental effect on the individual and society; compare with *dependence*

**adduction** turning inward or medially—*ant: abduction*

**Aδ pain fibers** pain-conducting nerve fibers 1 to 4 μm in diameter

**adenocarcinoma** malignant adenoma

**adenopathy** any disease of the glands, especially of the lymphatic system, usually characterized by enlargement

**adherence** binding, clinging, or sticking together of opposing surfaces

**adhesion** molecular attraction between adjacent surfaces in contact; the abnormal fibrous joining of adjacent structures following an inflammatory process or as the result of injury repair

   **capsular a.** fibrosis of the capsular tissues of a joint

   **fibrous a.** —*see* adhesion: intracapsular

   **intracapsular a.** fibrosis between intra-articular surfaces within a joint capsule, resulting in reduced mobility of the joint—*syn: fibrous ankylosis*

**adjunctive therapy** a supplemental procedure beyond the primary course of therapy

**affect** in psychology, the emotional reactions or feelings associated with an experience or mental state

**afferent neural pathway** nerve impulses transmitted from the periphery toward the central nervous system

**agenesis** defective development or absence of a body part

**agonist** muscle principally responsible for a particular movement; in pharmacology, a drug that acts at receptors on cells that are normally activated by a natural substance—*ant: antagonist*

**-al** [suffix] pertaining to

**-algia** [suffix] pain

**algogenic** causing pain

**algometer** instrument for measuring the degree of sensitivity to painful stimuli

   **pressure a.** instrument for reliably recording the pain pressure reaction point or pain pressure threshold

**allo-** [prefix] other

**allodynia** pain due to a stimulus that does not normally provoke pain

**allostasis** adaptation of neural, neuroendocrine, and immune mechanisms in the face of stressors

**alveolar** pertaining to the alveolar process of the mandible, including the tooth sockets, supporting bone, and associated connective tissues

**ameloblastoma** benign tumor of odontogenic epithelial origin—*syn: adamantinoma*

**analgesia** absence of pain in response to stimulation that would normally be painful

**analgesic** agent that removes pain without loss of consciousness; relieving pain or insensitive to pain

**anamnestic** pertaining to medical and psychosocial history and past or current symptom state as recalled by the patient

**Anamnestic Dysfunction Index** epidemiologic symptom severity scale based on history of disease or injury (Helkimo)

**anastomosis** a connection between two separate structures

**anatomic** pertaining to the structure of an organism

**anesthesia** absence of all feeling or sensation, especially pain

   **a. dolorosa** pain in an area or region that is anesthetic

   **block a.** regional anesthesia resulting from an anesthetic injected into or near a nerve trunk

**central a.** anesthesia due to central blocking of nerve impulses or due to a disease of the nerve centers

**general a.** drug-induced unconscious state typically used for surgical procedures

**local a.** anesthesia due to local blocking of nerve impulses in a limited part of the body

**regional a.** analgesia of a body part due to proximal blocking of nerve impulses by local anesthetic

**aneurysm** a sac filled with fluid or clotted blood formed by widening of the wall of an artery, a vein or the heart

**saccular a.** an unusual, localized widened area affecting only part of the circumference of the arterial wall

**Angle classification of occlusion** classification of occlusion based on the relationships of the maxillary and mandibular molar and incisor teeth

**class I** minor dental irregularities but a correct anteroposterior relationship of the maxillary to the mandibular teeth—***syn:*** *neutrocclusion*

**class II** mandible and its teeth are in a posterior or retruded relationship to the maxillary teeth—***syn:*** *distocclusion*

**division 1** maxillary anterior teeth have a normal or excessive forward inclination, often with excessive horizontal overjet

**division 2** maxillary incisors are upright or inclined backward, often with an excessive overbite

**class III** mandible and its teeth are positioned forward in relationship to the maxilla—***syn:*** *mesiocclusion*

**angular cheilitis** inflammation of the corners of the mouth usually due to candidiasis

**ankylosing spondylitis** ossification of the spinal ligament resulting in a bony encasement of the joint; more common in males; onset most often between 9 and 12 years of age—***syn:*** *spondylosis*

**ankylosis** stiffening or immobilization of a joint as the result of disease, trauma, or congenital process with bony union across the joint; *also,* fibrosis without bony union; compare with adhesion

**bony a.** osseous union of adjacent, usually movable, body parts—***syn:*** *synostosis, true ankylosis*

**dental a.** fusion of the tooth to the surrounding bony alveolus due to ossification of the periodontal membrane

**extracapsular a.** rigidity of the periarticular tissues resulting in joint stiffness or immobilization—***syn:*** *false ankylosis*

**false a.** —***see*** *ankylosis: extracapsular*

**fibrous a.** —***syn:*** *pseudoankylosis;* ***see*** *adhesion: intracapsular*

**intracapsular a.** bony adhesions of articular structures within a joint

**true a.** —***see*** *ankylosis: bony*

**anorexia** diminished appetite or aversion to food

**a. nervosa** psychiatric disorder characterized by distortions in body image and aversion to food, resulting in extreme weight loss and amenorrhea in women; usually occurring in young women

**ANS** autonomic nervous system

**ansa hypoglossi** *also* known as the *ansa cervicalis;* a nerve loop supplying the infrahyoid muscles formed by descending fibers of the hypoglossal nerve, the superior nerve root to C1 and C2, and inferior root to C2 and C3

**antagonist** muscle whose function is opposite the agonist or prime mover; in pharmacology, a drug that diminishes the effect of another drug or naturally occurring substance through stimulation at the same receptor sites—***ant:*** *agonist*

**anterior** toward the front or in the forward part of an organ—***ant:*** *posterior*

**anterior bite plate** a hard acrylic resin appliance that provides for occlusal contact only between the anterior teeth

**anterior guidance** —***see*** *anterior-guided occlusion*

**anterior-guided occlusion** a form of occlusion in which the vertical and horizontal overlap of the anterior teeth causes the posterior teeth to disengage in all mandibular excursive movements—***syn:*** *anterior guidance*

**anterior repositioning appliance, mandibular** intraoral device that guides or positions the mandible to a position forward of maximum intercuspation

**anticholinergic** an agent that blocks the action of acetylcholine in the central and peripheral parasympathetic nerves; the action of that agent

**anticonvulsant** an agent used to control or prevent convulsions; the action of that agent

**antidepressant** an agent used to treat depression; the action of that agent

**antidromic** conducting impulses in the opposite direction of normal

**antidromic release** secretion of chemicals and neurotransmitters at the receptor that occurs with antidromic nerve activity

**antinuclear antibody (ANA)** antibody directed against nuclear antigens, found primarily in the serum of patients with systemic lupus erythematosus but also in patients with rheumatoid arthritis, scleroderma, and other connective tissue disorders

**antipyretic** an agent that brings about fever reduction; the action of that agent

**anxiety** feeling of apprehension, uncertainty, or dread of a future threat or danger, accompanied by tension or uneasiness

    **a. disorder** a category of mental illness that includes obsessive compulsive disorder, posttraumatic stress disorders, phobia, and panic disorder, the symptoms of which are not relieved by reassurance, with resulting limitations in adaptive functioning

**aphasia** inability to speak or comprehend written or spoken language; caused by brain injury or lesions or of psychogenic origin

**aplasia** incomplete or arrested development of a structure due to failure of normal development of the embryonic primordium

**apnea** temporary cessation of breathing

**aponeurosis** flat, fibrous tendon sheath that invests and attaches muscle to bone or other tissue

**appliance** device or prosthesis used to provide or facilitate a particular function or therapy

**arteriovenous malformation** altered morphology, weakening, or distension of an artery or vein; arteritis; inflammation of an artery

**arteritis** cranial manifestation of giant cell arteritis characterized by fever, anorexia, loss of weight, leucocytosis, tenderness over the scalp and along facial and temporal arteries, headache, and jaw claudication; may lead to blindness; uncommon before the age of 60 years; associated with significantly elevated erythrocyte sedimentation rate—*syn: cranial arteritis, giant cell arteritis, temporal arteritis*

**arthralgia** pain felt in a joint

**arthritis** [*pl:* **arthritides**] inflammation of a joint, usually accompanied by pain

**arthrocentesis** puncture of a joint with a needle or a catheter, followed by removal of fluid

**arthrodial** pertaining to gliding movement by two adjacent surfaces

**arthrodial joint** joint that allows gliding movement of the parts

**arthrogenous pain** pain originating from joint structures

**arthrogram** radiograph of a joint

**arthrography** visualization of a joint by radiography

    **double-contrast a.** similar to single-contrast arthrography but with injection of a small amount of radiopaque contrast agent followed by inflation of the joint with air

    **double-space a.** contrast arthrography with injection of a radiopaque contrast agent into both the upper and lower synovial joint compartments of the TMJ

    **single-contrast a.** arthrography following injection of a radiopaque contrast agent into the joint space(s) to determine the location and integrity of intra soft tissue structures, including disc position, soft tissue contours, presence of perforations, joint motion, intra-articular free bodies, and adhesive capsulitis

    **single-space a.** contrast arthrography with injection of a radiopaque contrast agent into either the upper or the lower synovial joint compartment of the TMJ

**arthrogryposis** fixation of a joint in a flexed or contracted position that may be related to innervation, muscles, or connective tissue

**arthrokinematics, TMJ** the description of the movement between joint surfaces

**arthrokinetics, TMJ** temporomandibular joint motion—*syn: arthrokinematics, TMJ*

    **depression of mandible** movement of the mandibular alveolar process away from the maxilla

    **distraction of mandible** separation of surfaces of the TMJ by extension without injury or dislocation of the parts

**elevation of mandible** movement of the mandible alveolar process toward the maxilla

**lateral excursion of mandible** —*see arthrokinetics, TMJ: laterotrusion of mandible*

**laterotrusion of mandible** movement of the mandible away from the median or toward the side

**mediotrusion of mandible** movement of the mandible toward the median or center

**protrusion of mandible** anterior mandibular movement with bilateral forward condylar translation

**retrusion of mandible** posterior mandibular movement with bilateral retrusive condylar translation

**arthropathy** any disease or disorder that affects a joint

**arthroplasty** surgical repair or plastic reconstruction of a joint

**arthroscopy** direct visualization of a joint with an endoscope

**arthrosis** disease of a joint evidenced by bony alterations of a joint or articulation

**arthrotomography** tomographic radiography of a joint

**arthrotomy** surgical incision of a joint

**articular** pertaining to a joint

**articular capsule** fibrous connective tissue sac that encloses a synovial joint and limits its motion

**articular disc** —*see disc: intra-articular*

**articular remodeling** —*see remodeling*

**articulate** in dentistry, the state of the teeth being brought together into occlusion

**articulation, TMJ** —*see temporomandibular joint*

**articulator** mechanical device for attachment of dental casts that allows movement of the casts into various eccentric relationships to represent jaw movement

**asthen-** [prefix] weakness

**asymmetry** lack of symmetry due to inequality in size, shape, movement, or function between two corresponding parts on opposite sides of the body

**ataxia** impaired ability to coordinate movement or neuromuscular dysfunction

**atrophy** progressive decline in size or wasting away of tissue, organ, or body part, often due to denervation, disease, aging, lack of use, or malnutrition—**ant:** *hypertrophy*

**attrition** wearing away by friction or rubbing; a wearing away of tooth structure due to tooth-to-tooth contact

    **a. bruxism** tooth grinding with frictional wear of opposing teeth in excursive movements, in contrast with *clenching*

**atypical facial pain** —*see facial pain of unknown origin*

**atypical odontalgia** —*see idiopathic odontalgia*

**atypical tooth pain** —*see idiopathic odontalgia*

**aura** subjective sensation or phenomenon that precedes and marks the onset of a seizure or paroxysmal attack

**auricle** visible portion of the external ear—**syn:** *pinna*

**auriculotemporal nerve** sensory branch of the mandibular division of the trigeminal nerve; innervates the external acoustic meatus, the tympanic membrane, the lateral aspect of the TMJ capsule, the parotid sheath, the skin of the auricle, and the temple

**auriculotemporal neuralgia** —*see neuralgia: auriculotemporal*

**auscultation** the diagnostic technique of listening for sounds within the body

**autogenous graft** graft using one part of a patient's body for another

**autoimmune disorder** disease in which the body produces a disordered immunologic response against itself, causing tissue injury; eg, rheumatoid arthritis, scleroderma

**autologous** occurring naturally or normally within a structure or tissue

**autonomic effects of central excitation** secondary stimulation of internuncial neurons during pain, leading to transmission of efferent autonomic impulses that produce effects that differ from those normally associated with the physiology of pain

**autonomic nervous system (ANS)** a division of the peripheral nervous system distributed to smooth muscle and glands throughout the body, comprising the sympathetic and parasympathetic nervous systems, involved in motor (efferent) transmission, functioning independently of conscious control

**avascular** lacking in blood vessels

**avascular necrosis (AVN)** bone infarction not associated with asepsis but with circulatory impairment (vascular occlusion), leading to bone necrosis and collapse of joint surface into underlying infarction

**axon** long myelinated or unmyelinated portion of a nerve cell that transmits information from the nerve cell body

## B

**balancing occlusal contact** misnomer—*see nonworking occlusal contact*

**balancing interference** misnomer—*see nonworking occlusal contact*

**behavior** actions or reactions under specific circumstances

**behavior modification** psychotherapy that attempts to modify observable patterns of behavior by the substitution of a new response to a given stimulus

**Bell palsy** peripheral facial paralysis due to lesion of the facial nerve (CN VII)

**benign** mild, nonprogressive and nonrecurrent, nonmalignant character of a tumor

**benign masseteric hypertrophy** nonmalignant increase in size or bulk of masseter muscles of unknown etiology, usually bilateral

**benign migratory glossitis** —*see geographic tongue*

**Bennett angle** the angle between the condylar path and the median-sagittal plane

**Bennett mandibular movement** the lateral bodily offset of the mandible during asymmetric movement

**bilateral** pertaining to or having two sides—**ant:** *unilateral*

**biobehavioral** behavioral factors as they contribute to the functioning of biologic systems

**biofeedback training** therapy that teaches the voluntary modification of physiologic activity or autonomic function using equipment that gives a visual or auditory representation of the activity or function

**biomechanical** pertaining to the application of mechanical laws, such as those relating to intrinsic or extrinsic force, to living structures, in particular, the locomotor system

**biopsychosocial** the complex interactions between biology, psychologic states, and social conditions that bring about and/or maintain (dys)function

**bite** the interocclusal relationship or the registration thereof

> **closed b.** misnomer—*see posterior overclosure*
>
> **deep b.** misnomer—*see overbite: deep*
>
> **dual b.** discrepancy of greater than 2 mm between two intercuspal occlusal relationships
>
> **edge-to-edge b.** an intercuspal occlusion in which the incisal edge of the maxillary incisors meets the incisal edge of the mandibular incisors
>
> **open b.** an intercuspal occlusion where the anterior teeth do not occlude in any mandibular position
>
> **overclosed b.** contrast with *posterior bite collapse*—*see posterior overclosure*
>
> **scissor b.** an interocclusal relationship whereby the maxillary teeth are totally lingual to the mandibular teeth

**bite guard** misnomer—*see stabilization appliance*

**blepharospasm** tonic spasm of the orbicularis oculi producing more or less complete closure of the eyelid

**body dysmorphic disorder (BDD)** preoccupation with a defect in appearance that is either imagined, or, if a slight physical anomaly is present, the individual's concern is markedly excessive

**body section roentgenography** —*see tomography*

**bony ankylosis** —*see ankylosis: bony*

**border movements** movements of the mandible at the boundary or margin of the envelope of movement as determined by the joint anatomy, joint capsule, ligaments, and associated muscles

**brachycardia** —*see bradycardia*

**brachycephalic** head form that is rounded and short in the anteroposterior direction and broad in width;

**bracing** —*see clenching*

**bradycardia** abnormally slow pulse rate (< 60 beats/min)

**bradykinesia** abnormally slow movement

**bradykinin** plasma kinin that is a potent vasodilator and incites pain

**brainstem** neural tissue that connects cerebral hemispheres with the spinal cord, comprising the medulla oblongata, pons, and the midbrain

**breathing-related sleep disorder** disorder characterized by interruptions of sleep due to breathing-related medical conditions such as obstructive or central sleep apnea or central alveolar hypoventilation syndrome

**Briquet syndrome**—*see somatization disorder*

**bruxism** diurnal or nocturnal parafunctional activity including clenching, bracing, gnashing, and grinding of the teeth; in the absence of subjective awareness, past bruxism can be inferred from the presence of clear wear facets that are not interpreted to be the result of masticatory function, and contemporary bruxism can be observed through sleep laboratory recordings

> **b. appliance** intraoral device used for limiting the harmful effects of bruxism activity, such as associated discomfort or damage to the dentition

**buccally** toward the cheek

**buccolingual relationship** a positional reference relative to the tongue and the cheek

**buccoversion** pertaining to a tooth position that is buccal to the line of occlusion

**bulimia** an exaggerated craving for food, often resulting in episodes of binge eating

> **b. nervosa** psychiatric disorder usually seen in young women, characterized by bouts of overeating followed by intentional, self-induced vomiting, with resulting chemical erosion of teeth from stomach acids and sometimes bilateral enlargement of the parotid glands

**burning mouth syndrome (BMS)** dysesthesia described as a burning sensation in the oral mucosa occurring in the absence of clinically apparent mucosal abnormalities or laboratory findings and often perceived as painful

**bursa** sac-like cavity found in connective tissue at places where friction would otherwise develop; lined with synovial membrane and filled with viscous synovial fluid—*see synovial joint*

**bursitis** inflammation of a bursa

# C

**calcified cartilage zone** calcified tissue between the articular soft tissue and the subchondral bone in synovial joints

**calcium pyrophosphate dehydrate crystals** mineral deposits in synovial fluid of joints with chondrocalcinosis

**canine disclusion** —*see canine-protected occlusion*

**canine guidance** —*see canine-protected occlusion*

**canine-protected articulation** —*see canine-protected occlusion*

**canine-protected occlusion** occlusion where the canine acts as the sole discluder in laterotrusion—*syn: canine-/cuspid-protected articulation*

**canine rise** —*see canine-protected occlusion*

**capsular** pertaining to the joint capsule

**capsular fibrosis** —*see adhesion: capsular*

**capsular ligament, TMJ** a ligament that separately encapsulates the upper and lower TMJ synovial membrane

**capsule, joint** —*see articular capsule*

**capsulitis** inflammation of a capsule, its associated capsular ligaments, or the disc attachments in response to mechanical irritation or systemic disease

> **adhesive c.** adhesion and restriction of joint motion due to reduced joint space volume and swollen synovial membranes during a joint capsulitis condition

**carotid artery** principal artery of the neck supplying the neck, face, skull, brain, middle ear, pituitary gland, orbit, and choroid plexus of the lateral ventricle; the paired common carotid divides at the upper border of the thyroid cartilage into the external and internal carotid arteries

**carotidynia** pain due to inflammation of the carotid artery, usually self-limiting

**cartilage** dense fibrous connective tissue covering most articular surfaces and some parts of the skeleton

> **articular c.** a thin layer of cartilage located on the joint surfaces of some bones

**cast, dental** a model or representation of the teeth and supporting bone, usually made of stone or plaster—*syn: diagnostic cast, study cast, study model*

**catecholamines** biogenic amines with a sympathomimetic action

**caudal** inferior, toward the tail—*syn: inferior; ant: cephalad*

**causalgia** —*see complex regional pain syndrome II (CRPS II)*

**cellulitis** a diffuse inflammatory process that spreads along fascial planes and through cellular tissue spaces, especially the subcutaneous tissues

> **acute c.** cellulitis accompanied by swelling, suppuration, and pain

> **chronic c.** cellulitis with little swelling or pain

**central excitation effects** —*see autonomic effects of central excitation*

**central nervous system (CNS)** the brain and spinal cord

**central pain** pain initiated or caused by a primary lesion or dysfunction in the central nervous system*; *also,* pain resulting from damage to the central nervous system, eg, thalamic syndrome and spinal cord injury pain

**centric occlusion (CO)** —*syn: maximum intercuspal position, maximum intercuspation;* **see** *intercuspal position*

**centric relation (CR)** —*syn: centric relation occlusion;* **see** *retruded contact position*

**centric relation occlusion (CRO)** —*see retruded contact position*

**cephalad** superior, toward the head—*syn: cranial rostrad, superior;* **ant:** *superior caudal*

**cephalalgia** pain or ache in the head—*syn: headache*

**cephalic** pertaining to the head or structure of the head

**cephalogram** radiograph of the head

**cerebral ischemia** deficiency in blood supply to part of the brain due to constriction or actual obstruction of blood vessel

**cerebral palsy** motor function disorder caused by a permanent, nonprogressive brain defect or lesion present at birth or shortly thereafter; deep tendon reflexes are exaggerated, fingers are often spastic, and speech may be slurred

**cervical** pertaining to the neck

**cervical plexus** network of nerves formed by the ventral branches of the upper four cervical nerves

**cervical spine disorder (CSD)** a category of disorders involving the muscles, facet joints, discs, and nerves of the cervical spine

**cervicalgia** pain of the structures of the neck, including referred pain from noncervical origin—*syn: cervicodynia*

**cervicodynia** —*see cervicalgia*

**cervicogenic** originating in the structures of the neck

**cervicogenic headache** headache characterized by a moderately severe, dull, dragging, unilateral headache without side-shift, provoked or aggravated by neck movements, and accompanied by any of the following symptoms: lacrimation, conjunctival hyperemia, dizziness, nausea, vomiting, and sensitivity to light and noise

**chewing cycle** the pattern of mandibular movement during a single opening and closing occlusal masticatory stroke—*syn: masticatory cycle*

**chewing force** the force registered at the teeth during chewing

**chief complaint (CC)** the patient's statement of the main problem or primary concern

**chondritis** inflammation of cartilage

**chondroblastoma** benign tumor, derived from precursors of cartilage cells, sometimes showing scattered areas of calcification and necrosis

**chondrocalcinosis** a recurrent arthritic disease in which calcified deposits of calcium hypophosphate crystals collect in synovial fluid, articular cartilage, and adjacent soft tissues, leading to gout-like attacks of pain and swelling of the involved joints—*syn: pseudogout, pyrophosphate arthropathy*

**chondroma** benign cartilaginous tumor

**chondromalacia** softening of cartilage, sometimes accompanied by swelling, pain, and degeneration

**chondron** cell cluster in the cartilaginous zone of the articular cartilage

**chondrosarcoma** malignant tumor of cartilaginous cells or their precursors that may contain nodules of calcified hyaline cartilage

**chorea** a convulsive nervous disease with involuntary and irregular jerking movements

**chronic** developing slowly and persisting for a long time—*ant: acute*

**chronic idiopathic orofacial pain** —*see idiopathic odontalgia*

**chronic pain** pain that persists when other aspects of disorder or disease have resolved, and typically lasts more than 6 months or beyond the normal time for healing of an acute injury or pain; may have associated unpleasant sensory, perceptual, and emotional experiences accompanied by behavioral and psychosocial responses

**chronic paroxysmal hemicrania** rare form of consistently unilateral headache centered around the eye and radiating to the cheek or temple, with attacks lasting 5 to 60 minutes and occurring 4 to 12 times per day for years without remission; like cluster headache, may include associated conjunctival congestion and clear nasal discharge

**cinefluoroscopy** —*see* *fluoroscopy*

**claudication** muscle ischemia due to decreased arterial blood flow to an area causing intermittent pain

**clenching** nonfunctional intermittent application of masticatory force, primarily from the elevator muscles, in a static occlusal relationship; may be diurnal or nocturnal, and the patient may not be aware of the muscle activity—*syn:* *bracing*

**clicking joint noise, TMJ** distinct snapping or popping sound emanating from the TMJ during joint movement or with joint compression

    **early-closing c.j.n., TMJ** a click that occurs at the initiation of retrusive condylar translation

    **early-opening c.j.n., TMJ** a click that occurs at the initiation of protrusive condylar translation

    **late-closing c.j.n., TMJ** a click that occurs just before the end of retrusive condylar translation

    **late-opening c.j.n., TMJ** a click that occurs just before the end of protrusive condylar translation

    **mid-opening c.j.n., TMJ** a click that occurs midway along the condylar translatory path

    **reciprocal c.j.n., TMJ** a pair of clicks, one of which usually occurs during opening at a different location than the second one, which occurs during closing movements of the jaw; associated with disc displacement with reduction

    **terminal closing c.j.n., TMJ** —*see* *late-closing c.j.n., TMJ*

    **terminal opening c.j.n., TMJ** —*see* *late-opening c.j.n., TMJ*

**closed lock** misnomer—*see* *disc displacement without reduction*

**cluster headache** severe unilateral head and facial pain, often accompanied by involuntary lacrimation, with localized extracranial vasodilatation in the periorbital region contributing to the pain and conjunctival congestion; occurs in bouts or clusters, sometimes with clockwork regularity, usually occurring during the night and lasting 30 to 120 minutes—*syn: Horton syndrome, Horton headache, histamine cephalalgia*

**CNS** central nervous system

**cocontraction** reflexive contraction of antagonist muscles resulting from noxious stimuli of a sensory field of a joint, soft tissue, or other structure to prevent movement or provide stabilization of the painful area tissues—*syn: protective muscle splinting*

**cognition** the mental process of knowing, thinking, learning, and judging

**cognitive behavioral therapy** therapy focused on changing attitudes, assumptions, perceptions, and patterns of thinking

**cold laser therapy** —*see* *infrared laser therapy*

**collagen disease** —*see* *connective tissue: connective tissue disorders*

**collateral ligaments, TMJ** paired supportive ligaments on the lateral and medial aspects of the TMJ capsule, attaching the articular disc to the mandibular condyle; the ligaments allow rotational disc movement in an anterior-posterior axis only

**complex regional pain syndrome I (CRPS I)** pain syndrome with onset often after traumatic event; symptoms are not limited to the distribution of a peripheral nerve and are disproportional to the injury; edema, decreased cutaneous blood flow, atrophy of the skin, hair, and nails, autonomic changes in the region of the pain, hyperalgesia, or allodynia may occur at some time in the course of development; formerly *reflex sympathetic dystrophy* (RSD)

**complex regional pain syndrome II (CRPS II)** a syndrome of persistent severe burning sensation, allodynia, and hyperpathia, usually following partial injury of a peripheral nerve and combined with vasomotor and pseudomotor dysfunction; later, the condition is usually accompanied by trophic changes to the skin, hair, and nails; formerly *causalgia\**

**compression of joint** pressing together of joint surfaces

**computed tomography (CT)** misnomer —*see* *tomography: computerized*

**computer-assisted tomography** misnomer—*see* *tomography: computerized*

**computerized axial tomography** misnomer — *see* tomography: computerized

**computerized transaxial tomography** misnomer—*see* tomography: computerized

**condylar agenesis** developmental abnormality characterized by the absence of a condyle

**condylar fracture** fracture of the head or neck of the mandibular condyle, further characterized as intracapsular or extracapsular, displaced or nondisplaced

**condylarthrosis** joint containing a condyle—*syn: condyloid joint*

**condyle** rounded, articular end of a bone

**condylectomy** surgical removal of the entire mandibular condyle—*syn: subcondylar osteotomy*

**condyloid** resembling a condyle in shape

**condyloid joint** —*see* condylarthrosis

**condylolysis** —*see* condylysis

**condylotomy** surgical division or reshaping of a condyle

**condylysis** idiopathic resorption or dissolution of condyle—*syn: condylolysis*

**congenital disorder** developmental disorder present at or before birth

**conjunctiva** mucous membrane covering the anterior surface of the eyeball and lining the eyelids

**conjunctival hyperemia** dilation of the vasculature of the conjunctiva

**connective tissue** tissue of mesodermal origin that supports and binds other tissues; includes elastic or collagenous fibrous connective tissue, bone, and cartilage; connective tissues are highly vascular with the exception of cartilage

    **c.t. disorders** a group of connective tissue diseases of unknown etiology sharing common anatomic and clinical features—*syn: mixed connective tissue disease, collagen disease*

**contact** the mutual touching of two bodies or parts

**continuous passive motion (CPM)** cyclic motion of a body part caused by another individual or machine that moves an articulation through a determined range of motion

**contraction** normal shortening, tightening, or reduction in size or length of a muscle fiber

**contracture** abnormal shortening

    **capsular c., TMJ** —*see* adhesion: capsular

    **muscular c.** sustained increased resistance to passive muscle stretch due to reduced muscle length

    **myofibrotic c.** muscular contracture resulting from excessive fibrosis of the muscle, usually as a sequela of trauma or infection

    **myostatic c.** muscular contracture resulting from reduced muscle stimulation

**contralateral** pertaining to the opposite side—*ant: ipsilateral*

**contrast medium** radiopaque material injected before imaging that renders certain tissues or spaces opaque

**contributing factor** condition or action that contributes to the occurrence or aggravation of a disease or disorder

**contusion of joint** traumatic joint bruising characterized by acute synovitis, effusion, and possible hemarthrosis, but without fracture

**convergence, neural** the synapsing of a neuron with several others

**conversion disorder** mental disorder characterized by disturbances in sensory and motor function, due to unconscious needs and conflicts, in the absence of organic disease

**coping mechanisms** cognitive and behavioral efforts to manage specific tasks, problems, or situations

**cordotomy** an operation to divide bundles of nerve fibers within the spinal cord to relieve chronic pain; usually performed in cases where pain has not responded to more conservative treatments

**coronal** pertaining to the crown of the head or tooth, or the coronal suture of the skull

**coronal plane** —*see* frontal plane

**coronoid hyperplasia** benign overgrowth of the coronoid process of the mandible that may result in limited jaw opening

**coronoid process** conical process on the anterosuperior surface of the mandibular ramus that serves as the attachment of the temporalis muscle

**coronoid process impingement** restricted jaw movement due to coronoid hyperplasia

**coronoplasty** —*see* occlusal equilibration

**cortical bone** dense, solid outer layer of a bone that surrounds the medullary cavity

**corticosteroid** a crystalline steroid found in the adrenal cortex

**Costen syndrome** syndrome of dizziness, tinnitus, earache, stuffiness of the ear, dry mouth, burning in the tongue and throat, sinus pain, and headaches that an otolaryngologist in 1934 attributed to overclosure of the bite and posterior displacement of the mandibular condyle

**cracked tooth syndrome** set of symptoms including sporadic, sharp, momentary pain on biting or releasing along with occasional pain from cold food or drink due to (incomplete) fracture of the tooth

**cranial** *—see cephalad*

**cranial arteritis** *—see arteritis*

**cranial nerves (CN)** twelve pairs of nerves that have their origin in the brain

**cranial neuralgia** *—see neuralgia: cranial*

**craniocervical** relating to both the cranium and the neck

**craniofacial** relating to both the face and the cranium

**craniomandibular** *—see temporomandibular*

**craniomandibular disorders (CMD)** *—see temporomandibular disorders*

**cranium** the bones of the skull that encase the brain

**crepitation** rough, sandy, diffuse noise, or vibration produced by the rubbing together of irregular bone or cartilage surfaces, usually identified with osteoarthritic changes when heard in joints—*syn: grating, crepitus*

**crepitus** *—see crepitation*

**crossbite** condition in which normal labiolingual or buccolingual relationship between the maxillary and mandibular teeth is reversed

**cryoanalgesia** application of extreme cold to an affected nerve to deliberately disrupt its ability to transmit pain signals

**cryotherapy** the therapeutic use of cold

**CT** *—see tomography: computerized*

**CT scan** *—see tomography: computerized*

**cuspid disclusion** *—see canine-protected occlusion*

**cuspid guidance** *—see canine-protected occlusion*

**cuspid-protected articulation** *—see canine-protected occlusion*

**cuspid-protected occlusion** *—see canine-protected occlusion*

**cuspid rise** *—see canine-protected occlusion*

**cutaneous** relating to the skin

**cycle** a succession of events or symptoms

# D

**deafferentation** partial or total loss of afferent neural activity to a particular body region through removal of part of the neural pathway

**deafferentation pain** usually constant pain perceived in a localized area resulting from the loss or disruption of afferent neural pathways

**debridement** excision of devitalized tissue and foreign matter from a diseased area or wound

**decompression of a joint** removal or release of pressure on a joint

**deep bite** misnomer *—see overbite: deep*

**deep brain stimulation (DBS)** a type of neurostimulation that uses electrical signals from an implanted generator to stimulate targeted nerves or structures in the brain to relieve neurologic symptoms such as motor dysfunction

**deep-heat therapy** diathermy and ultrasound

**deflection on mandibular opening** eccentric displacement of mandible away from a centered mandibular midline path on jaw opening, without return to the midline position on full opening

**degeneration** tissue deterioration with soft tissue, cartilage, and bone converted into or replaced by tissue of inferior quality; failure of articulation to adapt to loading forces, resulting in impaired function; degenerative arthritis—*see osteoarthritis*

**degenerative joint disease** *—see osteoarthritis*

**deglutition** the act of swallowing

**delayed-onset muscle soreness** muscle pain caused by interstitial inflammation after intermittent overuse

**delta sleep** stage IV deep sleep without rapid eye movement

**demyelination** loss of myelin from the sheath of a nerve

**denervation** resection or removal of nerve tissue

**dental** pertaining to a tooth or teeth

**dentition** the natural teeth

**dentofacial orthopedics** —*see* orthodontics

**dentulous** with teeth

**dependence** use of a chemical substance resulting in the development of a physiologic need to the extent that withdrawal symptoms occur when the substance is removed; to be distinguished from addiction, in which psychologic reliance also occurs

**depression, major** psychiatric disorder characterized by prolonged periods of depression and often with associated symptoms of poor appetite, overeating, insomnia, hypersomnia, low energy or fatigue, low self-esteem, poor concentration, and feelings of hopelessness

**depression of mandible** movement of the mandibular alveolar processes away from the maxilla; a component of normal jaw opening—*ant: elevation of mandible, mandibular closure*

**depression, psychologic** mood characterized by feelings of sadness, helplessness, hopelessness, guilt, despair, and futility—*syn: dysthymia*

**deprogrammer** an appliance used to interfere with the proprioceptive mechanism during chewing or mandibular closure

**derangement** a disturbed arrangement of body parts

**dermatome** superficial zone of reference on the skin where pain is felt with stimulation of a single posterior spinal nerve root or cranial neural segment

**determinants of mandibular movement** anatomic structures that dictate the mandibular movements; the anterior determinant is the dental articulation, and the posterior determinants are the TMJs and associated structures

**detrusion** downward movement—*ant: occlusion*

**developmental disorder** —*ant: acquired disorder; see* congenital disorder

**deviation in form** irregularities or aberrations in the form of soft and hard intracapsular articular tissues

**deviation on mandibular opening** eccentric displacement of mandible on opening, away from centered mandibular midline path, with correction to midline position on full opening

**diagnosis** distinguishing one disease from another or determining the nature of a disease from a study of the history, signs, symptoms, and physical examination results

**diagnostic cast** —*see* cast, dental

**diaphragm sellae** a fascial membrane forming a roof over the sella turcica and pituitary gland; within the sella turcica, the cranial dura, arachnoid, and pia mater connect with the pituitary capsule

**diarthrodial joint** a freely moving joint enclosed in a fluid-filled synovial cavity and limited variously by muscles, ligaments, and bone

**diathermy** deep-heat therapy from high-frequency electric current

**differential diagnosis** differentiation of two or more diseases with similar symptoms to determine which is the correct diagnosis

**diginglymoarthrodial joint** paired joint like the TMJ that is both a hinged (ginglymoid) and a gliding (arthrodial) joint

**disability** alteration of the patient's capacity to meet personal, social, and/or occupational responsibilities as determined by behavioral, psychologic, and psychosocial assessments; disability is a social and not a medical term

**disc** circular, rounded, flat plate

> **intra-articular d.** intra-articular, circular, rounded, platelike fibrocartilaginous structure in some synovial joints—*syn: articular disc; misnomer: meniscus*

**disc-condyle complex** in the TMJ, the articulation of the condyle with the disc, which functions as a simple hinge joint

**disc degeneration** degenerative changes within the articular disc

**disc derangement** —*see* disc displacement

**disc detachment** a peripheral separation of the disc from its capsular, ligamentous, or osseous attachments

**disc dislocation** —*see* disc displacement

**disc displacement** in the TMJ, an abnormal position of the intra-articular disc relative to the mandibular condyle and the temporal fossa—*syn: disc derangement, disc interference disorder, disc prolapse*

> **d.d. with reduction** in the TMJ, a disc displacement at the intercuspal position, with reestablishment of a normal anatomic relationship between the disc and condyle during condylar rotation or translation—*syn: reducing disc*

**d.d. without reduction** disc displacement at the intercuspal position, whereby the condyle is incapable of reestablishing a normal anatomic relationship with the disc during condylar translation or rotation—*syn: nonreducing disc*

**disc interference disorder** —*see disc displacement*

**disc locking** misnomer—*see disc displacement without reduction*

**disc perforation** a circumscribed tear in the articular disc permitting communication between the superior and inferior joint spaces, with no disruption at the peripheral attachments to the capsule, ligaments, or bone

**disc prolapse** —*see disc displacement*

**disc-repositioning surgery, TMJ** arthrotomy with intent of reestablishing normal anatomic disc-condyle relationship

**disc space** radiolucent area in a TMJ radiograph between the mandibular condyle and the articular fossa

**disc thinning** degenerative decrease in the thickness of the articular disc

**discectomy** arthrotomy with complete removal of the intra-articular disc

**disclusion** separation of mandible from maxilla through tooth-guided contact during mandibular excursive movements—*syn: disocclusion*

**discopexy, superior** suturing of articular disc to the fossa after severing the anterior attachments

**discoplasty** correction or improvement in the contour of an intra-articular disc

**disease** illness, sickness, body function disorder, or pathologic alterations characterized by an identifiable group of signs, symptoms, and physical findings

**disk** misnomer—*see disc*

**dislocation of condyle** nonreducible anterior displacement of the mandibular condyle in a forward direction anterior to the eminence—*syn: luxation, open lock*

**disocclusion** —*see disclusion*

**disorder** disturbance of function, structure, or mental state

**displacement** removal from the normal or usual position or place

**distal** away from a point of reference—*ant: proximal*

**distocclusion** —*see Angle classification of occlusion: class II*

**distraction of the condyle** separation or forced downward movement of the condyle from the articular fossa

**diurnal** pertaining to or occurring in the daylight hours—*ant: nocturnal*

**dizziness** a disturbed sense of relationship to space and unsteadiness with a feeling of movement within the head; to be distinguished from vertigo

**dolichocephalic** head shape that is oval and long anteroposteriorly, and narrow in width

**Doppler effect** the apparent change in the frequency of a wave resulting from relative motion of the source in relation to the receiver

**Doppler ultrasonography** the application of the Doppler effect to ultrasonic scanning, with ultrasound echoes converted to (amplified) sound or graphic waves

**dorsal column stimulator** electrical stimulation of nervous tissues to produce paresthesia in a specific portion of the spinal cord known as the dorsal column; *also* called *spinal cord stimulation*

**drug pump** a small device surgically placed under the skin to deliver microdoses of medication, usually to the intrathecal space (space surrounding the spinal cord containing fluid); because the drug is delivered directly to the spinal cord, a smaller dose is required, which helps minimize systemic side effects

**dys-** [prefix] bad, disordered, difficult

**dysarthria** defective articulation secondary to motor deficit involving the lips, tongue, palate, or pharynx

**dysarthrosis** deformity or malformation of a joint whereby there is impairment of joint motion

**dysautonomia** malfunctioning of the autonomic nervous system that hinders normal activities of daily living or causes total disability; dysautonomia can interfere with the ability of the cardiovascular system to compensate for changes in posture, especially when changing rapidly from a supine to standing posture, and dizziness or syncope results; systemic effects can also cause tachycardia or diabetes insipidus; dysautonomias can occur from trauma to the autonomic nervous system, viral infection, genetic disorders, chemical exposure, pregnancy, or autoimmune disorders

**dyscrasia** morbid condition referring to an imbalance of the component parts

**dysesthesia** an unpleasant abnormal sensation, whether spontaneous or evoked*

**dysfunction** abnormal, impaired, or altered function

**dysfunction index** system of quantifying the severity of dysfunction

> **Clinical D.I.** a severity index developed by Helkimo and based on the symptoms and signs found during a clinical examination

**dyskinesia** motor function disorder with impairment of voluntary movement, characterized by spontaneous, imprecise, involuntary, irregular movements with stereotypical patterns

> **tardive d.** drug-induced dyskinesia

**dysmasesis** difficulty with mastication

**dysostosis** abnormal condition characterized by defective ossification, especially involving fetal cartilage

**dysphagia** difficulty in swallowing

**dysphasia** speech impairment due to centrally induced lack of coordination, including failure to arrange words in proper order

**dysphonia** impairment of the voice; speaking difficulties

**dysphoria** emotional distress, disquiet, restlessness, or malaise

**dysplasia** abnormality of development

**dysthymia** —*see depression: psychologic*

**dystonia** abnormal tonicity, usually in reference to muscle tissue, that may result in altered movement and posture

> **focal d.** localized dystonia characterized by momentary sustained contracture of involved muscles

> **lingual d.** dystonia involving the tongue

> **mandibular d.** dystonia involving the mandible

> **perioral d.** dystonia involving the perioral tissues

**dystrophy** developmental change in muscles resulting from defective nutrition, characterized by fatty degeneration and increased size but decreased strength, and not involving the central nervous system

# E

**eccentric jaw relation** mandibular posture that is peripheral or away from a centered jaw position or intercuspal position

**edema** abnormal accumulation of fluid in cells, tissue spaces, or cavities

**edentulous** without teeth

**efferent neural pathway** neural impulse transmitted away from the central nervous system

**efficacy** ability of a drug or treatment to produce a result

**effusion** escape of fluid from blood vessels or lymphatics into a body cavity or tissue

**Ehlers-Danlos syndrome** autosomal dominant inherited disorder of connective tissues characterized by lax joints, skin elasticity and fragility, and pseudotumors

**elastic tissue** connective tissue with approximately 30% elastin, a yellow fibrous mucoprotein

**electrodiagnostic testing** use of electric devices to assist in diagnosis

**electrogalvanic stimulation (EGS)** electrotherapy using direct current (galvanism) to produce muscle fiber contraction; also used in iontophoresis and as a pain-relieving modality

**electromyography (EMG)** graphic recording of the intrinsic change in the electric potentials of muscles

**electrotherapy** treating disease by use of electrical direct current (galvanism) or alternating current (faradism)

**elevator masticatory muscles** paired masseter, medial pterygoid, and temporalis muscles, the main action of which is to elevate the mandible

**eminence** prominence or projection of a bone—*syn: tubercle*

**emission scintigraphy** imaging process to show areas of relatively rapid bone turnover by administration of radiolabeled material

**emotional motor system** theory contending that thoughts and emotions create neuroendocrine-mediated motor responses

**enarthrosis joint** joint with a ball and socket arrangement—*syn: spheroidal joint*

**end-feel** quality of resistance felt during joint manipulation from full active stretch to full passive stretch

**endocrine** secreting a hormone from a gland directly into the circulatory or lymphatic system

**endogenous** produced or originating from within a tissue or organism

**endorphin** endogenous antinociceptive opioid substance in the cerebral spinal fluid that is synthesized in the nerve cells and acts as an inhibiting neurotransmitter on nociceptive pathways—*syn:* enkephalin

**endoscope** instrument for examining the interior of a body cavity

**enkephalin** —*see* endorphin

**enophthalmos** posteriorly positioned eyeballs within the orbit

**envelope of motion** the three-dimensional space circumscribed by border mandibular movements and by the incisal and occlusal contacts of a given point of the mandible

**ephapsis** electric cross talk between nerve fibers

**epidemiology** science concerned with defining and explaining the interrelationships of factors that determine disease frequency and distribution

**epilepsy** group of neurologic disorders characterized by recurrent seizures, at times accompanied by sensory disturbance, abnormal behavior, alterations in level of consciousness, and electroencephalographic changes

**equilibration, occlusal** —*see* occlusal equilibration

**Erb palsy** a condition that is mainly due to birth trauma; it can affect one or all five primary cervical nerves that supply the movement and feeling to an arm; the paralysis can be partial or complete; the damage to each nerve can range from bruising to tearing; *also* called *brachial plexus paralysis*

**erosion of teeth** wearing away of the nonoccluding surfaces of the dentition, especially by chemical means

**erythema migrans** —*see* geographic tongue

**erythema multiforme** an acute skin and mucous membrane disease characterized by papules, tubercles, and macules lasting for several days, with burning, itching, and sometimes headache symptoms

**erythrocyte sedimentation rate (ESR)** rate at which red blood cells settle in a tube of unclotted blood, expressed in millimeters per hour; elevated ESR indicates the presence of inflammation but is not specific for any disorder

**etiology** cause of a specific disorder

**euryprosopic** having a facial form that is short, broad, and flat

**eustachian tube** opening from the middle ear cavity into the pharynx

**Ewing sarcoma** endothelial myeloma, a malignant bone tumor that develops from bone marrow; most frequently in long bones, with pain, fever, and leukocytosis

**exacerbating factor** factor that increases the seriousness of a disease or disorder as marked by greater intensity or frequency in the signs or symptoms

**excursion of mandible** movement of the mandible away from the median or intercuspal occlusion position

    **lateral e.o.m.** movement of the mandible to the side

    **protrusive e.o.m.** movement of the mandible forward

**extension of joint** a motion that increases the joint angle—*ant: flexion*

**exophthalmos** protrusion of eyeballs

**external** away from the center of the body or outside a structure

**external auditory meatus** —*see* acoustic meatus

**extracapsular** outside or external to the capsule, usually of a joint—*ant: intracapsular*

**extracranial** outside or external to the cranium

**extrinsic** originating outside of a part where it is found or on which it acts

**extrinsic trauma** trauma originating from outside an organ system or individual

**extrusion** expulsion by force, thrusting, or pushing out

## F

**facet** small, smooth planar area on a hard surface

    **f. joint** —*see* zygapophyseal

**facial** pertaining to the face or anterior part of the head from forehead to chin; direction of the outer surfaces of the teeth

**facial nerve** mixed sensory and motor cranial nerve (CN VII) that innervates the scalp, forehead, eyelids, muscles of facial expression, platysma muscle, posterior digastric muscle, stylohyoid muscle, lip, chin, and nose muscles, sub-maxillary and submandibular salivary glands, and the afferent fibers from taste buds of the anterior two-thirds of the tongue

**facial neuralgia** —*see facial pain of unknown origin*

**facial pain of unknown origin** idiopathic facial pain

**facial plane** —*see frontal plane*

**facial tic** any spasmodic movement or twitching of the face

**facilitation** intensification of response; diminished nerve tissue resistance after passage of an impulse so that a second stimulus will evoke a reaction more easily—*ant: inhibition*

**factitious disorder** mental disorder characterized by the compulsive, voluntary production of signs and symptoms of a disease, for the sole purpose of assuming a "patient's role" and in the absence of other secondary gain

**falx cerebelli** a small fascial membrane extending from the tentorium cerebelli to the posterior cranial cavity; it attaches posteriorly to the internal occipital crest and margins of the occipital sinus

**fascia** fibrous band or sheath of collagenous connective tissue that encloses muscles and certain organs and separates them subcutaneously into various groups

**fascicle** —*see muscle compartment*

**fasciculation** involuntary contraction of a group of muscle fibers supplied by a single nerve fiber; a coarser form of muscle contraction than fibrillation

**fibrillation** spontaneous, involuntary contraction of individual muscle fibers

**fibrocartilage** type of cartilage characterized by large amount of fibrous tissue in the cartilage matrix and an ability for adaptive remodeling; found in the intervertebral discs, pubic symphysis, mandibular symphysis, and certain regions of the TMJ

**fibrocartilaginous joint** —*see symphysis*

**fibromyalgia** a generalized pain syndrome with bilateral diffuse musculoskeletal aches and stiffness both above and below the waist, associated with exaggerated tenderness in at least 11 of 18 defined anatomic sites

**fibrosarcoma** a sarcoma that contains fibrous connective tissue

**fibrosis** formation of fibrous connective tissue to replace normal tissue lost through injury or infection

**fibrositis** misnomer—*see fibromyalgia*

**fibrous** composed of or containing fibers of connective tissue

**fibrous dysplasia** abnormal fibrous replacement of bone marrow with onset usually during childhood

**filiform** thread-shaped or extremely slender

**flat-plane appliance** misnomer—*see stabilization appliance*

**flexion** a motion that reduces the joint angle; the act of bending or the condition of being bent—*ant: extension*

**flexion-extension injury** traumatic, sudden, exaggerated movement of joints through the extremes of their range of motion in hyperflexion and then hyperextension, resulting in ligamentous sprain, muscular strain, inflammation, and subsequent reflex muscle splinting

**fluoroscopy** radiographic technique providing immediate dynamic images for visualizing the contours and function of a deep structure such as an organ or joint

**focal** highly localized

**focal plane tomography** —*see tomography: focal plane*

**foraminal encroachment** stenosis of the opening for the passage of the spinal nerve from the spinal cord to the periphery—*syn: foraminal stenosis*

**force** anything that originates or arrests motion

    **masticatory f.** force created by the dynamic action of the muscles during the acts of mastication or occluding against an object

    **occlusal f.** force created by the dynamic action of the muscles during occlusion of teeth

**fos** the cellular analog of a viral oncogene, which is composed of genetic protein within a cell (*c-fos*), designed to prevent abnormal growth leading to cancer; cellular oncogenes function as a molecular marker of pain in that their presence within the nociceptive transmission system is induced by noxious stimulation; *also* called *proto-oncogene*, representative of normal genetic expression

**fossa** [*pl: fossae*] hollow pit, concavity, or depression, especially on the surface of the end of a bone or a tooth—*syn: fovea*

**fovea** —*see* fossa

**fracture** a break or rupture of a part, especially a bone

**freeway space** interocclusal distance or separation between the dental arches when the mandible is in its rest position

**fremitus** vibration, especially when palpable

**frontal plane** vertical plane, perpendicular to sagittal plane, dividing the body into front to back portions—*syn: coronal plane, facial plane*

**functional mandibular disorder** a disorder relating to abnormal mandibular movements or actions

**functional mandibular movement** a natural, proper, or characteristic movement or action of the mandible made during speech, mastication, yawning, swallowing, respiration, and other proper activities

**fungiform** mushroom-shaped or bulbous

# G

**gamma knife surgery** precisely focused radiation of 40 to 90 Gy emitted from 201 photon beams applied to the trigeminal root entry zone—*syn: stereotactic radiosurgery, stereotactic neurosurgery*

**ganglion** a collection or mass of nerve cells serving as a center of nervous influence

**generalized anxiety disorder (GAD)** disorder characterized by persistent and excessive uncontrolled feelings of anxiety or worry for a period of 6 months or longer accompanied by at least three of the following symptoms: restlessness, fatigue, difficulty concentrating, irritability, muscle tension, and sleep disturbance, and not associated with another mental disorder, substance use, or medical condition***

**genetic** pertaining to reproduction, birth, origin, or heredity

**geniculate neuralgia** —*see* neuralgia: geniculate

**genioplasty** plastic surgery of the chin

**geographic tongue** occasionally symptomatic, inflammatory disorder of the tongue mucosa characterized by multiple, well-demarcated zones of erythema located on the dorsum and lateral border of the tongue—*syn: benign migratory glossitis, erythema migrans*

**giant cell arteritis** —*syn: giant osteoid osteoma; see* arteritis

**Gilles de la Tourette syndrome** —*see* Tourette syndrome

**ginglymoid joint** hinging joint with one convex and one concave surface, with movement in only one plane of space

**gliding of condyle** —*see* translation of condyle

**globus** the feeling that there is a lump in the throat without the presence of a physical object

**glossalgia** —*see* glossodynia

**glossodynia** painful or burning tongue—*syn: glossalgia*

**glossopharyngeal nerve** mixed cranial nerve (CN IX) carrying somatosensory information from the posterior pharyngeal tissues and somatosensory and taste information from the posterior one-third of the tongue; the motor fibers supply the pharyngeal muscles

**glossopharyngeal neuralgia** —*see* neuralgia: glossopharyngeal

**glossopyrosis** burning tongue

**gnathic** pertaining to the jaw or cheek

**gnathologic** pertaining to the science of the dynamics of the jaws

**gout** disorder of purine metabolism characterized by hyperuricemia and the deposition of monosodium urate crystals in joints, resulting in acute attacks of arthritis with red, hot, and swollen joints, especially the big toe; gout occurs primarily in men older than 30 years—*syn: arthritis urica*

**grating joint sound** —*see* crepitation

**grinding of teeth** —*see* attrition bruxism

**group function** multiple contact relations between the maxillary and mandibular teeth during lateral movements on the working side, with simultaneous distribution of occlusal forces among the several posterior and anterior contacts

**guidance** the contact pattern between teeth during gliding occluding mandibular movement away or toward maximum intercuspation

> **anterior g.** contact between anterior teeth during gliding occlusal movement away or toward maximum intercuspation

> **posterior g.** contact between posterior teeth during gliding occlusal movement away or toward maximum intercuspation

**gustation** taste or the act of tasting

## H

**hard tissue** relatively rigid skeletal tissue including bone, hyaline cartilage, and fibrocartilage

**headache** —*see cephalalgia*

**hemarthrosis** bloody effusion into cavity of a joint

**hematoma** swelling or mass of blood confined to a tissue or space

> **epidural h.** collection of blood in epidural space due to damage and leakage of blood from the middle meningeal artery

> **subdural h.** collection of blood in subdural space from laceration of the brain or rupture of the bridging veins

**hemifacial microsomia** condition in which one side of the face is abnormally small and underdeveloped, yet normally formed

**hemifacial spasm** involuntary unilateral sudden contraction of the muscles in the facial nerve distribution

**hemiparesis** unilateral muscular weakness or paralysis

**hemiplegia** loss of motor function and sensation on one side of the body

**hemorrhage** abnormal internal or external discharge of blood; bleeding

**herpes zoster** *Varicella zoster* virus infection of the cranial or spinal nerve ganglia and cutaneous areas they supply, causing acute inflammation, characterized by painful vesicular skin or mucosal eruptions—*syn: zoster, shingles*

**heterogenous** derived from different sources

**heterophoria** deviation of an eye only when it is covered

**heterotopic pain** pain occurring at a site different from that of the cause

**heterotropia** a constant lack of parallelism of the visual axes of the eyes—*syn: strabismus*

**high condylectomy** surgical removal of only a portion of the superior mandibular condyle

**hinge axis** the theoretical single horizontal axis for some rotational articulation; for the mandible, the axis for a theoretical pure rotary movement at the beginning of jaw opening

**hinge movement** misnomer—*see rotation of condyle*

**histaminic cephalalgia** —*see cluster headache*

**histochemical** pertaining to the chemical substances in the body tissues on a cytologic scale

**histology** anatomic study of the minute structure, composition, and function of the tissues

**history of present illness (HPI)** narrative report of each symptom or complaint, including the onset, duration, and character of the present illness

**holocephalic headache** headache that is felt in the entire head; from Greek *holos* (entire) and *cephale* (head)

**homogenous** having a similar structure or characteristic

**homolateral** —*see ipsilateral*

**homologous** corresponding or alike in critical attributes such as structure, position, and origin, but not necessarily function

**horizontal dental overlap** —*see overjet*

**horizontal plane** —*see transverse plane*

**Horner syndrome** neurologic condition characterized by unilateral miosis, ptosis, and facial anhydrosis, usually resulting from a cervical sympathetic paralysis

**Horton headache** —*see cluster headache*

**Horton syndrome** —*see cluster headache*

**human leukocyte antigen B27 (HLA-B27)** genetic marker usually present in individuals with ankylosing spondylitis

**humoral** relating to or arising from any of the body fluids

**hyaline cartilage** type of cartilage found on the articular surfaces of most bones, characterized by flexibility, glasslike appearance, and network of connective tissue fibers; forms a template for endochondral bone formation

**hydrocephalus** an excessive accumulation of cerebrospinal fluid in the brain, causing cerebral ventricular dilation, elevated intracranial pressure, and enlargement of the skull

**hypalgesia** diminished sensibility to pain—*syn: hypoalgesia*

**hyperactivity** exaggerated amount of functional movement

**hyperacusis** painful or abnormally acute sensitivity to sound

**hyperalgesia** an increased response to a stimulus that is normally painful*

> **primary h.** —*see primary hyperalgesia*

**secondary h.** —*see* secondary hyperalgesia

**hyperesthesia** increased sensitivity to stimulation, excluding the special senses*

**hyperextension** extreme extension of a limb or joint

**hyperextension-hyperflexion injury** —*see* flexion-extension injury

**hyperflexion** extreme flexion of a limb or joint

**hyperfunction of muscle** excessive function of muscle

**hypermobility** excessive mobility; defined by extreme ranges of joint movement or laxity in a specific minimal number of defined joints; —*syn:* hypermobility syndrome (misnomer); *ant:* hypomobility

    **monoarticular h.** involving only one joint

    **oligoarticular h.** involving two to four joints

    **polyarticular h.** hypermobility involving more than four joints

**hyperpathia** a painful syndrome characterized by an abnormally painful reaction to a stimulus, especially a repeated stimulus, as well as an increased threshold*

**hyperplasia** overdevelopment of tissue or structure with an increase in the number of normal cells in a normal arrangement

**hypertonicity of muscle** excess muscular tonus, tension, or activity

**hypertranslation** excessive or exaggerated gliding movement range of a body part, such as the mandibular condyle

**hypertrophic arthritis** —*see* osteoarthritis

**hypertrophy** increase in size of an organ or structure but not in the number of its constituent cells—*ant:* atrophy

**hyperuricemia** abnormal amount of uric acid in the blood, found in gout but also in many other conditions

**hypesthesia** —*see* hypoesthesia

**hypoalgesia** diminished pain in response to a normally painful stimulus*—*see* hypalgesia

**hypochondriasis** somatoform disorder marked by the preoccupation with and anxiety over one's health, with exaggeration of normal sensations and misinterpretation of normal physical signs and minor complaints as serious illness or disease

**hypoesthesia** decreased sensitivity to stimulation, excluding the special senses*—*syn:* hypesthesia

**hypogeusia** diminished sensibility to taste

**hypoglossal nerve** mixed cranial nerve (CN XII) carrying afferent proprioceptive impulses as well as efferent motor impulses to the intrinsic and extrinsic muscles of the tongue, with communication to the vagus nerve (CN X)

**hypomobility** reduced or restricted range of motion—*ant:* hypermobility

**hypoplasia** incomplete or defective development or underdevelopment of a tissue or structure; implies fewer than the usual number of cells

**hypoxia** deficiency of oxygen

**hysteria** —*see* somatization disorder

**hysterical trismus** severe restriction of mandibular motion due to acute psychologic distress

## I

**-iasis** [suffix] abnormal condition

**iatrogenic** condition caused by medical personnel during examination, diagnostic tests, or treatment procedures

**idioglossia** imperfect articulation, with meaningless vocalization

**idiopathic** of unknown etiology

**idiopathic continuous neuropathic pain** constant unremitting pain from dysfunction in the nervous system without obvious pathology and of unknown etiology

**idiopathic odontalgia** tooth pain without obvious pathology and of unknown etiology

**idiopathic pain** painful disease or disorder without obvious pathology and of unknown etiology

**illness** condition characterized by a pronounced deviation from a normal healthy state

**illness behavior** alterations in behavior in response to an actual or perceived illness

**imaging** hard-record representation or visual reproduction of a structure for the purpose of diagnosis, including radiographs, ultrasound, computerized tomography, and magnetic resonance imaging

**impairment** a medical determination of the amount of deterioration from a state of normal health; a measure of the loss of use or abnormality of psychologic, physiologic, or anatomic structure or function

**incidence** number of new cases of a condition that occur during a specified period of time; compare with *prevalence*

**incisor** the four front teeth of each dental arch, used mainly for cutting

**incoordination** inability to move in a smooth, controlled, symmetric, and harmonious motion

**infarct** area of tissue necrosis following cessation or interruption of blood supply

**infection** invasion of a tissue by pathogenic microorganisms that reproduce and multiply, causing disease by local cellular injury, secretion of toxin, or antigen-antibody reaction in the host

**infectious arthritis** acute inflammatory condition of a joint caused by bacterial or viral infection

**inferior** —*ant: superior, cephalad; see caudal*

**inferior retrodiscal lamina** the most inferior border of the retrodiscal tissues or posterior attachment; this tissue is predominantly dense fibrous connective tissue and functions as a ligament to restrict anterior rotation of the disc on the condyle

**inflammation** protective response of tissue to irritation or injury, characterized by redness, heat, swelling, and pain

**infrared laser therapy** deep-heat therapy using an infrared laser light device—*syn: cold laser therapy*

**inhibition** suppression or arrest of a process

**initiating factors** factors that cause the onset of a disease or disorder

**insidious onset** development of a disorder that is gradual, subtle, or imperceptible—*ant: acute onset*

**insomnia** abnormal wakefulness or inability to sleep during the period when sleep should occur

**interarch** —*see interocclusal*

**interceptive occlusal contact** —*see supracontact*

**intercondylar** situated between two condyles

**intercondylar distance** the distance between two condyles

**intercuspal position (ICP)** mandibular position with the most complete interdigitation of opposing teeth independent of condylar position—*syn: maximum intercuspal position, maximum intercuspation, centric occlusion*

**intercuspation** occlusion of the teeth—*syn: interdigitation*

> **maximum i.** —*see intercuspal position*

**interdigitation** —*see intercuspation*

**interdisciplinary** the coordinated effort of multiple clinical specialties

**interference of occlusion** —*see supracontact*

**intermaxillary** misnomer—*see interocclusal*

**internal** inside the body or within a structure—*ant: external*

**internal derangement** disturbed arrangement of intracapsular joint parts causing interference with smooth joint movement; in the TMJ it can relate to elongation, tear, or rupture of the capsule or ligaments, causing altered disc position or morphology

**interocclusal** between the opposing dental arches

**interocclusal orthosis** an intraoral device that provides an artificial occlusal surface, designed to fit over either the maxillary or mandibular teeth

**interstitial** pertaining to the space between tissues

**intra-arch** within either the mandible or the maxilla

**intra-articular** located within a joint

**intra-articular disc** —*see disc: intra-articular*

**intracapsular** located within the capsule of a joint—*ant: extracapsular*

**intracapsular adhesion** —*see adhesion: intracapsular*

**intracondylar** within the condyle

**intracranial** within the cranium or skull—*ant: extracranial*

**intractable** resistant to treatment

**intrameatal** within the auditory canal or meatus

**intraoral** within the oral cavity

**intrathecal drug infusion** medication delivered directly to the intrathecal space through a small catheter; because the drug is delivered directly to the spinal cord, a smaller dose is required, which helps minimize systemic side effects

**intrinsic** originating from or situated entirely within an organ, tissue, or part—*ant: extrinsic*

**intrinsic trauma** —*ant: extrinsic trauma; see trauma: microtrauma*

**intrusion** inward projection; movement of the tooth in an apical direction

**ionizing radiation** radiation created by dislocating negatively charged electrons from atoms by the application of an electrical current

**iontophoresis** introduction of ions of soluble salts into tissues through intact skin by means of direct electric current

**ipsilateral** pertaining to the same side—*syn: homolateral; ant: contralateral*

**ischemia** local and temporary inadequate blood supply to a specific organ or tissue

**isokinetic exercises** dynamic muscle activity performed at a constant angular velocity

**isometric exercises** active exercise performed against stable resistance without change in the length of the muscle

**isotonic exercises** active exercise that shortens the muscle without appreciable change in the force of muscle contraction

## J

**jabs and jolts syndrome** *—see primary stabbing headache*

**jaw** either the maxilla or mandible

**jaw tracking** *—see mandibular movement recording*

> **j.t. devices** instruments used to quantify mandibular movements

**joint** the place of union or junction between two or more bones

**juvenile rheumatoid arthritis (JRA)** idiopathic arthritis that begins before the age of 16 years, with rheumatoid factor found in 70% of cases; more common in females, with onset most often between ages 12 and 15 years—*syn: Still disease*

**juxtaposed** positioned adjacently or in apposition

## K

**kinesiograph** instrument used to record and provide graphic representation of movement

**kinesiography** used to detect and record three-dimensional motion of the mandible—*see mandibular movement recording*

**kinesiology** the science or study of human movement

**kinetic** pertaining to, characterized by, or producing motion

## L

**labial** of, pertaining to, or toward the lip

**labioversion** condition of being displaced labially from the normal line of occlusion

**lacrimation** secretion of tears by the lacrimal glands

**lallation** a babbling, infantile form of speech

**larynx** musculocartilaginous structure lined with a mucous membrane, located below the dorsal root of the tongue and the hyoid bone at the top of the trachea; the organ of voice

**latent disease** dormant condition existing as a potential disorder

**lateral** away from the midline of the body; to the side—*ant: medial*

**lavage** the process of washing out or irrigating a cavity or an organ

**leaf gauge** set of blades of increasing thickness used to provide a metered separation or measure of the distance between two parts, such as the incisors

**leptoprosopic** having a facial form that is long, narrow, and protrusive

**leukocytosis** increase in the number of circulating white blood cells

**lichen planus** an inflammatory skin disease with wide, flat, irregular, often persistent circumscribed papules, with keratotic plugging

**ligament** flexible band of fibrous tissue, slightly elastic and composed of parallel collagenous bundles, binding joints together, and connecting various bones and cartilages

> **l. laxity** excessive looseness in ligamentous attachment

**lingual** of, pertaining to, or toward the tongue

**linguoversion** condition of being displaced lingually from a normal line of occlusion

**loading, joint** increasing the compressive force on a joint

**locking of joint** misnomer—*see disc displacement without reduction*

**longitudinal plane** *—see sagittal plane*

**lupus erythematosus** *—see systemic lupus erythematosus*

**luxation** —*see* *dislocation of condyle*

**lys-** [prefix] break apart

**lysis** dissolution, decomposition, or loosening of tissues

**lytic** pertaining to lysis

## M

**macroglossia** excessive tongue size

**macrotrauma** —*see* *trauma: macrotrauma*

**magnetic resonance imaging (MRI)** noninvasive, nonionizing imaging method that uses the signals from resonating hydrogen nuclei after they have been subjected to a charge in a magnetic field; their relaxation and resultant resonant frequency is detected, measured, and converted by a computer into an image

**malformation** failure of proper or normal development, a primary structural defect, or deformity that results from a localized error of morphogenesis

**malinger** to voluntarily feign or exaggerate an illness, usually to deliberately escape responsibility, provoke sympathy, or gain compensation; deliberate attempt to deceive in the absence of any psychiatric disorder

**malocclusion** —*see* *occlusal variation*

**mandible** horseshoe-shaped lower jawbone, consisting of the horizontal body joined at the symphysis and two vertical rami with the anterior coronoid process and the posterior condylar process, separated by the mandibular notch; the superior border of the body, the alveolus, contains sockets for the mandibular teeth

**mandibular** pertaining to the mandible

**mandibular closure** —*see* *arthrokinetics, TMJ: elevation of mandible*

**mandibular movement recording** kinesiographic recording of the movement of the mandible

**mandibular nerve** the third division of the trigeminal nerve, which leaves the skull through the foramen ovale and provides motor innervation to the muscles of mastication, the tensor veli palatini, the tensor tympani, and the anterior belly of the digastric and mylohyoid muscles; it provides the general sensory innervation to the teeth and gingivae, the mucosa of the cheek and floor of the mouth, the epithelium of the anterior two-thirds of the tongue, the meninges, and the skin of the lower portion of the face

**mandibular trismus** —*see* *trismus*

**mandibular orthopedic repositioning appliance (MORA)** an interocclusal appliance that covers only the posterior mandibular teeth to temporarily alter the mandibular position

**Marfan syndrome** autosomal dominant connective tissue disorder, characterized by abnormal length of extremities, cardiovascular abnormalities, and other deformities

**mastication** process of chewing food in preparation for deglutition

**masticatory cycle** —*see* *chewing cycle*

**masticatory muscles** muscles responsible for masticatory motion, including the paired masseter, temporalis, lateral pterygoid, and medial pterygoid muscles

**masticatory pain** pain or discomfort about the face and mouth induced by chewing or other use of the jaws but independent of local disease involving the teeth and the mouth

**maxilla** paired upper jaw bone that inferiorly forms the palate and the alveolus with the upper teeth, superiorly forms part of the orbit, and medially creates the walls of the nasal cavity

**maxillary** pertaining to the maxilla

**maxillofacial** pertaining to the maxillary and mandibular dental arches and the face

**maxillomandibular** pertaining to the maxilla and mandible

**maximum intercuspal position** —*see* *intercuspal position*

**maximum intercuspation** —*see* *intercuspal position*

**medial** toward the midline of the body—*ant:* *lateral*

**mediate auscultation** listening to sounds with the use of an instrument

**mediation** bringing about a result, conveying an action, communicating information, or serving as an intermediary

**mediotrusion** movement of the mandible medially

**medullary dorsal horn** -*see* *spinal trigeminal nucleus*

**meniscectomy, TMJ** misnomer—*see* *discectomy*

**meniscus** crescent-shaped fibrocartilaginous structure found in some synovial joints, but not in the TMJ

**meniscus, TMJ** misnomer—*see* *disc: intra-articular*

**mental disorder** a disorder of cognition, affect, or behavior that impairs adaptive functioning that may be of organic or psychologic origin

**mesial** toward the median sagittal plane of the face following the curvature of the dental arch

**mesiocclusion** —*see* Angle classification of occlusion: class III

**mesocephalic** having a head shape that is neither long nor short, narrow nor wide, oval nor rounded

**mesoprosopic** having a facial form that is neither long nor short, narrow nor broad, protrusive nor flat

**metaboreceptor** receptor that responds to an increase in metabolic products

**metaplasia** conversion of one tissue type into a form that is not normal for that tissue

**metastatic** shifting of a disease or its manifestation from one part of the body to another; in cancer, the appearance of neoplasms in parts of the body remote from the seat of the primary tumor

**microglossia** abnormally small tongue

**micrognathia** abnormal smallness of the jaw, especially the mandible

**microstomia** abnormally small mouth

**microtrauma** —*syn:* intrinsic trauma; *see* trauma: microtrauma

**midline of teeth** interproximal contact zone between the central incisor teeth of the maxillary or mandibular dental arch

**migraine headache** periodic, recurrent, intense throbbing headache, frequently unilateral and often accompanied by phonophobia, photophobia, and nausea or vomiting, and aggravated by routine physical activity; classified by descriptive characteristics rather than by known physiologic mechanisms

    **basilar m.h.** disturbance of brainstem function with dramatic but slowly evolving neurologic events, often involving total blindness, altered consciousness, confusional states, and subsequent headache

    **chronic m.h.** migraine occurring for at least 15 days per month for more than 3 months, not related to medication over use

    **classic m.h.** —*see* m.h. with aura

    **common m.h.** —*see* m.h. without aura

    **hemiplegic m.h.** headache associated with oculomotor nerve palsy and partial to complete unilateral paralysis of motor function

    **m.h. with aura** headache with associated premonitory sensory, motor, or visual symptoms (prodrome)—*syn: classic migraine*

    **m.h. without aura** condition in which no focal neurologic disturbance precedes the headache, but all other migraine with aura characteristics are the same—*syn: common migraine*

    **ophthalmoplegic m.h.** extremely rare nonthrobbing orbital or periorbital pain that radiates to the hemicranium, often accompanied by vomiting, lasting 1 to 4 days; frequently accompanied by ipsilateral ptosis and sometimes by pupillary dilatation in the absence of demonstrable intracranial lesion; may not truly be related to migraine

    **probable m.h.** migraine-like headache not completely fulfilling all criteria for migraine headache

    **retinal m.h.** repeated attacks of monocular scotoma or blindness lasting less than 1 hour and associated with headache; normal findings on examination and MRI or CT

    **transformed m.h.** headache that changes from episodic to daily

**miosis** pupillar contraction

**mixed connective tissue disease** —*see* connective tissue disorders

**mobilization, joint** the process of restoring motion to a joint

**mononeuropathy** neuropathy in a single nerve, *also* called *mononeuritis*

**monosynaptic reflex** simplest and fastest reflex involving one motor and one sensory neuron with one synapse; eg, muscle stretch reflex

**mood disturbance** persistent disturbance of the emotional state

**morphology** form or structure of an organism

**motor neuron** neuron carrying efferent impulses that initiate muscle contraction

**mouth guard** plastic intraoral appliance that covers and protects the teeth during contact sports

**MRI** —*see magnetic resonance imaging*

**multidisciplinary** use of multiple specialties in coordinated treatment of a single patient

**multifactorial** resulting from the combined action of several factors

**multiple myeloma** malignant neoplasm of bone marrow

**multiple sclerosis** chronic, slowly progressive disease of the central nervous system of unknown etiology, characterized by demyelinated glial patches called *plaques*

**muscle** tissue composed of contractile fibers that effect movements of an organ or part of the body; muscle types include striated skeletal and cardiac muscles, and smooth nonstriated visceral muscles

**digastric m.** originates on the digastric notch of the mastoid process and inserts on the mandible near the symphysis; raises the hyoid bone and base of the tongue, and depresses the mandible

**lateral (external) pterygoid m.** muscle with two heads, with a single origin on the lateral pterygoid plate and greater wing of the sphenoid; insertion is on the fovea of the condyle and capsule of the TMJ, and the other insertion may be partially on the intra-articular disc; this muscle of mastication translates the mandible and is active in mouth opening and near final mouth closure

**masseter m.** originates on the superficial masseter on the zygomatic process and arch and inserts on the ramus and the angle of the mandible; the deep masseter originates on the zygomatic arch and inserts on the upper half of the ramus and the coronoid process of the mandible; powerful muscle of mastication that elevates the mandible

**medial pterygoid m.** originates on the maxillary tuberosity and medial surface of the lateral pterygoid plate and inserts on the medial surface of the ramus and angle of the mandible; during mastication, elevates and protrudes the mandible, and, during speech, is active in mandibular movements

**scalene m.** these three muscles originate on the transverse process of the cervical vertebrae and insert on the ribs; act to stabilize the cervical vertebrae or incline the neck to the side and are accessory muscles to respiration

**sternocleidomastoid m.** muscle with two heads, one originating on the sternum and the other on the clavicle, and inserting onto the mastoid process and superior nuchal line of the occipital bone; rotates and extends the head and flexes the vertebral column

**suboccipital m.** muscles situated below the occipital bone that act to stabilize the cervical vertebrae and head position and to extend or rotate the head and neck

**suprahyoid m.** digastric, geniohyoid, mylohyoid, and stylohyoid; all attach to the upper part of the hyoid bone and act to stabilize and elevate the hyoid bone and depress the mandible

**temporal m.** fan-shaped muscle with its origin on the temporal fossa and insertion on the coronoid process and anterior aspect of the ramus; elevates and retrudes the mandible during mastication

**trapezius m.** originates on the superior nuchal line of the occipital bone and spinous process of the seventh cervical and all of the thoracic vertebrae and inserts on the clavicle and scapula; elevates the shoulder and rotates the scapula

**muscle compartment** muscle bundle enclosed within a single sheath—**syn:** *fascicle*

**muscle compartment syndrome** pain and stiffness in a muscle due to oxygen deprivation within the muscle compartment

**acute m.c.s.** oxygen deprivation due to capillary compression from an acute increase in volume in the muscle compartment secondary to fracture, edema, or bleeding

**chronic m.c.s.** oxygen deprivation during muscle contractions secondary to reduced muscle relaxation time between contractions

**muscle contraction** the shortening or development of tension in muscle

**muscle contracture** —**see** *contracture: muscular*

**muscle cramp** misnomer—**see** *myospasm*

**muscle hypertonia** increased tone of skeletal muscle or increased resistance to passive stretch

**muscle hypertonicity** —**see** *muscle hypertonia*

**muscle relaxation appliance** misnomer—**see** *stabilization appliance*

**muscle splinting** —**see** *protective muscle splinting*

**muscular dystrophy** group of genetically transmitted diseases characterized by progressive atrophy of symmetric groups of skeletal muscles without evidence of degeneration of neural tissue

**musculoskeletal** relating to the muscles (including fascial sheaths and tendons) and joints

**musculoskeletal pain** deep somatic pain that originates in skeletal muscles, fascial sheaths, and tendons (myogenous pain), bones and periosteum (osseous pain), joint, joint capsules, and ligaments (arthralgic pain), and in soft connective tissues

**myalgia** pain in a muscle

**myelin** lipid that forms a major component of the sheath that surrounds and insulates the axon of some nerve cells

**myelomeningocele** a congenital developmental defect of the neural tube causing a malformation or incomplete closure; *also* known as a *spina bifida*; most commonly occurs in the lumbosacral region

**myelopathy** functional disturbance or change in the spinal cord

**myoclonus** clonic spasm or twitching that results from the contraction of one or more muscle groups

**myofascial** pertaining to muscle and its attaching fascia

**myofascial pain** regional pain referred from or emanating around active myofascial trigger points

**myofascial pain dysfunction syndrome** misnomer—*see myofascial pain*

**myofascial trigger point** hyperirritable spot, usually within a taut band of skeletal muscle or in the muscle fascia, that is painful on compression and can give rise to characteristic referred pain, tenderness (secondary hyperalgesia), and autonomic phenomena; subdivided into active and latent

**active m.t.p.** myofascial trigger point responsible for local or referred current pain or symptoms without stimulation through palpation

**latent m.t.p.** myofascial trigger point with all the characteristics of an active myofascial trigger point, including referred pain with palpation, but not currently causing spontaneous clinical pain or symptoms

**myofascitis** inflammation of muscle and its fascia

**myofibrosis** replacement of muscle tissue by fibrous tissue

**myofibrositis** inflammation of the perimysium, the connective tissue separating individual muscle fascicles

**myofunctional therapy** use of exercises to improve the function of a group of muscles

**myogenous** of muscular origin

**myogenous pain** deep somatic musculoskeletal pain originating in the skeletal muscles, fascial sheaths, or tendons

**myositis** inflammation of muscle tissue

**myositis ossificans** ossification of muscle tissue, usually after injury

**myospasm** spasmodic continuous involuntary contraction of a muscle, typically causing acute pain—*syn: trismus, muscle cramp*

**myxoma** neoplasm derived from primitive connective tissue, composed of a stroma-resembling mesenchyme

## N

**narcotic** any drug that produces sleep, insensibility, or stupor; more commonly, opium or any of its derivatives (morphine, heroin, codeine, etc)

**natural history of disorder** natural sequence, duration, transitional stages, and nature of change of a disease or disorder over time, without external interference such as trauma or treatment

**neck-tongue syndrome** rare disorder characterized by infrequent shortlasting attacks of unilateral pain in the upper neck radiating toward the ear and associated with numbness, paresthesia, or the sensation of involuntary movement of the ipsilateral half of the tongue

**necrosis** tissue death

**neoplasm** abnormal, uncontrolled, progressive growth of new tissue; designated as benign or malignant—*syn: tumor*

**nerve** a visible cordlike structure, made up of numerous nerve fibers, that conveys impulses from one part of the body to another

**nerve block** injection of local anesthetics or steroids into the epidural space for extended pain relief

**nervus intermedius** smaller root of the facial nerve that merges with the facial nerve at the level of the geniculate ganglion and innervates the lacrimal, nasal, palatine, submandibular and sublingual glands and the anterior portion two-thirds of the tongue

**neural** pertaining to one or more nerves

**neural pathway** the nerve structures through which an impulse is conducted

**neuralgia** paroxysmal or constant pain, typically with sharp, stabbing, itching, or burning character, in the distribution of a nerve or nerves—**syn:** *neurodynia*

> **auriculotemporal n.** paroxysmal pain with refractory periods involving the auriculotemporal branch of the trigeminal nerve

> **cranial n.** neuralgia along the course of a cranial nerve

> **geniculate n.** painful disturbance of the sensory portion of the facial nerve characterized by lancinating pain in the middle ear and the auditory canal—**syn:** *nervus intermedius neuralgia, Ramsay Hunt syndrome*

> **glossopharyngeal n.** severe, paroxysmal, lancinating pain due to a lesion in the petrosal and jugular ganglion of the glossopharyngeal nerve (CN IX) that radiates to the throat, ear, teeth, and tongue and is triggered by movement in the tonsillar region by swallowing or coughing; branches to the carotid artery can trigger a vasovagal response, including altered respiration, blood pressure, and cardiac output; rare, unilateral condition; usually in men older than 50 years

> **nervus intermedius n.** —*see geniculate neuralgia*

> **occipital n.** neuralgia involving the greater occipital nerve (C2 or C3)

> **postherpetic n.** neuralgia following outbreak of the herpes zoster virus

> **postsurgical n.** pain of neuralgic character secondary to inadvertent damage to sensory nerves during a surgical procedure

> **pretrigeminal n.** syndrome of dull aching or burning pain, often in the oral cavity or teeth, which precedes true paroxysmal trigeminal neuralgia; pain duration varies widely from hours to months, with variable periods of remission; onset of true neuralgic pain may be quite sudden

> **superior laryngeal n.** condition characterized by sharp, paroxysmal, unilateral submandibular pain that may radiate to the ear, eye, or shoulder—a distribution indistinguishable from glossopharyngeal neuralgia; the superior laryngeal nerve is a branch of the vagus nerve (CN X) and innervates the cricothyroid muscle of the larynx

> **traumatic n.** deafferentation pain secondary to disruption of normal sensory pathways from traumatic or surgical injury

> **trigeminal n.** disorder of the sensory divisions of the trigeminal nerve (CN V), characterized by recurrent paroxysms of sharp, stabbing pains in the distribution of one or more branches of the nerve, often precipitated by stimulation of specific trigger points—**syn:** *tic douloureux*

**neurasthenia** syndrome of chronic mental and physical fatigue and weakness—term virtually obsolete in Western medicine

**neurectomy** peripheral ablative procedure in which the offending trigeminal nerve branch is avulsed under local or general anesthesia

**neuritis** inflammation of a nerve or nerves*

**neuroablative procedures** nonreversible procedures performed to interrupt sensory pathways to the brain or in the brainstem by severing or destroying the appropriate pathology; examples include: cordotomy, rhizotomy, thalamotomy, or chemical destruction of neural structures

**neuroaugmentation** use of medications or electrical stimulation to supplement activity of the nervous system

**neurodynia** —*see neuralgia*

**neurogenic pain** pain initiated or caused by a primary lesion, dysfunction, or transitory perturbation in the peripheral or central nervous system*—**syn:** *neuropathic pain*

**neurogenous** arising from neural tissues, or from a lesion in neural tissues

**neurogenous pain** —*see neuropathic pain*

**neurolepsis** altered state of consciousness characterized by quiescence, reduced motor activity, anxiety, and indifference to surroundings, induced by a neuroleptic medication

**neuroleptic** drug with antipsychotic properties

**neurologic** pertaining to the nervous system and its disorders

**neurolysis** longitudinal surgical incision to free a nerve sheath, surgical loosening of fibrous nerve adhesions, or destruction of nerve tissue

> **sympathetic n.** —*see sympathectomy*

**neuromodulation** a group of medical therapies that use drugs or electricity to regulate pain or minimize dysfunction, including drug pumps and neurostimulation

**neuromuscular** concerning both nerves and muscles

**neuron** nerve cell

**neuropathic** pertaining to neuropathy

**neuropathic pain** pain initiated or caused by a primary lesion or dysfunction in the nervous system—**syn:** *neurogenic pain*

**neuropathy** disturbance of function or pathologic change in a nerve; in one nerve, *mononeuropathy*; in several nerves, *mononeuropathy multiplex*; if diffuse and bilateral, *polyneuropathy**

**neuroplasticity** dynamic ability of the central nervous system to alter central processing of impulses secondary to ongoing afferent impulses usually thought to be nociceptive

**neurostimulation** low-level electrical pulses delivered by an implanted pacemaker-type device that stimulate various tissues of the nervous system, including the spinal cord, peripheral nerves, and brain

**neurotransmitter** any biochemical substance that mediates the passage of an impulse across the synapse from one nerve cell to another

**neurovascular** concerning both the nervous and vascular systems

**neutrocclusion** —**see** *Angle classification of occlusion: class I*

**nightguard appliance** interocclusal appliance traditionally worn only at night to reduce adverse effects of bruxism

**NMRI** nuclear magnetic resonance imaging—**see** *magnetic resonance imaging*

**nocebo** negative treatment effects induced by a substance or procedure containing no toxic or detrimental substance

**nociception** stimulation of specialized nerve endings designed to transmit information to the central nervous system concerning potential or actual tissue damage

**nociceptive** capable of receiving and transmitting painful sensation

**nociceptive pain** pain resulting from tissue damage and the subsequent release of chemicals that act as noxious stimuli and are perceived by the brain as pain; *also* called *somatic pain*

**nociceptive pathway** an afferent neural pathway that transmits pain impulses to the central nervous system

**nociceptor** a specialized nerve ending that senses painful or harmful sensations

> **primary afferent n.** one of three major groups of peripheral nerves capable of transmitting the presence of a noxious stimulus to the skin or the spinal cord; these include the Aβ mechanosensitive nociceptors, the Aδ mechanothermal nociceptors, and the unmyelinated C-polymodal nociceptors

**nocturnal** pertaining to or occurring in the hours of darkness—**ant:** *diurnal*

**noma** rapidly progressive necrotizing infection of the mouth and face usually seen in malnourished children; may also affect immunocompromised individuals

**noninnervated** tissue that is lacking in sensory or motor nerve supply

**noninvasive** denoting diagnostic or therapeutic procedures that do not require penetrating the skin or entering a cavity or organ of the body

**nonodontogenic toothache** pain presenting as a toothache but originating from a source other than dental and periodontal tissues

**nonreducing disc** —**see** *disc displacement: without reduction*

**nonsteroidal anti-inflammatory drug (NSAID)** class of anti-inflammatory medications that also provide analgesia but lack the detrimental side effects associated with steroid use

**nonworking** contralateral to the functioning side

**nonworking condyle** condyle contralateral to the functioning side

**nonworking occlusal contact** tooth contact on the contralateral side during guided lateral excursive movement of the mandible

**noradrenalin** —**see** *norepinephrine*

**norepinephrine** biogenic amine released as a hormone by the adrenal medulla that acts as a neurotransmitter in the central nervous system and the sympathetic nervous system; differs from epinephrine in the absence of an *N*-methyl group

**norepinephrinergic** relating to any drug that stimulates the production of norepinephrine

**noxious stimulus** a stimulus that is potentially or actually damaging to tissues

**nuchal line** bony ridge at the nape or back of the skull

**nuchal rigidity** resistance to flexion of the neck; often seen in meningitis

**nuclear magnetic resonance imaging (NMRI)** —*see magnetic resonance imaging*

## O

**occipital** pertaining to the back of the head

**occlude** bringing the maxillary and mandibular teeth together; obstruct or close off

**occlusal** pertaining to the masticatory surfaces of teeth

**occlusal adjustment** —*see occlusal equilibration*

**occlusal appliance** —*see interocclusal orthosis*

**occlusal contact** —*see occlusion*

**occlusal equilibration** adjustment of the coronal portion of the tooth by abrasive instruments, usually to more evenly distribute the vertical and excursive forces of occlusion

**occlusal guidance** tooth-determined guidance of the mandible in eccentric movements, when the teeth remain in contact

**occlusal interference** —*see supracontact*

**occlusal slide** movement of the mandible into maximum intercuspation from the retruded contact position

**occlusal splint** —*see interocclusal orthosis*

**occlusal trauma** injury to the periodontium resulting from occlusal forces in excess of the reparative capacity of the attachment apparatus; contrast with *primary occlusal trauma, secondary occlusal trauma*—**syn:** *periodontal trauma, occlusal traumatism, periodontal traumatism*

**occlusal traumatism** —*see occlusal trauma*

**occlusal variation** unusual biologic or functional relationship between the maxillary and mandibular teeth

**occlusal vertical dimension** —*see vertical dimension of occlusion*

**occlusal wear** —*see attrition*

**occlusion** the act or process of closure or of being closed or shut off; the static relationship between the incising or masticating surfaces of the maxillary and mandibular teeth or tooth analogs

**ocular** pertaining to the eye

**oculomotor nerve** cranial nerve (CN III) arising in the midbrain and supplying the levator palpebrae, superior rectus, recti, and inferior oblique muscles of the eye, the sphincter pupillae and ciliary muscles of the orbit, and the nasal mucosa

**odontalgia** pain felt in a tooth or teeth

**odontogenic** derived from or produced in the teeth or tissues that produce the teeth

**odontogenic pain** deep somatic pain arising or originating in the teeth or periodontal ligaments

**olfactory nerve** sensory cranial nerve (CN I) supplying the nasal mucosa

**open bite** abnormal dental condition in which the anterior teeth do not contact when the posterior teeth are brought into occlusion

**open lock** —*see dislocation of condyle*

**ophthalmic** —*see ocular*

**optic nerve** sensory cranial nerve (CN II) supplying the retina of the eye

**oral** pertaining to the mouth

**oral apraxia** inability to carry out purposeful oral movements in the absence of paralysis or other motor sensory impairment

**oral orthopedics** analysis of usual and unusual postural jaw relationships and their effects on the oral structures, including diagnostic, therapeutic, and prophylactic considerations

**organic** related to the organs of the body; pertaining to an organized structure; arising from an organism

**orofacial** relating to the mouth and face

**orthodontic** pertaining to the proper occlusal and maxillomandibular relationships

**orthodontics** specialty of dentistry dealing with the development, prevention, and correction of occlusal maxillomandibular irregularities

**orthodromic** impulses conducted in normal directions along nerve paths

**orthognathic** pertaining to malposition of the bones of the jaws

**orthognathic surgery** —*see surgery: orthognathic*

**orthopedic** relating to correction of form and function of the locomotor structures, especially the extremities, spine, and associated structures, including bones, joints, muscles, fascia, ligaments, and cartilage

**orthopedic appliance** —*see orthosis*

**orthosis** orthopedic appliance or splint used to support or improve function of moveable parts of the body—*syn: orthopedic appliance*

**orthostatic** relating to an erect or upright position

**orthotic** acting to support or improve function; pertaining to an orthosis

**osseous** bony

**ossification** development or formation of bone

**osteoarthritis** chronic disease that produces degenerative changes in the articular cartilage, fibrous connective tissue, and disc within a joint, resulting in joint deformity; the late stage is characterized by proliferation of new bony tissue at the margins of the joint surface, known as *marginal osteophytes, lipping,* or *spurs*; although the fibrillation and breakdown of cartilage is not an inflammatory process, the breakdown is accompanied by inflammation—*syn: degenerative arthritis, degenerative joint disease, hypertrophic arthritis*

**osteoarthrosis** chronic arthritis of noninflammatory character

**osteoblast** bone-forming cell derived from mesenchyme

**osteoblastoma** benign, vascularized tumor of poorly formed bone and fibrous tissue that causes resorption of native bone—*syn: giant osteoid osteoma*

**osteochondral junction** the interface between the calcified cartilage zone and the subchondral bone in synovial joints

**osteochondritis dissecans** inflammation of both bone and cartilage, resulting in the splitting of pieces of cartilage into the joint

**osteoclast** multinucleated cell that causes absorption and removal of bone

**osteoma** benign slow-growing mass of mature bone, usually found on a bone and sometimes on another structure

**osteomyelitis** inflammation of bone, especially of the marrow, caused by pathogenic organisms

**osteophyte** bony outgrowth

**osteoporosis** thinning of bone

**osteosarcoma** malignant bone tumor composed of anaplastic cells derived from mesenchyme

**osteotomy** surgical incision or cutting through a bone

**otolaryngology** division of medical science concerned with diseases of the ear, larynx, upper respiratory tract, and other associated head and neck structures

**otologic** pertaining to the ear

**overbite** vertical overlap of anterior teeth

>   **deep o.** excessive overlap of the anterior teeth

>   **excessive o.** —*see overbite: deep*

**overeruption, tooth** occlusal relationship whereby an unopposed or nonoccluding tooth extends beyond the normal occlusal plane

**overjet** horizontal overlap of anterior teeth

# P

**Paget disease** disorder of unknown etiology with inflammation of one or many bones, resulting in thickening and softening of bones with unorganized bone repair; *also* called *osteitis deformans*

**pain** an unpleasant sensory and emotional experience associated with actual or potential tissue damage, or described in terms of such damage\*\*

>   **p. behavior** visible actions that communicate suffering or pain to others

>   **p. detection threshold** —*see pain threshold*

>   **p. disorder** —*see somatoform pain disorder*

>   **p. map** a diagram showing the areas of pain on a patient

>   **p. mediators** neurovascular substances activated by noxious stimuli that trigger or sustain pain

>   **p. modulation** the suppression of pain within a nervous system network

>   **p. pathway** —*see nociceptive pathway*

>   **p. receptor** a specialized nerve ending that senses painful or harmful sensations and transmits them to a nerve

>   **p. threshold** the least experience of pain that a subject can recognize\*

>   **p. tolerance level** the greatest level of pain that a subject can tolerate\*

**palatal** pertaining to the roof of the mouth

**palate** the roof of the mouth

**palliative** mitigating, reducing the severity of, or denoting the elimination of symptoms without curing the underlying disease

**pallidotomy** a surgical procedure in which a wire probe is inserted into the globus pallidus of the brain to heat the surrounding tissue and destroy nerves with the goal of helping reduce uncontrollable movements caused by neurologic conditions such as Parkinson disease

**palpation** examination by feeling with the hands or fingers; perceiving by the sense of touch

**palsy** paralysis or paresis

**panic disorder** an anxiety disorder associated with recurrent, unexpected panic attacks characterized by intense apprehension, fearfulness, or terror and often accompanied by palpitations, accelerated heart rate, sweating, tremulousness, sensations of shortness of breath, choking, chest pain, abdominal distress, nausea, dizziness, derealization, fear of dying, and fear of losing control or going crazy; at least 1 month of persistent concern about having recurrent panic attacks and a significant alteration in adaptive functioning due to such worry are included in the criteria***

**panoramic radiograph** circular tomography that images the jaws and related structures

**pantograph** dental device that incorporates a pair of facebows fixed to the jaws, used for recording mandibular movement patterns and intercuspal jaw relationships

**parafunction** nonfunctional activity; in the orofacial region, clenching and bruxing, nail biting, lip or cheek chewing, etc

**paralysis** palsy, loss of power, or voluntary movement in muscle through injury or disease of its nerve supplies

**parasympathetic nervous system** division of the autonomic nervous system arising from preganglionic cell bodies in the brainstem and the middle three segments of the sacral cord; cranial nerves III, VII, and IX distribute parasympathetics to the head; cranial nerve X distributes to the thoracic and abdominal viscera via the prevertebral plexuses; and the pelvic nerve (nervus erigens) distributes its autonomic fibers to most of the large intestine and to the pelvic viscera and genitalia via the hypogastric plexus—*syn: craniosacral division*

**paratrigeminal syndrome** —*see Raeder syndrome*

**paravertebral** alongside or near the vertebral column

**paresis** partial or incomplete paralysis

**paresthesia** abnormal sensation, whether spontaneous or evoked; unlike dysesthesia, paresthesia includes all abnormal sensations whether unpleasant or not; dysesthesias are a subset of paresthesia specifically including those abnormal sensations that are unpleasant*

**parotid gland** paired salivary gland located superficial to the masseter muscle and extending from in front of the ear to down below the angle of the mandible

**paroxysm** sudden sharp spasm, convulsion, or attack

**paroxysmal** referring to a spasm, convulsion, or sudden short-lasting onset or change in symptoms

**passive range of motion** motion imparted to an articulation, associated capsule, ligaments, and muscles by another individual, machine, or outside force

**passive resistive stretch** activity designed to increase muscle length by activating the reciprocal muscle against an opposing force and then stretching

**pathogenic condition** giving rise to pathology

**pathogenic occlusion** occlusal relationship capable of producing pathologic changes in the stomatognathic system

**pathognomonic** specifically distinctive or characteristic of a disease or pathologic condition; a sign or symptom on which a diagnosis can be made

**pathologic** indicative of or caused by a disease

**pathologic condition** diseased state or condition

**pathophysiologic derangement of function** alteration of function due to disease and not due to structural alteration

**pathophysiology** the study of how normal, physiologic processes are altered by disease

**pathosis** misnomer—*see pathologic condition*

**pemphigus** a group of skin diseases characterized by successive crops of bullae that may leave pigmented spots after resolution and are often accompanied by itching and burning

**percutaneous** performed through the skin

**percutaneous balloon microcompression** neurosurgical procedure in which the trigeminal nerve is compressed by inflating a tiny balloon in the area of the involved nerve fibers

**percutaneous glycerol rhizotomy** neurosurgical procedure in which nerve fibers are destroyed by injection of anhydrous glycerol

**percutaneous radiofrequency thermocoagulation** neurosurgical procedure in which nerve fibers are destroyed by thermal lesioning

**periarticular** surrounding a joint

**pericranium** fibrous membrane surrounding the cranium; periosteum of the skull

**periodontal trauma** —*see occlusal trauma*

**periodontalgia** pain that emanates from the periodontal ligaments

**periodontium** the investing tissue surrounding the teeth, including the connective tissues, alveolar bone, and gingiva; anatomically used to denote the connective tissue between the tooth and the alveolar bone; *also* called *periodontal ligament*

**peripheral nerve stimulation** a type of neurostimulation that uses electrical signals from an implanted generator to stimulate targeted nerves that lie outside the spine to relieve pain; eg, sacral nerve stimulation

**peripheral nervous system** the motor, sensory, sympathetic, and parasympathetic nerves and the ganglia outside the brain and spinal cord

**peripheral neurogenic pain** pain initiated or caused by a primary lesion, dysfunction, or transitory perturbation in the peripheral nervous system*

**peripheral neuropathic pain** pain initiated or caused by a primary lesion or dysfunction in the peripheral nervous system*

**personality disorder** disorder characterized by a long-term pattern of thinking and acting that is significantly different from the general population and results in significant adverse consequences to the individual and those around the individual

    **antisocial p.d.** disorder characterized by a pervasive pattern of disregard for and violation of the rights of others described by the presence of at least three of the following: doing things that could lead to arrest, lying, not planning ahead, being irritable and aggressive to the point of getting into fights, disregarding safety of self and others, being irresponsible, and not expressing remorse or sorrow for behavior that hurts others***

    **avoidant p.d.** disorder characterized by a pervasive pattern of social inhibition, feelings of inadequacy, and hypersensitivity to any criticism***

    **borderline p.d.** disorder characterized by a pervasive pattern of instability of interpersonal relationships, self-image, affects and impulsivity in action***

    **dependent p.d.** disorder characterized by a pervasive and excessive need to be taken care of leading to submissive and clinging behaviors and separation anxiety***

    **histrionic p.d.** disorder characterized by pronounced emotional expression and attention seeking behavior of often inappropriate, provocative and sexually seductive nature***

    **narcissistic p.d.** disorder characterized by a pervasive pattern of grandiosity, an intense need for the admiration by, while displaying little empathy for others***

    **obsessive-compulsive p.d.** disorder characterized by a drive for perfection, orderliness, and interpersonal control, and limited openness and flexibility***

    **paranoid p.d.** disorder characterized by pervasive distrust and suspiciousness of others such that their motives are interpreted as malevolent***

    **schizoid p.d.** disorder characterized by a pervasive pattern of detachment from social relationships and very limited emotional expression in interpersonal settings***

    **schizotypal p.d.** disorder characterized by substantial distortions of thought and very unusual behavior in addition to pervasive pattern of detachment from social relationships and very limited emotional expression***

**perpetuating factor**s factors that interfere with healing or exacerbate a disease process

**PET scan** —*see tomography: positron emission*

**phantom limb pain** a condition in which a patient senses that the missing body part is still attached and subsequently feels pain in that area

**pharmacotherapy** drug treatment of a disease or disorder

**pharyngeal plexus** comprises cranial nerves IX-XI and provides innervation of the pharynx as well as the upper trapezius and sternocleidomastoid

**pharynx** musculomembranous sac between the mouth, nasal cavities, and esophagus

287

**Phoenix abscess** abscess originating from a suddenly symptomatic previously dormant chronic periapical granuloma

**phonophobia** abnormal fear of or exaggerated sensitivity to sound

**photophobia** abnormal fear of or exaggerated sensitivity to light

**physical dependence** pharmacologic property of a drug resulting in the occurrence of an abstinence syndrome following abrupt discontinuation of the agent

**physical therapy** treatment of disease or disorder with physical and mechanical means such as massage, manipulation, exercise, heat, cold, ultrasound, and electricity; includes (re)education in correct posture, body mechanics, and movement—*syn: physiotherapy*

**physiologic** pertaining to normal function of a tissue or organ—*ant: pathologic*

**physiologic rest position of mandible** —*see rest position of mandible*

**physiotherapy** —*see physical therapy*

**pinna** —*see auricle*

**pivot appliance** hard acrylic resin appliance with a single unilateral or bilateral posterior contact designed to provide condylar distraction

**placebo** substance, device, or behavior that superficially resembles and is believed by the patient to be an active substance, material, or behavior, but has no influence

**placebo effect** physical or emotional change in a patient occurring after a placebo is provided, with the change not directly attributable to any specific property or effect of the substance, behavior, or therapeutic agent

**planar scintigraphy** two-dimensional imaging process in which the area of interest is scanned with a gamma camera 2 to 4 hours after the administration of a radioactive material; increased uptake of the radioisotope in the tissue scanned indicates an increase in cellular activity—*syn: scintigraphy, scintiscan*

**plane of reference** plane that guides the location of other planes

**platelet-aggregating factor (PAF)** substance produced in the blood by the action between an antigen and immunoglobulin E–sensitized basophiles; PAF aggregates platelets and is a factor in producing inflammation

**plication** the stitching of folds or tucks in a tissue to reduce its size, as in the retrodiscal tissues of the TMJ or the walls of a hollow viscus

**polyarthritis** simultaneous inflammation of several joints

**polymyalgia rheumatica** self-limiting syndrome in elderly people characterized by progressive pain and stiffness of the proximal limbs after acute onset, with myalgia, fever, and an elevated ESR; onset may be unilateral but invariably becomes bilateral, resulting in successive involvement of muscle groups with morning stiffness

**polyneuropathy** disease involving several nerves, usually bilateral and diffuse

**polysynaptic reflex** a reflected movement resulting from neural conduction along a pathway formed by a chain of synaptically connected nerve cells

**positron emission tomography (PET)** —*see tomography: positron emission*

**posterior** relating to the back or dorsal side of the human body—*ant: anterior*

**posterior attachment, TMJ** loose connective tissue attached to the posterior region of the fibrous portion of the articular disc and extending to and filling the posterior capsule, rich in interstitial collagen fibers, adipose tissue, arteries, and elastin, and possessing a venous plexus—*syn: retrodiscal tissue*

**posterior bite collapse** intercuspal relationship with reduction of occlusal vertical dimension through loss, partial loss, or drifting of the posterior supporting dentition, often accompanied by compensating protrusion of the anterior teeth

**posterior cranial fossa** the largest cranial fossa, formed by the basilar, lateral, and squamous sections of the occipital, the petrous section of the temporal, the mastoid sections of the temporal and parietal, and the posterior body of the sphenoid

**posterior ligament** misnomer—*see posterior attachment, TMJ*

**posterior open bite** lack of posterior tooth contact in the intercuspal position

**posterior overclosure** a presumed subnormal vertical dimension of occlusion due to factors such as attrition, erosion, or intrusion of posterior teeth or developmental irregularities, preventing full eruption of posterior teeth—*syn: overclosed bite*

**postganglionic** situated posterior or distal to a ganglion

**postherpetic neuralgia** —*see* neuralgia: postherpetic

**postsurgical neuralgia** —*see* neuralgia: postsurgical

**posttraumatic stress disorder (PTSD)** disorder characterized by the development of a specific set of symptoms following exposure to a traumatic event involving direct personal experience or witnessing of an event that involves actual or threatened death or serious injury, or the threat to one's physical and psychologic integrity***

**postural** pertaining to the attitude or position of the body

**preauricular** located in front of the ear

**predisposing** indicating a tendency or susceptibility to develop a disease or condition

**predisposing factors** factors that increase the risk of developing a disease or condition

**preganglionic** situated anterior or proximal to a ganglion

**premature occlusal contact** —*see* supracontact

**prematurity** —*see* supracontact

**pretreatment records** any records made for the purpose of diagnosis, recording of patient history, or treatment planning in advance of therapy

**pretrigeminal neuralgia** —*see* neuralgia: pretrigeminal

**prevalence** number of cases of a disease or disorder for a given area and population at a given point in time, usually measured as the percentage of positive cases; compare with *incidence*

**primary afferent nociceptor** —*see* nociceptor: primary afferent

**primary hyperalgesia** hypersensitivity to noxious stimuli at a site of primary nociception and tissue damage

**primary occlusal trauma** injury to the periodontium from excessive occlusal forces in teeth with normal supporting structures

**primary pain** pain located over the true source of nociceptive input

**primary stabbing headache** spontaneous short-lasting stabs of pain felt in the head, not usually unilateral or localized to one area—*syn: jabs and jolts syndrome*

**prodrome** symptom indicating the onset of a disorder

**prognathic** having a forward-projecting jaw—*syn: prognathous*

**prognosis** a prediction of the course of the outcome of a disease or condition

**progressive supranuclear palsy** spastic weakness of facial, masticatory, and oropharyngeal muscles due to a lesion in the corticospinal tract; may cause spontaneous laughing or crying—*syn: pseudobulbar paralysis, supranuclear paralysis, spastic bulbar palsy*

**projected pain** neurogenic pain that is felt in the anatomic peripheral distribution of a nerve while the stimulus occurs along the pathway from the nerve to the cortex

**proprioception** reception and interpretation of stimulation of sensory nerve terminals within the tissues of the body that provides information concerning movements and positions of the body

**prostaglandins** fatty acids that serve as extremely active biologic substances, with effects on the cardiovascular, gastrointestinal, respiratory, and central nervous systems

**prosthesis** cosmetic or functional artificial substitute of a missing body part, including teeth, eyes, and limbs

**prosthetic** pertaining to the replacement of a missing body part or augmentation of a deficient part by an artificial substitute

**protective muscle splinting** reflexive contraction of adjacent muscles resulting from noxious stimuli of a sensory field of a joint, soft tissue, or other structure to prevent movement or provide stabilization to the painful surrounding tissues; differs from muscle spasm in that the contraction is not sustained when the muscle is at rest—*syn: reflex muscle splinting, protective cocontraction, muscle guarding*

**proteoglycan** mucopolysaccharides bound to protein chains in covalent complexes within the extracellular matrix of connective tissue

**protrusion** state of being thrust forward or projected; in the head and neck area, reflects movement of the mandible forward of the intercuspal position

**provisional appliance** any appliance for time-limited use

**provocation test** diagnostic method of attempting to induce a disease episode or aggravate a symptom by provoking a tissue or system

**proximal** closer to a point of reference—***ant:*** *distal*

**pseudoaddiction** phenomenon resembling typical behaviors associated with addiction but due to undermedication of an identifiable pain complaint; behaviors will cease when pain is adequately controlled

**pseudoankylosis** a false ankylosis—***see*** *adhesion: intracapsular*

**pseudobulbar paralysis** —***see*** *progressive supranuclear palsy*

**pseudogout** —***see*** *chondrocalcinosis*

**psoriatic arthritis** polyarticular, progressive erosive joint inflammation with associated scaly, red skin lesions and usually involving the distal interphalangeal joints

**psychic trauma** an actual or perceived acute or protracted emotional shock, injury, or stress that exceeds the individual's psychologic coping capabilities

**psychoactive medication** drug that affects the mental functioning of an individual

**psychogenic pain disorder** —***see*** *pain disorder*

**psychomotor retardation** a slowing of both thoughts and physical activity often seen with depression and other psychiatric disorders

**psychosocial** involving both psychologic and social aspects of functioning

**psychosomatic** referring to both mind and body; pertaining to the influence of the mind or higher functions of the brain (emotions, fears, desires, etc) on the functions of the body, especially in relation to bodily disorders or disease—***syn:*** *somatopsychic*

**psychotic** pertaining to severe mental disorders characterized by disorganized thought processes and loss of reality-testing; such illnesses typically include hallucinations, delusions, disorganized speech, and grossly impaired adaptive functioning

**psychotropic medication** —***see*** *psychoactive medication*

**ptosis** prolapse or drooping of an organ or part; for example, the upper eyelid due to altered third cranial nerve function or cervical sympathectomy

    **eyelid p.** droopiness of the upper eyelid as seen in *Horner syndrome*; functional deficit of the levator palpebrae superior due to palsy of the oculomotor nerve; ptosis may also be a sign of other syndromes

**pulpal pain** odontogenic pain that emanates from the dental pulp

**pulpitis** inflammation of the dental pulp

**pumping procedure** passive joint mobilization after intracapsular addition of fluid into the joint

**pyrophosphate arthropathy** —***see*** *chondrocalcinosis*

## R

**radiculalgia** pain in the distribution of one or more sensory nerves

**radiculitis** inflammation of one or more nerve roots\*\*—***see*** *radiculopathy*

**radiculopathy** a disturbance of function or pathologic change in one or more nerve roots\*\*; disease of a nerve that results from mechanical nerve root compression and may lead to pain, numbness, weakness, and paresthesia

**radiofrequency lesioning** uses high-frequency energy to produce heat and thermal coagulation of affected nerves to disrupt their ability to transmit pain signals

**radiograph** image of internal structures produced by radioactive rays striking a sensitized film after passing through a body part—***syn:*** *roentgenogram*

**radionucleotides** atoms that disintegrate with emission of electromagnetic radiation, used in radiographic studies

**radiopaque** not permitting the passage of radiation energy and registering white or light on radiograph

**RadioVisioGraphy (RVG)** digital imaging technique using radiation but not film, with computer storage of images

**Raeder syndrome** characterized by severe, unilateral craniofacial pain or dysesthesia that is usually in the V1 or V2 distribution—***syn:*** *paratrigeminal syndrome*

**Ramsay Hunt syndrome** —***see*** *neuralgia: geniculate*

**range of motion (ROM)** the range, typically measured in degrees of a circle, through which a joint can be extended or flexed; with reference to the TMJ, usually reported as millimeters of interincisal distance

**rapid eye movement (REM)** active stage of deep sleep, characterized by prominent increase in the variability of heart rate, respiration, and blood pressure, including periods of rapid eye movements and muscle twitching; the stage of sleep during which dreaming occurs

**reciprocal clicking** —*see clicking joint noise, TMJ: reciprocal*

**recruitment of muscle** gradual increase in the number of active muscle units to a maximum in response to prolonged stimulus

**reducing disc** —*see disc displacement: with reduction*

**reduction** restoration of a part to its normal anatomic location by surgical or manipulative procedures, for example a fracture or dislocation

**reference zone** —*see referral zone*

**referral zone** site at which referred (heterotopic) pain or symptoms are perceived—*syn: reference zone*

**referred pain** pain perceived in a site distant from the nociceptive source—*syn: heterotropic pain*

**reflex** the sum total of any particular involuntary activity

**reflex splinting of muscle** —*see protective muscle splinting*

**reflex sympathetic dystrophy (RSD)** sympathetically maintained burning and hyperesthesic deafferentation pain typically initiated by trauma or surgical procedure, often accompanied by vasomotor, sudomotor, and later trophic changes in the skin; preferred term *complex regional pain syndrome*—*syn: causalgia, Sudeck atrophy, shoulder-hand syndrome*

**refractory** resistant to treatment

**Reiter syndrome** triad of polyarticular arthritis, urethritis, and conjunctivitis that usually follows nonspecific nongonococcal urethritis, predominantly in men; may be associated with stomatitis and ulceration of the glans penis

**relaxed position of mandible** —*see rest position of mandible*

**remodeling** adaptive alteration of tissue form in response to functional demands through a cellular response of articular fibrocartilage and subchondral bone

**repositioning appliance** —*see anterior repositioning appliance, mandibular*

**repositioning, jaw** the changing of any relative position of the mandible to the maxilla, usually through alteration of the occlusion of the natural or artificial teeth, or through the use of an orthosis

**resorption** loss of tissue substance by physiologic or pathologic processes

**rest position of mandible** postural relationship of the mandible to the maxilla when the patient is resting comfortably in an upright position, with the condyles in a neutral, unstrained position in the glenoid fossa and the mandibular musculature in a state of minimum tonic contraction to maintain the posture—*syn: relaxed position of mandible, physiologic rest position of mandible*

**restorative dentistry** area of dental science pertaining to the repair, reconstruction, or replacement of the dentition

**retrodiscal pad** misnomer—*see posterior attachment, TMJ*

**retrodiscal tissue** —*see posterior attachment, TMJ*

**retrodiscitis** inflammation of the retrodiscal tissues within the TMJ

**retrognathia** facial disharmony in which the jaw, usually the mandible, is receded posterior to normal in their craniofacial relationship

**retruded contact position (RCP)** point of initial tooth contact when the condyles are guided along the posterior slope of the articular eminence into their most superior position on jaw closure—*syn: centric relation, centric relation occlusion*

**retrusion** posterior location or movement; in the orofacial region, posterior positioning of a tooth or mandible from normal

**reversible treatment** any therapy that does not cause permanent change

**review of systems (ROS)** system-by-system review of body functioning while completing the health history and physical examination

**rheumatic** pertaining to rheumatism

**rheumatism** a group of disorders characterized by degeneration, metabolic change, or inflammation of the connective tissues, particularly those associated with muscles and joints

**rheumatoid arthritis** chronic polyarticular erosive inflammatory disease, more common in women, characterized by bilateral involvement with proliferative synovitis, atrophy, and rarefaction of bones

**rheumatoid factor (RhF)** anti–gamma globulin antibodies found in the serum of most patients with rheumatoid arthritis, but also found

291

in a small percentage of apparently normal patients as well as patients with other collagen vascular diseases, chronic infections, and noninfectious diseases

**rhizotomy** an operation to cut or destroy nerve fibers close to the spinal cord to relieve chronic pain or treat movement disorders that have not responded to more conservative treatments

**risk factor** factor that causes an individual or a group to be vulnerable to a disease or disorder, resulting in increased incidence or severity for the susceptible population

**roentgenogram** —*see radiograph*

**rostral** —*syn: superior; **ant:** caudal; **see** cephalad*

**rostrum** beaklike appendage or part

**rotation** to move about an axis

**rotation of condyle** the part of mandibular condylar movement that occurs primarily between the condyle and inferior surface of the disc and that does not involve translation

## S

**sagittal** pertaining to an anteroposterior plane or section parallel to the long axis of the body

**sagittal plane** vertical reference plane parallel to the long axis of the body, situated in an anterior-posterior direction, dividing the body into right and left halves

**saline** solution containing sodium chloride and purified water

**sarcoidosis** chronic progressive disease of unknown cause marked by granulomatous lesions in the skin, lymph nodes, salivary glands, eyes, lungs, and bones

**scintigraphy** —*see planar scintigraphy*

**scintillation** perception of twinkling light of varying intensity that can occur during a migraine aura

**scintillation detector** device for measuring radioactivity that relies on the emission of light or ultraviolet radiation from a crystal subjected to ionizing radiation

**scintiscan** —*see planar scintigraphy*

**scleroderma** disease characterized by thickening and hardening of connective tissue in any part of the body, including skin, heart, lungs, and kidneys; skin may be thickened and hard with pigmented patches

**scotoma** isolated area of varying size and shape within the visual field in which vision is absent or depressed

**secondary gain** indirect benefit, usually obtained through an illness or debility, that allows an individual to avoid responsibility or an activity that is noxious to him or her and/or to obtain support from others that would not ordinarily be forthcoming

**secondary hyperalgesia** increased sensitivity to normally painful stimuli outside and surrounding a zone of primary hyperalgesia

**secondary occlusal trauma** injury to the periodontium from excessive occlusal forces in teeth already affected with periodontal disease

**secondary pain** —*see referred pain*

**sedimentation rate** —*see erythrocyte sedimentation rate*

**sella turcica** a saddle-shaped section of the sphenoid bone located in the middle cranial fossa that houses the pituitary gland

**sensitization** the increased sensitivity of afferent receptors following repeated application of a noxious stimulus; a lowering of the pain threshold; psychologically, a defensive hyperarousal, induced by repetitive exposure to a noxious stimulus; *also,* development of lowered pain threshold in unstimulated undamaged regions adjacent to an area of primary nociception and hyperalgesia—*syn: secondary hyperalgesia*

**sensory nerve** afferent fibers of a peripheral nerve that conduct sensory impulses from the periphery of the body to the brain or spinal cord

**serology** study of in vitro antigen-antibody reactions

**serotonergic** encouraging the production of serotonin; cells that contain or are activated by serotonin

**serotonin** biogenic amine produced from tryptophan; found in serum and many other tissues, including mucosa, pineal body, and the central nervous system; acts as a vasoconstrictor, neurotransmitter, and pain-sensitizing agent—*syn: 5-hydroxytryptamine, 5-HT*

**shingles** misnomer—*see herpes zoster*

**shoulder-hand syndrome** —*see reflex sympathetic dystrophy*

**sialography** radiographic technique in which a salivary gland is filmed after an opaque substance is injected into its duct

**sign** any objective evidence of a disease

**silent period, masticatory muscle** momentary electromyographically observable decrease in elevator muscle activity on initial tooth contact, presumably the inhibitory effect of stimulated periodontal membrane receptors

**single-photon emission computerized tomography (SPECT)** —*see* tomography: single-photon emission computerized

**sinusitis** inflammation, either purulent or nonpurulent, of the mucosa of the sinuses

**sinuvertebral nerve** formed by mixed spinal and sympathetic branches that anastomose contralaterally; provides innervation to the vertebral periosteum, outer fibers of the annulus fibrosus, posterior longitudinal ligament, dura mater and epidural blood vessel walls—*syn: recurrent meningeal nerve*

**Sjögren syndrome** idiopathic collagen disorder, more common in middle-aged or older women, that is characterized by atrophic changes of the lacrimal and salivary glands, resulting in dryness of the eyes and mouth, sometimes associated with polyarthritis

**skeletal** pertaining to bony, hard framework of the animal body

**sleep apnea** breathing abnormality during sleep, characterized by cessation of airflow secondary to a lack of respiratory effort; commonly related to upper airway obstruction but may be related to central causes

**sliding condylar movement** misnomer—*see* translation of condyle

**SNOOP** mnemonic tool of the American Headache Society that outlines aspects of a patient's signs and symptoms that indicate a severe or life threatening disorder; aspects include: systemic symptoms/disease, neurologic signs/symptoms, onset sudden, older age, pattern change of headache

**soft tissue** nonbony or noncartilaginous tissue including muscles and their fascial envelopes, tendons, tendon sheaths, ligaments, joint capsule, bursae, fat, skin, etc

**somatic** pertaining to the body as distinct from the mind or psyche; pertaining to the structures of the body wall, eg, skeletal tissue in contrast with visceral structures

**somatic pain** pain resulting from tissue damage and the subsequent release of chemicals that act as noxious stimuli that are perceived by the brain as pain; *also* called *nociceptive pain*

**somatization** in psychiatry, the process whereby a mental condition is experienced as a bodily symptom

**somatization disorder** a polysymptomatic disorder that begins before age 39, extends over a period of years, and is characterized by a combination of pain, gastrointestinal sexual, and pseudoneurologic symptoms***—*syn: Briquet syndrome, hysteria*

**somatoform disorder** psychogenic condition in which symptoms suggest physical disease in the absence of organic findings and cause clinically significant impairment in adaptive functioning; the *DSM-VI* recognizes seven disorders in this group: somatization disorder, undifferentiated somatoform disorder, conversion disorder, pain disorder, hypochondriasis, body dysmorphic disorder, and somatoform disorder not otherwise specified***

> **s.d. not otherwise specified** disorder with somatoform symptoms that does not meet the criteria of any specific somatoform disorder***

> **undifferentiated s.d.** unexplained physical complaints lasting at least 6 months that are below the threshold for a diagnosis of somatization disorder***

**somatoform pain disorder** clinical condition in which complaints of pain are prominent, in the absence of adequate physical findings, and in association with evidence of psychologic factors having a role in the onset, severity, exacerbation, and maintenance of pain—*syn: psychogenic pain disorders*

**somatosensory** related to somatic afferent neural systems

**sonography** —*see* ultrasonography

**space-occupying lesion** abnormal mass or tumor that distends adjacent tissue as it enlarges

**spasm, muscle** involuntary, sudden movement or convulsive contraction of muscle or groups of muscles, usually associated with pain and dysfunction—*syn: myospasm*

**spastic bulbar palsy** —*see* progressive supranuclear palsy

**SPECT** —*see* tomography: single-photon emission computerized

**speculum** appliance that allows for opening a body cavity or passage for inspection

**sphenoid bone** compound, unpaired wedge-shaped bone at the base of the cranium, separating the frontal and ethmoid bones, and maxilla frontally from the temporal and occipital bones—*syn: sphenoid*

**spheroidal joint** —*see enarthrosis joint*

**spinal accessory cranial nerve** motor cranial nerve (CN XI) comprising cranial and spinal branches that supply the trapezius and sternomastoid muscles and the pharynx

**spinal anesthesia** a type of medication that produces temporary loss of sensation below the area of injection into the spinal cord without loss of consciousness; *also* called *epidural anesthesia*

**spinal cord stimulation** electrical stimulation of nervous tissues on a specific portion of the spinal cord to produce paresthesia

**spinal nerves** nerves that emerge from the spinal cord and innervate the organs and tissues; there are 31 pairs of spinal nerves, each attached to the cord by two roots, ventral and dorsal

**spinal trigeminal nucleus** one of the nuclei of the trigeminal nerve, consisting of three subnuclei: subnucleus oralis, subnucleus interpolaris, and subnucleus caudalis—*syn: medullary dorsal horn*

**spine** —*syn: vertebral column, spinal column*

**splint** —*see interocclusal orthosis*

**splinting, muscle** —*see protective muscle splinting*

**spondyloarthropathy** disease of the spinal or intervertebral articulations

**spondylosis** —*see ankylosing spondylitis*

**spontaneous remission** resolution of signs or symptoms of disease occurring unaided and without treatment

**spray and stretch** physical therapy technique using vapocoolant spray followed by passive muscle stretch

**Spurling test** used in confirming the diagnosis of cervical radiculopathy; involves side bending and extending the patient's head to the side of involvement, and pressure may or may not be applied; the finding is positive if the patient's upper extremity paresthesia or pain is intensified or reproduced

**stabilization appliance** hard acrylic, flat plane intraoral appliance fitted over either the maxillary or mandibular teeth without significant mandibular repositioning, used to control joint or muscle symptoms or the harmful effects of bruxism

**standard of care** established model or guidelines of diagnostic and therapeutic management in a given community or setting

**status migrainosus** severe unrelenting migraine headache associated with nausea and vomiting that lasts longer than 72 hours; may not be manageable under outpatient care

**stellate ganglion** star-shaped sympathetic ganglion located between the transverse process of the seventh cervical vertebra and the head of the first rib, with postganglionic fibers running to the carotid, middle ear, salivary and lacrimal glands, and the ciliary ganglion via CN IX, X, and XI, and the upper three cervical nerves

**stenosis** narrowing or stricture of a duct or canal

**stent** device used to hold a skin or mucosal graft in place or provide support for tubular structures; may also be used to facilitate radiation therapy

> **antihemorrhagic s.** controls bleeding during surgery
>
> **burn s.** minimizes contraction of burned tissue during healing
>
> **medication s.** holds topical medication in contact with a mucosal site
>
> **nasal s.** supports the form of the nose
>
> **palatal s.** protects a palatal surgical site during healing, or to keep a mucosal flap or skin graft in close apposition to the surgical bed
>
> **radiation s.** used in the process of delivery of radiation therapy; protects healthy tissues, displaces such tissues away from the field of radiation, or directs the radiation beam to the target site

**stethoscope** instrument for performing mediate auscultation

**stereotactic neurosurgery** —*see: gamma knife surgery*

**stereotactic radiosurgery** —*see: gamma knife surgery*

**Still disease** seronegative arthritis, often accompanied by fever and lymphadenopathy, representing 70% of cases of arthritis that begin before the age of 16 years—*syn: juvenile rheumatoid arthritis*

**stimulation** the action of a stimulus on a receptor

**stimulation coverage** the amount of a patient's pain pattern that is converted by stimulation

**stimulus** anything that arouses action in the muscles, nerves, or other excitable tissue

**stomatognathic** denoting the mouth and jaws collectively

**stomatognathic system** the functional and anatomic relationships among the teeth, jaws, TMJs, and muscles of mastication

**stomatology** study of structures, functions, and diseases of the mouth

**strabismus** —*see* heterotropia

**stress** the challenge for adaptation created by the sum of physical, mental, emotional, internal, or external stimuli that tend to disturb the homeostasis of an organism; inappropriate reactions can lead to disease states

**stressor** cause of stress; any factor that disturbs homeostasis

**study cast** —*see* cast, dental

**study model** —*see* cast, dental

**stump pain** pain located in the amputated limb's remaining stump

**subchondral** beneath cartilage

**subchondral bone** bone beneath cartilage

**subcondylar osteotomy** —*see* condylotomy

**subcutaneous** beneath the skin

**sublingual** pertaining to the regions or structures beneath the tongue

**subluxation, TMJ** the partial or incomplete condylar dislocation during wide jaw opening, usually accompanied by a joint sound and during which the joint surfaces remain in partial contact

**submandibular** situated below the mandible

**subnucleus caudalis** one of the subnuclei of the spinal trigeminal nucleus; the main terminus for most slow first-order neurons conveying potential pain impulses from trigeminal receptive fields

**subnucleus interpolaris** one of the subnuclei of the spinal trigeminal nucleus that receives some peripheral nociceptive input but mostly relays temperature and touch impulses

**subnucleus oralis** one of the subnuclei of the spinal trigeminal nucleus that receives some peripheral nociceptive input but mostly relays temperature and touch impulses

**Sudeck atrophy** —*see* reflex sympathetic dystrophy

**suffering** a state of severe distress associated with events that threaten the intactness of the person; may be associated with pain

**summation** progressive increase of pain intensity with repeated noxious stimulation; depends on activity in unmyelinated nociceptors

**SUNCT syndrome** short-lasting, unilateral, neuralgiform pain with conjunctival injection and tearing

**superior** —*see* cephalad

**superior laryngeal neuralgia** —*see* neuralgia: superior laryngeal

**superior retrodiscal lamina** the most superior surface of the retrodiscal tissues or posterior attachment

**superior sagittal sinus** one of a series of venous sinuses situated between the meningeal and endosteal layers of the dura mater that drain blood from the brain and cranial bones; the superior sagittal sinus attaches to the falx cerebri and enlarges posteriorly at the internal occipital protuberance to form the confluence of sinuses

**supraclusion** occlusal relationship where an occluding surface extends beyond the normal occlusal plane—*syn:* overeruption of teeth

**supracontact** posterior occlusal contact before maximum intercuspation—*syn: prematurity, premature occlusal contact;* **misnomers:** *occlusal interference, interceptive occlusal contact*

**supranuclear paralysis** —*see* progressive supranuclear palsy

**surgery, orthognathic** surgical repositioning of all or parts of the maxilla or mandible to correct malpositions or deformities

**symmetry** correspondence in size, shape, and relative position around an axis or on each side of a plane of the body—**ant:** asymmetry

**sympathectomy** excision or interruption of some portion of the sympathetic nervous system pathway—*syn: sympathetic neurolysis*

**sympathetic** pertaining to the sympathetic nervous system

**sympathetic nervous system** division of the autonomic nervous system originating in the thoracic and upper three or four lumbar segments of the spinal cord, responsible for the regulation of vasomotor tone, temperature, blood sugar levels, and other aspects of the "flight or fight" reaction to stress—*syn: thoracolumbar division*

**sympathetic neurolysis** —*see* sympathectomy

**sympathetically maintained pain** pain sustained through activity of the sympathetic nervous system; may accompany disorders such as *complex regional pain syndrome, reflex sympathetic dystrophy* and possibly *idiopathic odontalgia*

**symphysis** the fused immovable cartilaginous junction between two originally distinct bones—*syn: fibrocartilaginous joint*

>   **mandibular s.** the midline symphysis of the right and left halves of the fetal mandible

**symptom** any subjective experience perceived as evidence of a disease by a patient

**Symptom Checklist-90-Revised (SCL-90-R)** 90-item multidimensional self-report measure of nine dimensions of psychologic functioning

**synapse** junction between the processes of two adjacent neurons where a neural impulse is transmitted from one neuron to another—*syn: synaptic junction*

**synaptic junction** —*see* synapse

**syndrome** set of symptoms or signs that together define a disorder

**synkinesis** unintentional movement accompanying a volitional movement

**synostosis** —*see* ankylosis: bony

**synovia** clear, thick lubricating fluid in a joint, bursa, or tendon sheath secreted by the membrane lining the cavity or sheath—*syn: synovial fluid*

**synovial** pertaining to or secreting synovia

**synovial chondromatosis** rare condition in which cartilage nodules develop in the connective tissue below the synovial membranes; the cartilage foci on the surface of the synovium may detach and result in loose bodies within the joint—*syn: synovial osteochondromatosis*

**synovial fluid** —*see* synovia

**synovial joint** joint possessing a synovial lining

>   **s.j. lining** membrane lining synovial joints that secretes synovia

**synovial osteochondromatosis** —*see* synovial chondromatosis

**synovitis** inflammation of the synovial lining of a joint due to infection, an immunologic condition, or secondary to cartilage degeneration or trauma; usually painful, especially with movement

**syringomyelia** characterized by longitudinal cavities (syrinx) within the spinal cord that cause pain and paresthesia, atrophy of the hands and lower extremities, and spastic paralysis

**systemic disease** disease affecting the entire organism as distinguished from any of its individual parts

**systemic lupus erythematosus (SLE)** generalized connective tissue disorder affecting primarily middle-aged women, causing among other things, lesions of the skin, vasculitis, arthralgia, and leukopenia; usually associated with evidence of autoimmune dysfunction such as elevated antinuclear antibodies

# T

**tachycardia** excessively rapid pulse rate (ie, >100 beats/min)

**tardive dyskinesia** involuntary, repetitious movements of the muscles of the face, limbs, and trunk, most often related to the use of neuroleptic medications and persisting after withdrawal

**temporal** pertaining to the temples; *also,* limited in time

**temporal arteritis** —*see* arteritis

**temporal bone** paired, irregular bone forming part of the lower and lateral surfaces of the cranium; consists of four portions: mastoid, squama, petrous, and tympanic; contains the hearing apparatus

**temporomandibular** relating to the TMJ

**temporomandibular disorders (TMDs)** a number of clinical problems that involve the masticatory muscles, the TMJ, or both

**temporomandibular joint (TMJ)** paired synovial joint capable of both gliding and hinge movements, articulating the mandibular condyle, articular disc, and squamous portions of the temporal bone

>   **t.j. dysfunction** abnormal, incomplete, or impaired function of the TMJ(s)

>   **t.j. hypermobility** excessive mobility of the TMJ

>   **t.j. syndrome** misnomer—*see* temporomandibular disorders

**tender point** in rheumatology, specifically in fibromyalgia, one of nine paired sets of anatomic sites that may be painful to palpation; a diagnosis of fibromyalgia is made if, with an appropriate history, 11 of these 18 sites are tender

**tendomyositis** inflammatory condition of a tendon and its associated muscle

**tendon** strong, flexible, and inelastic fibrous band of tissue attaching muscle to bone

**tendonitis** inflammatory condition of a tendon or tendon-muscle junction

**TENS** *—see transcutaneous electrical nerve stimulation*

**tension** act or condition of being stretched, strained, or extended—*syn: stress* (psychiatry)

**tension-type headache** dull, aching, pressing, usually bilateral headache of mild to moderate intensity; when severe, may include photophobia or phonophobia and, rarely, nausea; may be intermittent, lasting minutes to days, or chronic without remission

> **chronic t.h.** average of 15 or more headaches per month for at least 3 months

> **frequent episodic t.h.** number of headaches average more than 1 but less than 15 days per month for at least 3 months

> **infrequent episodic t.h.** number of headaches average less than 1 day per month

> **probable t.h.** headaches fulfilling all but one of the criteria for specified type

**tentorium cerebelli** fascial membrane that separates the cerebellum from the cerebral hemispheres and forms a crescent-shaped tent or roof to the posterior cranial fossa

**therapeutic** relating to treatment or the art of healing; producing improvement or cure of an illness

**therapeutic prosthesis** prosthesis used to transport and retain some agent for therapeutic purposes

**thermography** technique using an infrared camera that provides a graphic representation of the skin temperature variations between adjacent tissues or between the same area on two sides of the body

**thoracic outlet syndrome (TOS)** condition in which pressure exerted on nerve roots in the thoracic area (including the brachial plexus) causes pain

**threshold** smallest stimulus that can be perceived; the minimum level required to produce a result

**thunderclap headache** abruptly starting headache, reaching most severe intensity usually within 1 minute and lasting from 1 hour to 10 days

**tic douloureux** *—see neuralgia: trigeminal*

**tidemark** the demarcation line between the calcified cartilage zone and the fibrocartilaginous zone of synovial joints

**time-contingent basis** prescription of medication or provision of treatment at regular intervals rather than on the patient's perceived need for medication or treatment because of symptom severity

**tinnitus** presence of any subjective noise, such as a ringing, buzzing, or roaring sound in the ear or head

**tissue** the various cellular combinations that make up the body; an aggregation of similarly specialized cells united in the performance of a particular function

**TMJ** *—see temporomandibular joint*

**tolerance** physiologic state requiring increasing doses of agents to produce a sustained desired effect

**tomography** radiographic technique that shows structural images of the internal body lying within a predetermined plane of tissues, while blurring or eliminating images of structures lying in other planes—*syn: body section roentgenography*

> **computerized t. (CT)** imaging method that uses a narrowly collimated radiographic beam that passes through the body and is recorded by an array of scintillation detectors; the computer calculates tissue absorption, with the film images reflecting the densities of various structures—***misnomers:*** *CAT scan, computed tomography, computer-assisted tomography, computerized axial tomography, computerized transaxial tomography*

> **corrected cephalometric t.** tomography of structures of the head, in particular, the condyle of the mandible, with the radiographic section oriented to the precise location and angulation of the structure of interest

> **focal plane t.** imaging method that shows a detailed cross section of a body part at a predetermined depth and thickness of cut; accomplished by moving the film and the x-ray source in opposite directions during the ex-

posure, blurring the structures in front of and behind the area of interest

**positron emission t. (PET)** imaging method based on detection of positron emission from decaying radionucleotides within a patient; provides information on both tissue density and metabolism

**single-photon emission computerized t. (SPECT)** imaging method based on detection of single gamma photons emitted by radionucleotides within a patient; provides information on location of these radionucleotides, which, depending on the type of scan desired, are taken up by inflammatory cells or metabolizing bone cells, etc

**torticollis** contracted state of cervical muscles producing twisting of the neck and an unnatural head posture

**spasmodic t.** intermittent torticollis due to tonic, clonic, or tonicoclonic spasm in cervical muscles

**Tourette syndrome** syndrome with juvenile onset and including facial tics; purposeless, uncoordinated, voluntary movements; and involuntary vocalisms—*syn: Gilles de la Tourette syndrome*

**Towne radiograph** fronto-occipital plain film projection of the skull, with the patient supine and chin depressed; allows visualization of the occipital and petrous bones as well as condyles of the mandible

**transcranial radiograph** plain-film projection of the contralateral TMJ condyle from a supero-posterior angulation

**transcutaneous electric nerve stimulation (TENS)** low-voltage electric stimulation used as therapy

**translation of condyle** mandibular condylar movement that occurs during protrusion, lateral excursion, or mouth opening, primarily involving the superior aspect of the disc and the articular tubercle; usually mixed with some degree of condylar rotation—*syn: gliding of condyle, sliding condylar movement*

**transverse plane** horizontal plane dividing the body into upper and lower portions

**trauma** an injury or wound to a part of the living body; *also*, acute or chronic psychologic shock that exceeds the individual's coping capacities and that may cause lasting deleterious effects on the personality

**macrotrauma** injury to the body from an external source, involving large or excessive force

**microtrauma** repetitive, low-level, potentially injurious force to the body, usually internal to the organism, as with chronic habits such as poor posture or clenching of the teeth

**traumatic arthritis** arthritis that is the direct result of a macrotrauma, affecting normal joints or aggravating existing joint disease or derangement

**Treacher Collins syndrome** inherited disorder characterized by mandibular and facial dysostosis

**treatment plan** the sequence of procedures planned for a patient's treatment after a diagnosis

**tremor** involuntary trembling or quivering, repetitive and rhythmic

**essential t.** benign hereditary familial extrapyramidal tremor; worsens with age and stress

**movement-induced t.** tremor triggered by a particular body movement

**parkinsonian t.** slow tremor associated with Parkinson disease; worse with cold, fatigue, and stress

**resting t.** tremor at rest that disappears with body movement—*syn: static tremor*

**static t.** —*see resting tremor*

**trigeminal nerve** mixed cranial nerve (CN V) comprising three main branches: ophthalmic ($V_1$), maxillary ($V_2$), and mandibular ($V_3$); responsible for somatosensory innervation of structures embryologically derived from the first brachial arch, including the oral cavity and the face; the motor fibers principally supply the muscles of mastication as well as the mylohyoid, anterior belly of the digastric, the tensor veli palatini, and the tensor tympani muscles

**trigeminal neuralgia** —*see neuralgia: trigeminal*

**trigger point** a hypersensitive area in muscle or connective tissue that, when palpated, produces pain—*see myofascial trigger point*

**trismus** myospasm of masticatory muscles specifically causing limited jaw opening; early symptom of tetanus—*syn: mandibular trismus*

**trochlear nerve** motor cranial nerve (CN IV) supplying the superior oblique muscle of the eye

**trophic** pertaining to nutrition or nourishment

**tubercle** characteristic lesion of tuberculosis; nodule on skin or bone—*see* eminence

**tumor** —*see* neoplasm

## U

**ultrasonic** referring to ultrasound

**ultrasonography** visualization of deep structures of the body by directing ultrasonic waves into the tissues and recording the reflections—*syn:* sonography

**ultrasound** sound waves (mechanical radiant energy) beyond the upper frequency limit of the human ear (>20,000 vibrations per second Hz)

**uncinate processes** located in the cervical region of the spine between C3 and C7 and formed by uncinate processes that are located laterally on the vertebral body, which project upward from the vertebral body below and downward front the vertebral body above, and allow for flexion and extension and limit lateral flexion in the cervical spine; though referred to as *joints*, they are not true diarthrodial joints—*syn:* joints of Luschka

**unilateral** occurring on one side only—*ant:* bilateral

**urate crystal** salt of uric acid that may be deposited in gouty joints

## V

**vagus nerve** mixed cranial nerve (CN X) that exits the cranium via the jugular foramen and supplies sensory fibers to the ear, tongue, pharynx, and larynx, parasympathetic and visceral afferents to the viscera, as well as motor fibers to the muscles of the pharynx, esophagus, and larynx

**vapocoolant spray** highly volatile liquid that evaporates quickly when sprayed on warm skin, causing immediate cooling; used in spray-and-stretch therapy

**vapocoolant spray–stretch procedure** —*see* spray and stretch

**vascular** pertaining to a blood vessel

**vascular pain** deep somatic pain of visceral origin that emanates from the afferent nerves that innervate blood vessels

**vasculitis** inflammatory condition of a blood vessel

**vasoconstriction** narrowing of blood vessels, causing reduced blood flow to part of the body

**vasodilatation** widening of blood vessels, causing increased blood flow to part of the body

**vasomotor** effecting changes in the diameter of a blood vessel

**vasospasm** sudden decrease in the internal diameter of a blood vessel, caused by the contraction of the muscle within the wall of the vessel, resulting in decreased blood flow

**vertical dimension of occlusion (VDO)** vertical distance between any two arbitrary points when the teeth are in intercuspal position; one point is on the mandible and the other is on the face

**vertical plane** sagittal or frontal plane; perpendicular to the transverse plane

**vertigo** hallucination of movement; a sensation as if the external world were revolving around the patient (objective vertigo) or as if the patient were revolving in space (subjective vertigo; sometimes erroneously used as a synonym for *dizziness*; vertigo may result from disease of the inner ear; from cardiac, gastric, or ocular disorders; from organic brain disease; or from other causes

**vestibular nucleus** a cluster of nerve cells within the medulla that has extensive neuronal connections to and from the head, neck, trunk, eyes, and ears, serving to coordinate reflexive control of balance, gaze, equilibrium, and posture; descending tracts synapse within the cervical spine and represent another aspect of the relationship between the head and neck

**vibration analysis** method to measure minute vibrations of the condyle on translation to aid with the diagnosis of internal derangements

**visceral pain** deep somatic pain that originates in visceral structures, such as mucosal linings, walls of hollow viscera, parenchyma of organs, glands, dental pulps, and vascular structures

## W,X,Y,Z

**Waldeyer tonsillar ring** ring of lymphoid tissues surrounding the upper airway, consisting of adenoid, tubal, palatine and lingual tonsils

**whiplash** misnomer—*see* flexion-extension injury

**windup** repetitive nerve stimulation leading to exuberant response in the central nervous system

**working interference** misnomer—*see* working occlusal contact

**working occlusal contact** tooth contact on the ipsilateral side during guided lateral excursive movement of the mandible

**working side** ipsilateral to the functioning side of the oral cavity

**xerostomia** dryness of the mouth

**x-ray** —*see radiograph*

**zoster** —*see herpes zoster*

**zygapophyseal** the articulation (moving) of facet joints of the spine that enable extension, flexion, and rotation—*syn: facet joint*

**zygoma** area formed by the union of the zygomatic bone and the zygomatic process of the temporal bone and the maxillary bone

## Terms to Avoid/Preferred Terms

**arthritis deformans** Use **rheumatoid arthritis**

**balancing interference** Use **nonworking occlusal contact**

**balancing occlusal contact** Use **nonworking occlusal contact**

**bilaminar zone** Use **posterior attachment**

**bite guard** Use **stabilization appliance**

**closed bite** Use **posterior overclosure**

**closed lock** Use **disc displacement without reduction**

**computer-assisted tomography** Use **computerized tomography**

**computerized axial tomography** Use **computerized tomography**

**computerized transaxial tomography** Use **computerized tomography**

**CT scan** Use **computerized tomography**

**deep bite** Use **deep overbite**

**disc locking** Use **disc displacement without reduction**

**disk** Use **disc**

**fibrositis** Use **fibromyalgia**

**flat-plane appliance** Use **stabilization appliance**

**interdigitation** Use **intercuspation**

**intermaxillary** Use **interocclusal**

**locking of joint** Use **disc displacement without reduction**

**meniscectomy, TMJ** Use **discectomy**

**meniscus, TMJ** Use **intra-articular disc**

**muscle cramp** Use **myospasm**

**muscle relaxation appliance** Use **stabilization appliance**

**myofascial pain dysfunction syndrome** Use **myofascial pain**

**pathosis** Use **pathologic condition**

**posterior ligament** Use **posterior attachment**

**psychogenic pain disorder** Use **somatoform disorder**

**reflex sympathetic dystrophy** Use **complex regional pain syndrome**

**retrodiscal pad** Use **posterior attachment**

**shingles** Use **herpes zoster**

**sliding condylar movement** Use **translation of condyle**

**temporomandibular joint syndrome** Use **temporomandibular disorders**

**whiplash** Use **flexion-extension injury**

**working interference** Use **working occlusal contact**

---

\* International Association for the Study of Pain, Task Force on Taxonomy. Scheme for coding chronic pain diagnoses. In: Merskey H, Bogduk N (eds). Classification of Chronic Pain. Descriptions of Chronic Pain Syndromes and Definitions of Pain Terms, ed 2. Seattle: IASP Press, 1994:3–4.

\*\* Loeser JD (ed). Bonica's Management of Pain, ed 3. Philadelphia: Lippincott Williams & Wilkins, 2001.

\*\*\*Diagnostic and Statistical Manual of Mental Disorders, ed 4. Washington, D.C. American Psychiatric Association, 1994.

Dorland's Illustrated Medical Dictionary, ed 30. Philadelphia: Saunders, 2003.

# Index

Figures followed by *"f"* denote figures; those followed by *"b"* denote boxes; those followed by *"t"* denote tables.

## A

Abducens nerve
  characteristics of, 32t
  palsy of, 67
Aβ fibers, 6, 12
Abscess
  combined periodontal–endodontic abscess, 109–110
  gingival, 106
  microabscesses, 103
  pericoronal, 108–109
  periodontal, 106–107, 110
  periradicular, 107–108, 110
  Phoenix, 108
Accessory nerve, 8, 32t, 210
Acoustic vestibular nerve, 32t
Active range of motion, for mandible, 33
Acupuncture, 167
Acute pseudomembranous candidiasis, 117–118
Acute atrophic candidiasis, 118
Acute ischemic cerebrovascular disease, 63–64
Acute necrotizing ulcerative gingivitis, 113–114
Acute pain
  characteristics of, 16
  periodontal, 110–111
Acute pseudomembranous candidiasis, 117–118
Addiction, 242
Aδ fibers, 3, 6, 10, 102–103
Aggravating factors, 30

AIDS, 122
Alcohol injections, 87
Allodynia
  definition of, 12
  with postherpetic neuralgia, 92
Allostasis, 15
Allostatic load, 15
α-Amino-3-hydroxy-5-methyl-4-isoxazole-propionic acid receptors, 11–12
Amitriptyline, 164
Amlexanox, 115
Analgesics, 162
Anesthesia
  blockade uses of, 166–167, 209
  diagnostic uses of, 40–41, 41t
Anesthesia dolorosa, 93
Angular cheilitis, 119
Ankylosis, 152
Ansa cervicalis, 8
Anterior capsular ligament, 130f
Anterior positioning appliances, 169–171
Anterior teeth, referred pain from, 104
Anteroposterior radiography, 39
Anticonvulsants
  glossopharyngeal neuralgia treated with, 89
  trigeminal neuralgia treated with, 86
Antidepressants. *See* Tricyclic antidepressants.
Antifungal agents, 118
Antisocial personality disorder, 244
Anxiety/anxiety disorders, 35, 57, 239–241, 245
Aphthous ulcers. *See* Recurrent aphthous stomatitis.
Aplasia, 143
Appliances. *See* Orthopedic appliances.
Arnold-Chiari syndrome, 219

301